FIFTH EDITION

WHEATER'S
Basic Pathology

A TEXT, ATLAS AND REVIEW
OF HISTOPATHOLOGY

Commissioning Editor: Kate Dimock
Development Editor: Ben Davie
Project Manager: Alan Nicholson
Design: Erik Bigland/Louis Forgione
Illustration Manager: Bruce Hogarth
Illustrator: Phil Deakin
Marketing Manager(s) (UK/USA): Tim Jordan/Allan McKeown

FIFTH EDITION

WHEATER'S
Basic Pathology

A TEXT, ATLAS AND REVIEW OF HISTOPATHOLOGY

Barbara Young BSc Med Sci (Hons), PhD, MB BChir, MRCP, FRCPA
Consultant Pathologist
Department of Anatomical Pathology
Hunter Area Pathology Service
Newcastle
NSW, Australia

William Stewart BSc (Hons), MBChB, PhD, DipFMS, FRCPath
Consultant Neuropathologist & Honorary Clinical Senior Lecturer
Department of Neuropathology
Institute of Neurological Sciences
Southern General Hospital
Glasgow, UK

Geraldine O'Dowd BSc(Hons), MBChB(Hons), FRCPath
Consultant Diagnostic Pathologist
Lanarkshire NHS Board
Honorary Clinical Senior Lecturer
University of Glasgow
Glasgow, UK

CHURCHILL
LIVINGSTONE

ELSEVIER

CHURCHILL
LIVINGSTONE
ELSEVIER
an imprint of Elsevier Limited.

Main Edition ISBN: 978-0-443-06797-6
  Reprinted 2012 (twice)
International Edition ISBN: 978-0-443-06802-7

British Library Cataloguing in Publication Data
A catalogue record for this book is available from the
British Library

Library of Congress Cataloging in Publication Data
A catalog record for this book is available from the Library
of Congress

Notice
Medical knowledge is constantly changing. Standard safety
precautions must be followed, but as new research and
clinical experience broaden our knowledge, changes in
treatment and drug therapy may become necessary or
appropriate. Readers are advised to check the most current
product information provided by the manufacturer of each
drug to be administered to verify the recommended dose,
the method and duration of administration, and
contraindications. It is the responsibility of the practitioner,
relying on experience and knowledge of the patient, to
determine dosages and the best treatment for each individual
patient. Neither the Publisher nor the author assume any
liability for any injury and/or damage to persons or property
arising from this publication.

      The Publisher

ELSEVIER   your source for books,
journals and multimedia
in the health sciences
www.elsevierhealth.com

Working together to grow
libraries in developing countries
www.elsevier.com | www.bookaid.org | www.sabre.org

ELSEVIER   BOOK AID International   Sabre Foundation

The
publisher's
policy is to use
paper manufactured
from sustainable forests

Printed in China

CONTENTS

PREFACE TO THE FIFTH EDITION

In writing this new edition of Basic Pathology (Basic Histopathology in previous editions) we have aimed to maintain the ethos of previous editions, i.e. to provide a clear and comprehensible text and atlas for beginners in Pathology and a succinct treatment of the major pathological processes and diseases for the slightly more advanced trainee either in Pathology or in other specialities. First to explain the name change: we found that the term Histopathology in the old name was often confused with Histology and that the book was confused with Histology texts. Our companion work Wheater's Functional Histology covers the normal microscopic structures of the body, while this work deals only with the pathological.

Along with the name change, we also have 2 new authors on the team. Professor James Lowe and Dr Alan Stevens, both of Nottingham, have left the authorship team due to overwhelming commitments in other areas for the former and retirement for the latter. Our two new authors (Drs Stewart and O'Dowd) are both enthusiastic and knowledgeable and bring great ability to this work. However, those familiar with the previous editions will realise that the book has maintained the same general format as previously. The book has been comprehensively updated with complete rewrites of some chapters and less comprehensive but important updates added to others. Many illustrations have been added or old ones replaced with better. We have greatly expanded the clinical components of the book and highlighted many clinical correlations in text boxes for easy access. Likewise, we have highlighted new research in molecular and cell biology that illuminates disease processes. Another new feature in this edition is the Key to Figures for each double page spread, allowing the reader to easily identify the labelled structures in the images. We hope the students will also find the new Glossary of Pathological Terms (Appendix 2) useful to clarify commonly used descriptive terms. The Review section at the end of each chapter is intended as a revision aid to highlight the main points of the conditions covered in the chapter in a brief but comprehensible fashion.

Many features of the book, however, remain the same: we have aimed this Text, Atlas and Review squarely at medical students but hope it will also be useful to those beginning speciality training in Pathology and in other areas such as surgery. Indeed, we would argue that a grounding in Pathology is vital for all practising doctors, whatever their speciality. Knowing the ever increasing demands on students and doctors in speciality training, we have kept this volume as short as possible, while covering all of the major topics. There are many resources available for those who develop an interest and want to delve deeper into the subject. We have also aimed to make the information easily accessible. The book is designed to be read in any order although it is also a good read from beginning to end. We hope that this Text, Atlas and Review of Histopathology will stimulate your interest and perhaps lead some of you to a career in this area.

Barbara Young

Willie Stewart

Geraldine O'Dowd

PREFACE TO THE FIRST EDITION

Histopathology is an essential component of pathology teaching in all medical and dental courses, nevertheless the scope, content and emphasis on microscopy vary considerably between different centres. Adding to this diversity are the different stages in the preclinical and/or clinical years when the subject matter is presented. This book has been designed to meet as closely as possible the requirements of these many differing courses. We believe that practical microscopy is an important part of pathology teaching, and therefore we have chosen to centre our discussion around appropriate colour photomicrographs as might be done in the lecture room or microscope laboratory. The text has been designed as a series of amplified captions explaining not only the features visible in the labelled colour plates, but also providing some background text in order to relate the subject matter to the theoretical and clinical implications of the pathological processes. Consequently this book should not be regarded as a copiously illustrated introductory textbook of pathology, but rather it is intended as a histopathology companion to any of the many excellent standard pathology textbooks; the text, though more than normally found in an atlas, is thus by no means comprehensive.

The subject matter has been divided into two sections, the first covering basic pathological processes and the second encompassing the common diseases encountered in systems pathology. In general, our material has been taken from both surgical and necropsy specimens of common clinical conditions. Uncommon conditions have been included only where they illustrate important pathological principles. The haematoxylin and eosin staining method has mainly been employed as is standard practice in pathology laboratories, but special staining methods have been occasionally used where appropriate. Rather than specifying numerical magnification factors, each micrograph has been designated as low power, medium power or high power by the abbreviations LP, MP and HP respectively as this is probably more relevant to student needs.

It is our hope that this book will be useful both as a guide in formal practical classes, as well as assisting the student in private study. Although the book is primarily aimed at preclinical and clinical medical and dental students, it would also prove useful for other groups such as veterinary science students, medical laboratory scientists specialising in histopathology, and candidates for post-graduate examinations in surgery and pathology.

Nottingham, 1985
P.R.W.
H.G.B.
A.S.
J.L.

ACKNOWLEDGEMENTS

As with previous editions, we have relied on the help of a great many people in the production of this new edition of Basic Pathology. Our colleagues in our various departments generously allowed us access to their glass slides for photography. Particular thanks are due to the following for loan of glass slides for the photography for particular Figures: Dr Lorna Cooper of the Department of Pathology, Glasgow Royal Infirmary for Fig. 13.5, Dr Robin Reid of the Department of Pathology, Western Infirmary, Glasgow for Figs 13.14a&b, Dr Julie McAdam of the Department of Forensic Medicine and Science, The University of Glasgow for Figs 10.4 and 11.16, Dr Maria Benkovicova of the Department of Pathology, Wishaw General Hospital for Fig. 4.22 and Dr Gareth Bryson of the Department of Pathology, Southern General Hospital for Figs 20.7c&d. We thank the scientists and technical staff (far too many to name individually) in our laboratories (Departments of Pathology at the Western Infirmary, Glasgow and Wishaw General Hospital, Wishaw and the Department of Neuropathology, Institute of Neurological Sciences, Southern General Hospital, Glasgow). Without your high quality sections, none of this would have been possible. We also thank the many contributors who provided material for earlier editions as mentioned previously.

Finally, we would like to thank the staff of Elsevier for their help and support in the writing of this edition.

DEDICATION

For my children, Alex and Katie Burkitt, of whom I am infinitely proud.

Barbara Young

For Lucy and Katie

Willie Stewart

In loving memory of my grandparents, John and Veronica O'Dowd and James and Mary Mallon.

Geraldine O'Dowd

PART I

BASIC PATHOLOGICAL PROCESSES

1 Cellular responses to injury

Introduction to pathology

Pathology, which is also sometimes called histopathology, anatomical pathology or morbid anatomy, is the study of abnormal or diseased tissues and organs. This book is intended for the student approaching histopathology for the first time and aims to give a thorough but concise grounding both in basic pathological processes and in specific diseases of the various organs and systems. Pathology is fundamental to the study, understanding and diagnosis of disease and therefore to successful treatment. We assume in this text that the student has already studied histology, the microscopic appearances of normal tissues, and has a basic understanding of the workings of the microscope. Most student doctors who use this text will not become specialist pathologists, but almost all will have regular interactions with pathologists as part of their normal work and a basic understanding of pathology, even if only an ability to understand written pathology reports, is vital. For instance, what is the difference between adenocarcinoma, adenomatoid tumour and carcinoid tumour? These are three very different tumours with different behaviours requiring very different treatments and the non-pathologist receiving such a report needs to understand the difference.

As part of the diagnostic process, the pathologist uses a range of techniques. Many pathological changes can be identified by routine histopathological staining methods (see Appendix 1). If these do not allow specific identification of the disease then the pathologist has at his or her disposal a range of ancillary techniques, including immunohistochemistry, electron microscopy and various molecular methods. These allow precise diagnosis of many conditions that otherwise have similar clinical manifestations. For this reason a biopsy is often carried out to obtain tissue for diagnostic purposes. This may be an incisional biopsy, i.e. removing a sample of a lesion, or an excisional biopsy, which removes the entire lesion and may also be a curative procedure. Cytopathology is also a branch of pathology, but in this case the pathologist examines single cells from a lesion rather than intact tissue. A specimen for cytopathology may be obtained by fine needle aspiration biopsy (FNAB) when a needle is inserted into the lesion, such as a breast lump, and cells obtained by suction. Cells may also be obtained by scraping them from a surface (exfoliative cytology) which is the technique used for cervical screening. Fluid from collections of liquid such as a pleural effusion can also be obtained by aspiration for cytological examination. The pathologist's role may also include autopsies or post-mortem examinations, some of which may be forensic, i.e. investigation of suspicious or unexplained deaths.

Fig. 1.1 Types of biopsy used in diagnostic histopathology and cytopathology

Branch of pathology	Type of biopsy	What exactly is done	Examples
Histopathology	Core biopsy	Sample of a lesion removed by insertion of a needle to take a core biopsy (often uses a 'biopsy gun')	Core biopsy of breast mass Core biopsy of kidney in glomerulonephritis
	Incisional biopsy	Removes part of a lesion	Biopsy of skin rash
	Excision biopsy	Removes entire lesion	Benign breast lump
	Radical excision	Removes entire lesion plus additional tissues as required for cure or staging	Radical nephrectomy for malignant kidney tumour removes surrounding fat, adrenal gland and lymph nodes
Cytopathology	Aspiration cytology	Aspiration of a collection of fluid through a needle – may be part of a drainage procedure	Aspiration of pleural fluid to determine if the pleural fluid contains malignant cells
	Fine needle aspiration biopsy (FNAB)	Aspiration of a solid lesion using a very small diameter needle and suction	Aspiration of cells from a breast lump
	Exfoliative cytology	Removal of cells from the surface of tissue	Cervical screening

Normal cells exhibit a considerable degree of cellular adaptability in response to the constantly changing environment. For instance, over the course of a day most normal bodies are exposed to varying levels of hydration, nutrition, temperature and energy expenditure, to name but a few variables. Most of these adaptations take place at a biochemical level and represent fine regulation of metabolic function, a process known as **homeostasis**. However, some adaptations are also accompanied by structural changes that are visible microscopically. Many such structural changes fall within the normal pattern of growth of a tissue; for example, the thyroid gland enlarges in pregnancy owing to the action of increased thyroid-stimulating hormone on thyroid epithelial cells. This is an example of physiological cellular adaptation to a stimulus within the normal range. In contrast, certain environmental changes lie outside the normal physiological range and result in cellular malfunction, damage or even cell death: these stimuli are termed **pathological**. Pathological stimuli may simply be a more extreme form of a normal physiological event, e.g. exposure to extremes of temperature compared to normal day to day variations, or may be intrinsically pathological agents such as poisons, toxins or infective organisms.

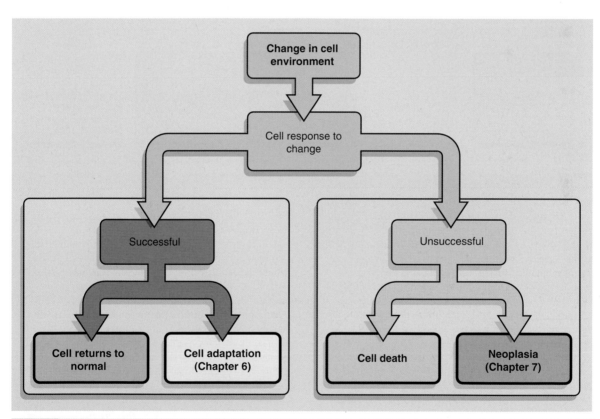

Fig. 1.2 Cellular adaptation

This diagram outlines the ways in which cells respond to changes in their environment. If a cell makes a successful response to an environmental change, then it will either return to normal or it may make an adaptive change. Adaptive changes, such as **hyperplasia** and **atrophy** are discussed in Chapter 6. This chapter will consider the morphological changes that occur when cells are exposed to pathological stimuli leading to cell damage and/or cell death. There is a further consequence of unsuccessful adaptation to an environmental change, the development of **neoplasia**, which will be discussed in Chapter 7.

The fate of a cell exposed to a harmful stimulus depends on the type, duration and magnitude of the injury, and partly on how vulnerable the cell is to the injury. For example, a cerebral neuron is much more vulnerable to damage following hypoxia than a fibroblast. Host factors also contribute to the overall response: an individual who has an immunodeficiency disorder or poor nutrition is more likely to succumb to overwhelming infection than a well-fed individual with a normal immune response.

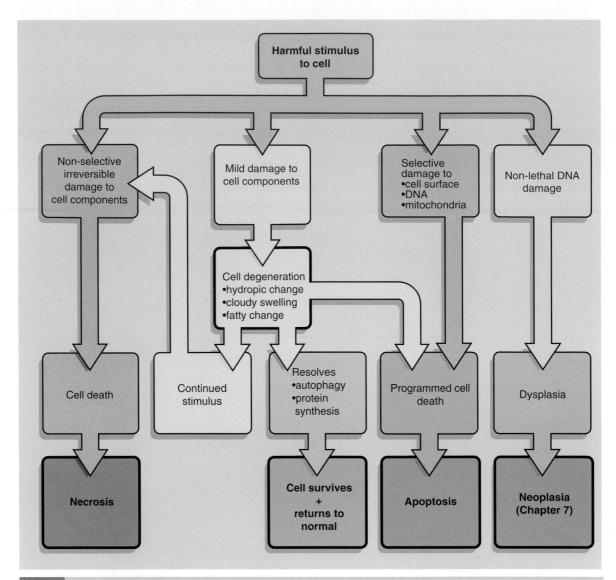

Fig. 1.3 **Response of cells to injury**

The ultimate fate of a cell, once exposed to a harmful stimulus, depends on the type, severity and duration of the stimulus and also on the type of cell. If there is mild damage to cell components, including the energy supply, then a cell may develop morphological changes termed *cellular degeneration*. The commonest structural changes are *cloudy swelling*, *hydropic degeneration*, and *fatty change* (see Figs 1.5 and 1.6). Importantly, such morphological changes are reversible if the causative harmful stimulus is removed or abates. Under such circumstances, a cell may return to normal after removal of damaged organelles through autophagy and the synthesis of new proteins. However, the outcome is not always successful and the damaged cell may still die.

If a cell develops severe, irreversible damage, usually involving many cellular components, then it is unable to respond and dies. Following cell death, a series of morphological changes take place, termed *necrosis* (Figs 1.7 and 1.8). Necrosis may also take place if, following development of the changes of cell degeneration, the harmful stimulus does not abate.

A variety of different triggers may initiate a process

of programmed cell death, known as *apoptosis* (Fig. 1.9). This is a highly organised process whereby intracellular signalling systems bring about destruction of the cell. Damage to DNA, cell surface membrane, or mitochondria are potent stimuli for apoptosis. Additionally, some cells that have initially responded by showing signs of cell degeneration (sublethal cell injury) may enter programmed cell death and die through apoptosis. Apoptosis is not always pathological: it is an important mechanism in embryonic development, in regression of normal tissues such as during the normal menstrual cycle and during the maintenance and renewal of normal cells and tissues. It is still uncertain why a cell is triggered to undergo apoptosis rather than necrosis, but certain types of pathological stimuli typically initiate apoptosis, e.g. radiation damage, certain viral infections. Necrosis, on the other hand, is the usual pattern of cell death in severe hypoxia.

Although discussed later in Chapter 7, it is important to note here that some harmful stimuli to cells can cause non-lethal DNA damage that leads to mutations and development of *dysplasia* and *neoplasia*.

Mitochondria – supply energy by oxidative phosphorylation

Rough endoplasmic reticulum studded with ribosomes

Free ribosomes in cytoplasm

Internal membrane systems

(a)

Mitochondria become dilated with disturbance of cristae

Rough endoplasmic reticulum becomes dilated with the loss of surface ribosomes

Loss of cytoplasmic free ribosomes

Internal membrane systems are dilated

(b)

(c)

Fig. 1.4 Early cellular responses to injury (a) Normal cell **(b)** Reversible cell damage **(c)** EM

Reversible cell damage involves injury to one or more vital cell systems including mitochondria, (leading to inability to produce energy in the form of ATP), cell membranes (causing loss of fluid and ion homeostasis) and accumulation of free radicals. The first ultrastructural evidence of sublethal cell damage is swelling of membrane-bound organelles, particularly endoplasmic reticulum and mitochondria as shown in (b).

In micrograph (c), an electron micrograph of a renal tubular epithelial cell damaged by hypoxia, most of the mitochondria are swollen. Instead of regular stacks of cristae (inner mitochondrial membrane), several of the mitochondria now contain spaces or vacuoles **V**, pushing the cristae apart. This is probably a result of accumulation of electrolytes and water owing to early damage to the enzymes of the membrane sodium pump. This change is potentially reversible but further insult leads to destruction of the cristae, more severe swelling of the mitochondria and formation of electron-dense bodies. At this stage, the changes are probably not reversible and cell death occurs.

Another manifestation of early cell injury is loss of ribosomes from both cytosol and the surface of the rough endoplasmic reticulum. Inner cell membrane systems, particularly the endoplasmic reticulum, become dilated and, in time, form vacuoles visible by light microscopy (see Fig. 1.5). Lethal injury is marked by progressive disintegration of other organelles, particularly lysosomes, which release hydrolytic enzymes causing autodigestion of the cell (*autolysis*). The cell membranes lose specialised structures such as microvilli and may form blebs that separate off from the cell.

KEY TO FIGURES
V vacuole

Fig. 1.5 **Hydropic degeneration** (*caption opposite*)

The earliest light microscopic evidence of cellular injury is loss of normal staining intensity of the cytoplasm owing to swelling of membrane-bound organelles. Normal cytoplasm stained with haematoxylin and eosin is light pink with a faint tint of blue; the blue tint (basophilia) is mainly due to the presence of ribosomal RNA. With sublethal cellular damage, ribosomes are reduced in number and the normal blue cytoplasmic tint is lost. Swelling of endoplasmic reticulum and mitochondria contributes to further cytoplasmic pallor. This is described as cloudy swelling and may be subtle and difficult to identify. With further swelling of organelles, the cell becomes waterlogged and true vacuoles appear in the cytoplasm, which now stains faintly with total loss of basophilia. At this stage, cells are said to exhibit *hydropic degeneration*. Micrograph (b) shows a section of kidney (cortex) with inadequate blood flow owing to severe hypotension. The cytoplasm of the epithelial cells of the cortical tubules is pale and vacuolated and exhibits hydropic degeneration **H**. The nuclei **N** are enlarged indicating increased protein synthesis as the cells attempt to recover and restore normal functions. Compare these tubular epithelial cells with Figure 1.5(a), a micrograph of normal renal cortex taken at similar magnification. These cells are very susceptible to hypoxia due to the very high energy demands required to produce urine. Such damage to the renal tubules may lead to acute renal failure, known as *acute tubular necrosis (ATN)*. With proper supportive measures, patients can make a full recovery.

Cloudy swelling and hydropic change reflect failure of membrane ion pumps, because of lack of cellular ATP, allowing the cell to accumulate fluid.

Fig. 1.6 **Fatty change: liver** (HP)

Fatty change (or *steatosis*) is another manifestation of sublethal metabolic derangement seen in certain cell types with high energy demand. It is most common in the liver, as in this example, but also occurs rarely in the myocardium and skeletal muscle. The common causes of fatty change in the liver are toxins (particularly alcohol and halogenated hydrocarbons such as chloroform), chronic hypoxia, diabetes mellitus and obesity. Impaired metabolism of fatty acids leads to accumulation of triglycerides (fats) that form non-membrane-bound vacuoles in cells, which may displace the nucleus from its usual location.

This example of liver from an alcoholic shows large vacuoles **V** in the hepatocytes with displacement of the nucleus **N**. In conventionally prepared tissue, organic solvents used in processing dissolve out the fat to leave empty, non-staining spaces. If necessary, frozen sections can be prepared to preserve the fat, which can then be specifically stained.

KEY TO FIGURES
H hydropic degeneration   **N** nucleus   **V** vacuoles

Fig. 1.7 Cell necrosis (a) Liver (HP) (b) Renal cortex (HP)

When a cell has sustained irreversible damage, a succession of histological changes occur which are grouped under the term *necrosis*. By definition, necrosis can only occur in a living organism.

Micrograph (a) is a section of liver from a person poisoned by paracetamol, an hepatic toxin in overdose. Many of the hepatocytes are pale-stained and a few exhibit early cytoplasmic vacuolation, indicating hydropic degeneration. Several cells also show early histological features of necrosis **N**. The dead cells stain a bright pink (eosinophilia) and stand out from the other cells; this is due to degeneration of structural proteins which form a compact homogeneous mass. Compared to living cells, the nucleus of each necrotic cell is smaller, condensed and intensely stained with haematoxylin (basophilia). This nuclear condensation is termed *pyknosis* and is due to progressive chromatin clumping, possibly as a result of reduced pH resulting from terminal anaerobic metabolism.

In micrograph (b), which is a micrograph of necrotic kidney, the changes of necrosis are more developed. Pyknotic nuclei **Py** stand out as intensely basophilic, round bodies. Note that the nuclear changes are accompanied by cytoplasmic changes. The cytoplasm has lost definition and the cell margins (plasma membranes) are indistinct. In time, the pyknotic nuclei become fragmented into several particles which represent pieces of degenerate nuclear material, a change termed *karyorrhexis* **K**.

Complete breakdown of nuclear material then takes place by release of cellular hydrolytic enzymes, leading to loss of the groups which bind haematoxylin. This process is termed *karyolysis* and, when complete, leaves the dead cell as an anucleate, homogeneous, eosinophilic mass.

Many of the structural changes seen in necrosis are mediated through the action of lysosomal enzymes, liberated through breakdown of internal cell membranes.

Fig. 1.8 **Patterns of tissue necrosis** (a) Coagulative necrosis: kidney (MP) (b) Colliquative necrosis: brain (HP)

Traditionally, three main patterns of tissue necrosis are described: *coagulative*, *colliquative* and *caseous*. Each term describes the macroscopic appearance of necrotic tissue. In coagulative necrosis, the tissue appears firm, as if cooked. In colliquative necrosis, the dead tissue appears semi-liquid, while in caseous necrosis, the dead tissue has a soft consistency, reminiscent of cream cheese. These gross patterns correlate closely with histological appearances.

In areas of coagulative necrosis, much of the cellular outline and tissue architecture can be discerned histologically even though the cells are dead. The commonest cause of this pattern of necrosis is ischaemia owing to loss of arterial oxygenated blood, such as in myocardial infarction.

In areas of caseous necrosis, cells die and form an amorphous proteinaceous mass in which no semblance of original architecture can be discerned. Caseous necrosis is typically seen in tuberculosis, several examples of which are shown in Chapter 4.

The term colliquative necrosis was originally used to describe the macroscopic appearance of necrosis in the brain as a result of arterial occlusion (cerebral infarction) at a stage when the necrotic area was occupied by semi-liquid material. This appearance, however, is not a specific form of necrosis, but results from dissolution of tissue after an initial coagulative phase, which is common to all tissues immediately following cell death. The subsequent liquefaction of

dead tissue reflects both tissue composition and the cause of necrosis. In brain, the relative lack of extracellular structural proteins (reticulin and collagen) leads to rapid loss of tissue architecture as autolysis occurs, resulting in the early formation of a semi-liquid mass of dead cells. Otherwise, liquefaction of dead tissues is virtually confined to cases of necrosis associated with *pyogenic* (pus-producing) bacteria such as in an abscess (Fig. 2.13).

Micrograph (a) is an example of coagulative necrosis in an area of kidney subject to infarction. Note that the architecture of a glomerulus **G** and surrounding tubules is still recognisable despite the dissolution of nuclear material, except for a few pyknotic and karyorrhectic remnants.

Micrograph (b) illustrates the liquefaction phase in a cerebral infarct where no residual tissue architecture is preserved; the earlier phase of coagulative necrosis in brain can be seen in Figure 23.2. The necrotic brain is now largely replaced by wisps of pink-staining cellular debris, with phagocytic cells **P** engulfing degenerate material. Some of these contain haemosiderin pigment **H** which is a breakdown product of haemoglobin and is indicative of haemorrhage into the tissue.

A fourth type of necrosis, known as *fibrinoid necrosis*, is principally seen in the walls of blood vessels and is discussed in Chapter 11.

KEY TO FIGURES
G glomerulus   **H** haemosiderin pigment   **K** karyorrhexis   **N** necrotic cells   **P** phagocytic cells   **Py** pyknosis

(a)

(b)

(c)

Fig. 1.9 Apoptosis (a) Early stage **(b)** Later stage **(c)** Apoptosis in colonic glands (HP)

Certain stimuli to cells lead to their controlled elimination by programmed cell death in a process called *apoptosis*. Although apoptosis is a normal physiological process, for example in embryonic development and normal cell turnover, it is also an important mechanism for elimination of damaged or diseased cells. Apoptosis may be triggered by the *intrinsic* or *extrinsic pathways*: for example, absence of a necessary growth factor triggers the intrinsic pathway, while binding of signalling molecules such as tumour necrosis factor to its receptor (one of the 'death receptors') on the cell surface, triggers the external pathway. Increased permeability of mitochondrial outer membranes and release of cytochrome c into the cytoplasm is a common step in apoptosis whatever the trigger. Cytochrome c is able to activate the early or initiation members of the caspase cascade. Caspases which are proteases, cleave cellular proteins, and activate endonucleases that break down chromatin. Caspases are present in all cells as proenzymes and form an enzymatic cascade system analogous to the blood clotting system or the complement system. They represent the final effector mechanism of apoptosis.

When apoptosis is triggered, cells undergo a distinct set of structural changes that correspond to the biochemical changes occurring in the cell. Diagram (a) illustrates how the cell loses specialised surface features and attachments to other cells and structures, becoming 'rounded up'. The nucleus becomes shrunken with dense condensation of chromatin beneath the nuclear membrane.

Diagram (b) illustrates the rapid fragmentation of the cell into multiple small *apoptotic bodies*, each one being membrane-bound and many containing nuclear remnants. Each fragment is still a vital entity. The surface membranes express factors that facilitate phagocytosis by adjacent cells and macrophages.

Many stimuli can activate apoptosis. Cell membrane damage, damage to mitochondria, damage to DNA, viral infection, and immune-mediated attack are all common triggers. The benefit of eliminating cells by apoptosis is that individual cells can be removed in a way that does not stimulate an inflammatory response.

Micrograph (c) shows apoptosis in colonic glands in a patient who had a bone marrow graft and is suffering from graft-versus-host disease, in which donor immune cells attack host tissues, in this case the colonic epithelial cells. At least three late apoptotic cells represented by multiple dot-like *apoptotic bodies* A are seen.

In tumour pathology, apoptosis is a major factor that limits the growth of a neoplasm. The production by tumour cells of factors that prevent apoptosis is an important mechanism in the development of uncontrolled growth.

KEY TO FIGURES
A apoptotic bodies

Fig. 1.10 Chapter review

Pathological process	Causes	Clinical presentation	Main histological features	Figure
Acute reversible cell damage	Acute ischaemia Toxins	Acute failure/malfunction of organ, e.g. acute renal failure	Swelling of cell cytoplasm Vacuolation of cells	1.5
Fatty change	Toxins, e.g. alcohol,	Initially normal Later develop organ failure to varying degrees	Clear vacuole within cells containing excess lipid May expand to completely fill cytoplasm	1.6, 14.4, 14.7(a)
Necrosis – coagulative	Ischaemia	Organ malfunction e.g. myocardial infarction	Maintenance of tissue architecture, loss of cell nuclei, cytoplasm becomes eosinophilic, eventually develops fibrous scar	1.8(a)
Necrosis – colliquative	Ischaemia – only affects brain	Organ malfunction e.g. cerebral infarction ('stroke')	Damaged area replaced by cyst filled with fluid, surrounding brain has increased glial cells (gliosis)	1.8(b)
Necrosis – caseous	Mycobacterial infection (tuberculosis)	Low grade fever, malaise, organ malfunction – can affect any organ, very variable clinical presentation	Classical epithelioid granulomas with central featureless necrotic material, surrounded by a zone of lymphocytes; later there is fibrosis and scarring	Ch. 4
Necrosis – fibrinoid	Damage to blood vessel walls due to accelerated hypertension or immune mechanisms	Vessel malfunction – blockage due to thrombosis and/or haemorrhage due to rupture	Deposition of plasma proteins within the vessel wall- appears as an eosinophilic deposit, may be associated with inflammation and/or thrombus	11.2, 11.7
Apoptosis (programmed cell death)	May be physiological or pathological	Destruction of virus-infected cells, graft versus host disease, elimination of old/ worn-out cells	Drop-out of individual cells often surrounded by lymphocytes, apoptotic bodies	1.9

2 Acute inflammation, healing and repair

Introduction

Inflammation is an almost universal response to tissue damage by a wide range of harmful stimuli, including mechanical trauma, tissue necrosis and infection. The purpose of inflammation is to destroy (or contain) the damaging agent, initiate repair processes and return the damaged tissue to useful function. Inflammation is somewhat arbitrarily divided into ***acute*** and ***chronic inflammation*** but, in reality, the two often form a continuum. Many causes of tissue damage provoke an acute inflammatory response but some types of insult may bring about a typical chronic inflammatory reaction from the outset (e.g. viral infections, foreign body reactions and fungal infections). Acute inflammation may ***resolve*** or ***heal by scarring*** but may also progress to chronic inflammation, and it is common for a mixed acute and chronic response to coexist. This chapter describes acute inflammation and its sequelae, while chronic inflammation is discussed in Chapter 3. Many examples of acute and chronic inflammation are illustrated throughout this book.

There are three major and interrelated components of acute inflammation:

■ **Vascular dilatation**

- Relaxation of vascular smooth muscle leads to engorgement of tissue with blood (***hyperaemia***)

■ **Endothelial activation**

- Increased endothelial permeability allows plasma proteins to pass into tissues

- Expression of adhesion molecules on the endothelial surface mediates neutrophils adherence

- Production of factors that cause vascular dilatation

■ **Neutrophil activation and migration**

- Expression of adhesion molecules causes neutrophils to adhere to endothelium

- Increased motility allows emigration from vessels into surrounding tissues

- Increased capacity for bacterial killing

Fig. 2.1 Outline of acute inflammation (*illustration opposite*)

Acute inflammation may develop over minutes or hours, depending on the type and severity of the tissue damage, and generally lasts hours to days. Vascular dilatation, increased vascular permeability and neutrophil activation and migration are interdependent processes and all three are required for the full response. Immediately after the tissue damage has occurred there may be a brief phase of constriction of arterioles, but this is followed within seconds by arteriolar and capillary dilatation, increasing blood flow to the area. This is mediated by histamine and nitric oxide, released by tissue mast cells and endothelial cells respectively. At much the same time, gaps form between endothelial cells of the post-capillary venules, allowing protein-rich plasma to leak into the tissue. The dilated capillaries and venules become engorged with red cells and blood flow slows and then stops. The slowing of blood flow brings neutrophils into contact with the endothelial cells, which have been activated to increase expression of ***adhesion molecules*** on their surface membranes. These include selectins and integrin receptors. As the neutrophils come into contact with the endothelium, adhesion molecules on the neutrophil cell membrane bind to their complementary molecules on the endothelial cells and become stuck. Activation of neutrophils plays a role here, in that activated neutrophils are more likely to stick. The neutrophils pass through the basement membrane of the endothelium and move along a concentration gradient of ***chemotactic factors***. When they arrive at the site of injury, the activated neutrophils phagocytose necrotic tissue debris and any pathogenic organisms. The activation of the neutrophils makes them more efficient at phagocytosis and bacterial killing. ***Opsonisation*** of bacteria by complement and immunoglobulins renders them more readily phagocytosed.

Meanwhile, in the tissues, the plasma-derived proteins undergo various changes. The ***complement cascade*** is initiated (alternative pathway) forming components, such as C5a and C3a, with a wide range of activities. ***Immunoglobulins*** bind to any causative organisms, immobilising them and forming immune complexes that further activate complement (classical pathway). ***Fibrinogen*** is cleaved to form monomers which then polymerise to form a network of ***fibrin*** that impedes the movement of any pathogenic organisms present and also provides a framework for the movement of neutrophils. The increased fluid in the tissue causes an increased flow of lymph to carry immune complexes and antigenic material to the lymph nodes, where a specific immune response is initiated over the next few days. This entire process is orchestrated by a plethora of chemical mediators derived from injured tissues, bacteria, plasma proteins and leukocytes. The most important of these mediators are indicated at their sites of action. Note that some mediators have multiple actions.

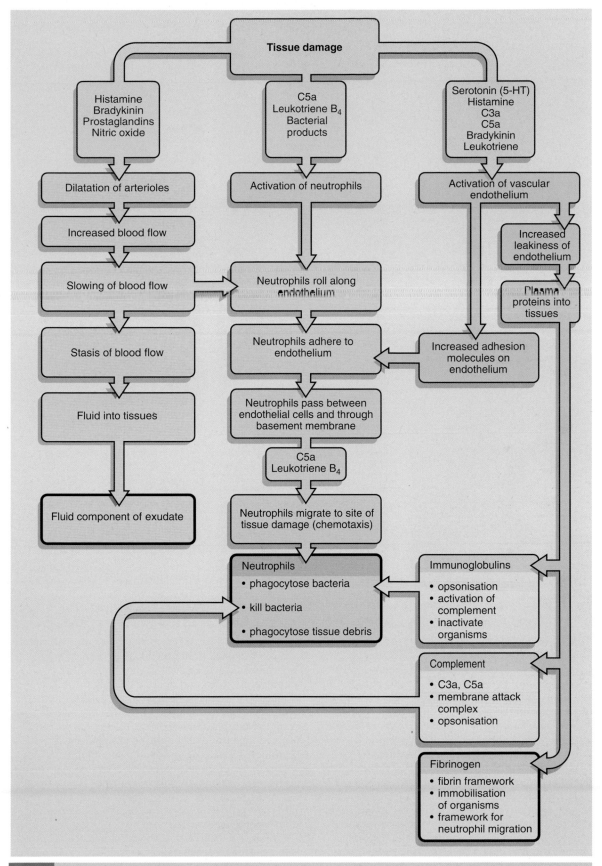

Fig. 2.1 **Outline of acute inflammation** (*caption opposite*)

Fig. 2.2 **Formation of the acute inflammatory exudate** **(a)** Early vascular changes (HP) **(b)** Migration of neutrophils (HP) **(c)** Early formation of exudate (LP)

This set of micrographs illustrates the sequence of events during the initial phases of the acute inflammatory response described in Figure 2.1. In micrograph (a), two small capillaries are shown. Both vessels are dilated and in the larger, neutrophils **N** line up around the periphery of the vessel, a process termed *pavementing*. Neutrophils are easily identified in tissue sections by their lobulated nuclei and inconspicuous cytoplasm. These neutrophils are adherent to the endothelium, a process facilitated by increased expression of adhesion molecules on the endothelium and on the neutrophils. The surrounding fibrous connective tissue contains clear spaces owing to the accumulation of fluid (*oedema*) between the collagen bundles. Plasma proteins, although not visible, are also found free within the tissue. These include components of the blood coagulation cascade, acute phase reactants, complement proteins and circulating immunoglobulins.

The neutrophils pass through the vessel wall by extending a pseudopodium between adjacent endothelial cells. The neutrophils then penetrate the endothelial basement membrane and move into the perivascular connective tissue as shown in micrograph

(b). Once in the extravascular tissues, the neutrophils **N** are attracted to the site of tissue damage by chemotactic agents, such as the complement component *C5a*, and migrate actively towards higher concentrations of these agents (*chemotaxis*); this is shown in micrograph (c). At the site of tissue damage, neutrophils play an important role in destruction of microorganisms. Phagocytosis of organisms is promoted by a coating of immunoglobulin and complement (*opsonisation*) and activated neutrophils are more effective at killing pathogens. These three components, namely water, proteins (including fibrin **Fi**) and neutrophils **N**, form the typical *acute inflammatory exudate*.

Chemical mediators, although not visible, control this process. Vasodilatation is mediated by *histamine*, *prostaglandins* and *nitric oxide*. Increased vascular permeability is controlled by substances such as the vasoactive amines, serotonin (5-hydroxytryptamine (5-HT)) and histamine, complement components *C5a* and *C3a*, leukotrienes C_4, D_4, and E_4, and *platelet activating factor (PAF)*. Leukocyte activation and chemotaxis are influenced by *C5a*, *leukotriene B_4*, various *chemokines* and bacterial products.

KEY TO FIGURES

A alveolus   **C** alveolar capillary   **F** interlobar fissure   **Fi** fibrin   **M** alveolar macrophage   **N** neutrophils

Fig. 2.3 **Established acute inflammation: lobar pneumonia** (a) LP (b) MP

This is an example of an established acute inflammatory reaction in the lung parenchyma, namely lobar pneumonia. This pattern of pneumonia is most commonly caused by the pneumococcus (*Streptococcus pneumoniae*). In lobar pneumonia, which is less common now than previously, a whole lobe becomes solidified as a result of a massive outpouring of fluid, fibrin and neutrophils into the alveolar spaces. However, by far the most common type of pneumonia is bronchopneumonia (see Fig. 12.5), where infection spreads from the bronchi into adjacent lung tissue.

In micrograph (a), a portion of lung is shown with an interlobar fissure **F** running vertically. The lung tissue on the left shows obliteration of alveolar spaces by purple-staining masses of inflammatory cells (mainly neutrophils) with associated fibrin; this is termed *consolidation*. Alveolar walls can still be discerned. The dense inflammatory exudate is sharply limited by the interlobar fissure. The lung on the right of the fissure shows the earliest changes of acute inflammation, with faint pink-staining serous exudate in alveoli **A** and early neutrophil migration giving rise to a few scattered cells within the alveolar spaces.

At higher magnification in micrograph (b), alveolar wall capillaries **C** are seen engorged with blood. The alveolar spaces are obliterated by an acute inflammatory exudate rich in neutrophils and lesser amounts of wispy pink-stained fibrin. Occasional large, rounded mononuclear cells, macrophages **M**, can also be seen, but these are few in the acute phase of the disease.

If untreated, there are various possible outcomes to lobar pneumonia: death may occur (as in this patient), there may be complete resolution (see Fig. 2.8), or, very rarely, the exudate may become organised with consequent permanent fibrosis of the lung tissue, or lung abscess or empyema may develop.

Morphological types of acute inflammation

While the basic process of acute inflammation is the same in all tissues, there are frequently qualitative differences in the inflammatory response seen under different circumstances. Terms describing these variations are widely used in clinical practice and are summarised below:

■ *Suppurative inflammation (purulent inflammation)* refers to acute inflammation in which the acute inflammatory exudate is particularly rich in neutrophil leukocytes. Suppurative inflammation is most commonly seen as a result of infection by bacteria where the mixture of neutrophils (viable and dead), necrotic tissue, and tissue fluid in the acute inflammatory exudate form a semi-liquid material referred to as *pus*; hence the term *purulent inflammation* (see Fig. 2.4). Within tissues, a circumscribed collection of semi-liquid pus is termed an *abscess* (see Fig. 2.13). The destruction of tissue may be due as much to release of neutrophil lysosomal enzymes as to tissue destruction by bacteria. Bacteria which produce purulent inflammation are described as *pyogenic bacteria*. They initiate massive neutrophilic infiltration with subsequent destruction of infected tissues. Pyogenic bacteria include staphylococci, some streptococci *(S. pyogenes, S. pneumoniae), Escherichia coli* and the neisseriae *(N. meningitidis, N. gonorrhoeae)*.

■ *Fibrinous inflammation* refers to a pattern of acute inflammation where the acute inflammatory exudate has a high plasma protein content (see Fig. 2.4). Fibrinogen, derived from plasma, is converted to fibrin, which is deposited in tissues. This pattern is particularly associated with membrane-lined cavities such as the pleura, pericardium and peritoneum, where the fibrin strands form a mat-like sheet causing adhesion between adjacent surfaces.

■ *Serous inflammation* describes a pattern of acute inflammation where the main tissue response is an accumulation of fluid with a low plasma protein and cell content. This is often called a *transudate*, which by definition has a specific gravity of <1.012 or protein content of <25 g/L in contrast to an *exudate,* with a specific gravity >1.020 and protein content >25 g/L. This pattern of response is most commonly seen in the skin in response to a burn.

| Fig. 2.4 **Acute inflammatory exudate** (a) Neutrophilic exudate (HP) (b) Highly fibrinous exudate (HP) (c) Fibrinous inflammation: acute pericarditis (LP) |

These micrographs contrast purulent and fibrinous inflammation. Micrograph (a) shows a purulent acute inflammatory exudate in which neutrophils **N** are the main component (i.e. pus). This is the typical pattern of acute inflammation when the damaging stimulus is a pyogenic bacterial infection. After migration into the tissues, neutrophils phagocytose and kill the causative organisms. At the site of inflammation the activated neutrophils generate a *respiratory burst* to produce the hydrogen peroxide and other reactive oxygen species used to kill bacteria; the neutrophils then die by apoptosis. Mature neutrophils only survive for 3 days but their numbers are maintained in acute inflammation by new arrivals from the circulation; the systemic response to acute inflammation is release of neutrophils from bone marrow into the blood, resulting in a *neutrophil leukocytosis*. Apoptotic neutrophils can be recognised by condensation (pyknosis) and fragmentation (karyorrhexis) of their nuclei and,

eventually, cytoplasmic disintegration; the neutrophil debris is usually phagocytosed by macrophages. Good examples of purulent inflammation include lobar pneumonia (see Fig. 2.3), bronchopneumonia (see Fig. 12.5) and acute appendicitis (see Fig. 13.16) and many other examples are found throughout this text.

An acute inflammatory exudate on a serosal surface usually contains plentiful fibrin. Micrograph (b) shows an acute inflammatory exudate consisting of fibrin **F** with very few neutrophils *(fibrinous exudate)*, sometimes described as 'bread and butter pericarditis'. Macroscopically, a shaggy layer of fibrin coats the formerly smooth surface as in acute pericarditis (c). In this low-magnification micrograph, the exudate **Ex** is well established on the pericardial aspect of the pericardium **P**. No myocardium is seen in this micrograph, but epicardial fat **Fa** is readily identifiable. Acute pericarditis most commonly occurs after death of underlying cardiac muscle (*myocardial infarction*).

The vascular and exudative phenomena of acute inflammation are responsible for the clinical features and were described by Celsus in the first century AD. The *cardinal signs of Celsus* are:

■ **redness** (rubor) caused by hyperaemia

■ **swelling** (tumor) caused by fluid exudation and hyperaemia

■ **heat** (calor) caused by hyperaemia

■ **pain** (dolor) resulting from release of bradykinin and PGE_2.

Virchow later added:

■ **loss of function** (functio laesa) caused by the combined effects of the above.

Clinically, patients who have significant acute inflammation feel unwell and have a fever. This is mediated by cytokines released into the blood (*interleukins 1 & 6, tumour necrosis factor (TNF)* and prostaglandins), acting on the hypothalamus. Laboratory investigations commonly reveal a raised neutrophil count in the blood (neutrophil leukocytosis).The nomenclature used to describe inflammation in different tissues employs the tissue name (or its Greek or Latin equivalent) and the suffix '-itis'. For example, inflammation of the appendix is referred to as *appendicitis,* inflammation of the Fallopian tube is termed *salpingitis* and inflammation of the pericardium is termed *pericarditis*. Notable exceptions to this rule include *pleurisy*, for inflammation of the pleura and acute *cellulitis* for inflammation of subcutaneous tissues. Many examples of acute inflammatory diseases are presented in the systematic pathology chapters, which form the second half of this book.

Fig. 2.5	Nomenclature and aetiology of common types of inflammation

Tissue	Acute inflammation	Typical causes
Meninges	Meningitis	Bacterial and viral infections
Brain	Encephalitis	Viral infections
Lung	Pneumonia	Bacterial infections
Pleura	Pleurisy	Bacterial and viral infections
Pericardium	Pericarditis	Bacterial and viral infections, myocardial infarction
Oesophagus	Oesophagitis	Gastric acid reflux, fungal infection (*Candida albicans*)
Stomach	Gastritis	*Helicobacter pylori* infection, reflux/chemical gastritis
Colon	Colitis	Bacterial infections, inflammatory bowel disease
Rectum	Proctitis	Infections, ulcerative colitis
Appendix	Appendicitis	Faecal obstruction
Liver	Hepatitis	Alcohol abuse, viral infections
Gallbladder	Cholecystitis	Bacterial infections, chemical irritation
Pancreas	Pancreatitis	Obstructed pancreatic duct, alcoholism, shock
Urinary bladder	Cystitis	Bacterial infections
Bone	Osteomyelitis	Bacterial infections
Subcutaneous tissues	Cellulitis	Bacterial infections
Joints	Arthritis	Infections, autoimmune diseases
Arteries	Arteritis	Immune complex deposition
Kidney	Pyelonephritis	Bacterial infections
Peritoneum	Peritonitis	Spread from intra-abdominal inflammation, e.g. appendicitis, salpingitis Ruptured viscus, e.g. perforated peptic ulcer

KEY TO FIGURES
Ex exudate   **F** fibrin   **Fa** pericardial fat   **N** neutrophils   **P** pericardium

Outcomes of acute inflammation

The process of acute inflammation is designed to neutralise injurious agents and to restore the tissue to useful function. There are four main outcomes of acute inflammation (if the patient survives): *resolution*, *healing by fibrosis*, *abscess formation*, and *progression to chronic inflammation*. Three factors determine which of these outcomes occurs:

■ the severity of tissue damage

■ the capacity of stem cells within the damaged tissue to divide and replace the specialised cells required, a process termed *regeneration*

■ the type of agent which has caused the tissue damage.

Resolution involves complete restitution of normal tissue architecture and function. This can only occur if the connective tissue framework of the tissue is intact and the tissue involved has the capacity to replace any specialised cells that have been lost (regeneration). Neutrophils and damaged/dead tissue are removed by phagocytosis by macrophages which leave the tissue via the lymphatics. Regeneration of tissues plays an important part in resolution, for example regrowth of alveolar lining cells following pneumonia: this regrowth is dependent on the intrinsic ability of resident stem cells to divide and differentiate into mature tissue cells. Examples of resolution are recovery from sunburn (acute inflammatory response in the skin as a result of ultraviolet (UV) radiation exposure) and the restitution of normal lung structure and function following lobar pneumonia (see Fig. 2.3).

Healing by fibrosis (scar formation) occurs when there is substantial damage to the connective tissue framework and/or the tissue lacks the ability to regenerate specialised cells. In these instances, dead tissues and acute inflammatory exudate are first removed from the damaged area by macrophages (see Fig. 2.7), and the defect becomes filled by ingrowth of a specialised vascular connective tissue called *granulation tissue* (see Fig. 2.9). This is termed *organisation*. The granulation tissue gradually produces collagen to form a *fibrous (collagenous) scar*, constituting the process of *repair* (see Figs 2.9 and 2.10). Despite the loss of some specialised cells and some architectural distortion by fibrous scar, structural integrity is re-established. Any impairment of function is dependent on the extent of loss of specialised cells. Modified forms of fibrous repair occur in bone after a fracture when new bone is created (see Fig. 2.12), and in brain with the formation of an astrocytic scar (see Fig. 23.2).

Abscess formation takes place when the acute inflammatory reaction fails to destroy/remove the cause of tissue damage and continues, usually with a component of chronic inflammation. This is most common in the case of infection by pyogenic bacteria. As the acute inflammation progresses, there is liquefaction of the tissue to form *pus*. At the periphery of this acute abscess, a chronic inflammatory component surrounds the area and fibrous tissue is laid down, walling off the suppuration (see Fig. 2.13).

Chronic inflammation may result following acute inflammation when an injurious agent persists over a prolonged period, causing concomitant tissue destruction, inflammation, organisation and repair. Some injurious agents elicit a chronic inflammatory type of response from the outset. Chronic inflammation is discussed fully in Chapter 3.

INFLAMMATION OUT OF CONTROL

Inflammation can do harm as well as good. In most people, inflammation is activated appropriately in response to some kind of adverse stimulus and terminated promptly when the infective organisms have been eliminated and tissue damage repaired. In some individuals, control of the inflammatory process is lost for unknown reasons. One of the major stimuli to acute inflammation is the specific immune response where specific antibodies recruit components of the acute inflammatory response as effector mechanisms, thereby directing the non-specific components of the acute inflammatory system at specific targets. Normally, the immune system is programmed to ignore the potentially antigenic molecules that make up the individual's own body. In people who develop *autoimmune disease* this *self-tolerance* is lost for one or more antigens. This may be organ-specific antigens as in the organ-specific autoimmune disease Hashimoto's thyroiditis (see Ch. 20) or, at the other end of the spectrum, the antigens triggering the response may be widespread in many tissues, as in systemic lupus erythematosus (SLE), where the body reacts to double-stranded DNA as well as many other cellular antigens.

In many autoimmune disorders, inflammation and pain may cause major morbidity. Also, the misdirection of the immune response causes local tissue damage such as pain and swelling in the joints in people with rheumatoid arthritis (see Ch. 22) or renal failure due to damage to the kidney in SLE. Many anti-inflammatory drugs are available but almost all have potentially serious and quite common side effects. Therefore, the recent discovery of a range of naturally occurring mediators including lipoxins, resolvins and neuroprotectins that function normally to switch off the immune response has opened up new possible avenues of treatment of these conditions with potentially fewer side effects.

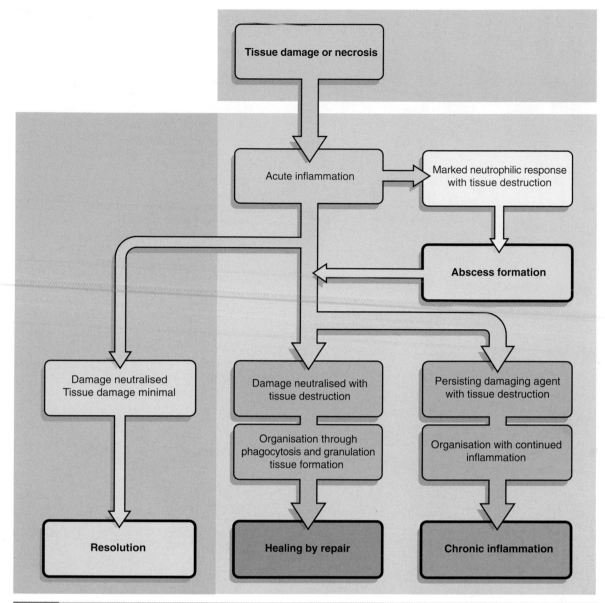

Fig. 2.6 **Outcomes of acute inflammation**

This flow chart summarises the main outcomes following acute inflammation. Complete restoration is uncommon, the most usual outcomes being either healing by fibrous repair (leaving a collagenous scar) or progression to chronic inflammation.

Fig. 2.7 Early outcome of acute inflammation: macrophage accumulation (HP)

As early as the second or third day of the acute inflammatory response, macrophages accumulate in increasing numbers. These enter the tissue in a similar fashion to neutrophils in response to chemotactic factors. Macrophages phagocytose cell debris, dead neutrophils and fibrin. At the same time, lymphocytes begin to enter the damaged area, reflecting an immune response to any introduced antigens.

This micrograph shows an area of cardiac muscle that has undergone necrosis following blockage of its arterial supply (*myocardial infarction*). The acute inflammatory response has almost run its course, and the neutrophils and fibrin predominant in the earlier stages have been removed by macrophages. All that remains is a soft, loose tissue containing a few necrotic myocardial remnants **My**, one of which is shown here being engulfed by macrophages **M**. The macrophages can be identified under these circumstances by the foamy appearance of their cytoplasm, which also often contains brownish pigment granules. These brown granules are iron-containing pigments (*haemosiderin*) derived from haemoglobin. Further details of the events following myocardial infarction are shown in Figure 10.2.

Fig. 2.8 Resolution of acute inflammation: lobar pneumonia (MP)

Occasionally, a damaging stimulus may excite a strong acute inflammatory response with minimal tissue damage. In such circumstances, resolution of the exudate may occur without any need for organisation and repair, thereby leaving no residual tissue scarring.

This phenomenon occurs in lobar pneumonia, in which the acute inflammatory response is due to infection by a bacterium, commonly the pneumococcus (see Fig. 2.3). The alveoli of one or more lobes of the lung are filled with acute inflammatory exudate and the loss of respiratory function may be so great as to cause fatal *hypoxia*. In the pre-antibiotic era this was a common cause of death in previously fit young people.

Bacteria are engulfed by neutrophils and fibrin strands are broken down by *fibrinolysins* derived from plasma and neutrophil lysosomes. Macrophages **M** are recruited and phagocytose apoptotic neutrophils, extravasated red cells and other cell debris. Fluid and degraded proteinaceous material **P**, together with the macrophages, are then resorbed into the circulation via alveolar wall vessels and interstitial lymphatics, or may be coughed up as brown-coloured sputum. Alveolar spaces are thus cleared of exudate and can participate in gas exchange. Regeneration of alveolar lining cells completes the return to normal structure and function.

Fig. 2.9 **Granulation tissue** **(a)** Vascular granulation tissue (HP) **(b)** Fibrous granulation tissue (MP)

Where there is significant damage to the connective tissue framework, the first phase of the healing process is the formation of *granulation tissue*, a mixture of proliferating capillaries, fibroblasts and inflammatory cells. Formation of a network of new capillaries **C** (*angiogenesis*) occurs by a combination of budding from vessels at the periphery of the damaged area and from endothelial precursor cells. This is stimulated by growth factors such as *vascular endothelial growth factor (VEGF)*. In this early form, termed *vascular granulation tissue* (micrograph (a)), the spaces between the capillaries are occupied by macrophages **M**, lymphocytes, proliferating fibroblasts and loose oedematous extracellular matrix. The capillaries are thin-walled and relatively leaky, leading to extravasation of erythrocytes and fluid into the tissue. Students often confuse granulation tissue with *granulomas* (see Ch. 3) but the two are quite different.

Over time, most of the vessels regress, collagen is laid down, and the inflammatory cells return to the circulation. The effect of this progression is seen in

micrograph (b), where numerous plump activated fibroblasts **F** can be seen with a few residual lymphocytes and relatively inconspicuous capillaries **C**. This is now termed *fibrous granulation tissue* in recognition of the presence of mature collagenous fibrous tissue. Collagen, laid down by the fibroblasts, becomes remodelled in an orderly pattern (upper left area of micrograph) and the fibrous granulation tissue takes on the characteristics of an early *fibrous scar* (see Fig. 2.11).

Granulation tissue is also involved in healing of wounds, whatever the cause and site of the tissue defect. In the case of a simple skin incision, where the wound edges are in close apposition and the actual defect is minimal, healing occurs quickly with a small amount of granulation tissue and is termed *healing by primary intention*. In other situations, the tissue defect will be large and filled with blood clot and a variable amount of tissue debris. In this case, described as *healing by secondary intention*, organisation and filling of the defect by granulation tissue take considerably longer (see Fig. 2.10).

DELAYED WOUND HEALING

Many factors can delay or stop healing. A common one is continuing inflammation where the initial stimulus to inflammation persists: a good example of this would be an infected wound or persistent peptic ulceration due to *Helicobacter pylori* infection (see Ch. 13). The presence of dead tissue or a foreign body in a wound can also slow healing. Host factors such as poor nutrition, poor circulation, pre-existing diabetes mellitus or medications such as steroids can also delay healing.

KEY TO FIGURES
C capillary **F** fibroblast **M** macrophage **My** myocardial remnant **P** proteinaceous debris

Wound healing by primary intention	Wound healing by secondary intention

Simple incision

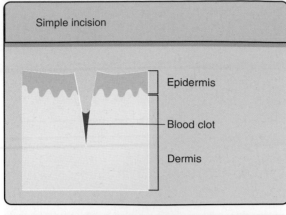

- Epidermis
- Blood clot
- Dermis

Ragged, dirty or infected wound (at 2–3 days)

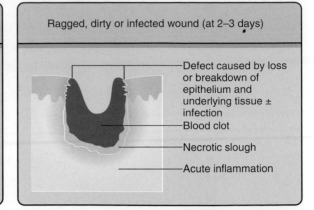

- Defect caused by loss or breakdown of epithelium and underlying tissue ± infection
- Blood clot
- Necrotic slough
- Acute inflammation

Sutured incision with acute inflammatory response (2–7 days)

- Redness and swelling
- Zone of acute inflammation Formation of granulation tissue

Phase of rapid proliferation of vascular granulation tissue (about 1–2 weeks)

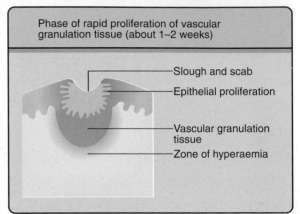

- Slough and scab
- Epithelial proliferation
- Vascular granulation tissue
- Zone of hyperaemia

Healing incision (early weeks)

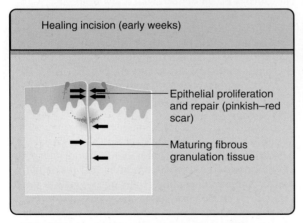

- Epithelial proliferation and repair (pinkish–red scar)
- Maturing fibrous granulation tissue

Phase of granulation tissue maturation and wound contraction (about 3–6 weeks)

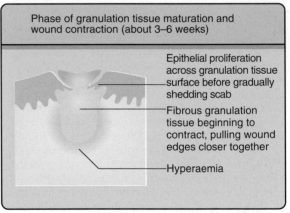

- Epithelial proliferation across granulation tissue surface before gradually shedding scab
- Fibrous granulation tissue beginning to contract, pulling wound edges closer together
- Hyperaemia

Linear fibrous scar (6–12 months)

- White scar

Healed wound

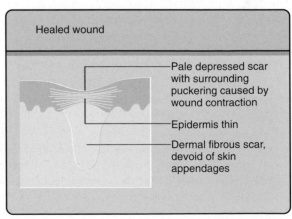

- Pale depressed scar with surrounding puckering caused by wound contraction
- Epidermis thin
- Dermal fibrous scar, devoid of skin appendages

Fig. 2.10 Wound healing

Fig. 2.11 **Fibrous scar** **(a)** Fibrous scar tissue (HP) **(b)** Skin scar (LP)

The deposition of collagen within fibrous granulation tissue occurs over a period of many weeks. Collagen is remodelled in an appropriate orientation to withstand the tensile stresses placed on the area of repair. With time, the previously plump and metabolically active fibroblasts regress and become relatively inconspicuous, as shown in micrograph (a) of a typical area of early fibrous scar. Note the condensed nuclei of inactive fibroblasts **F**. Some capillaries **C** persist, accounting for the red appearance of recent scars.

Micrograph (b) illustrates, at low magnification, a recent area of scarring in the skin after healing of a simple incision for biopsy of a skin tumour. Immature collagenous tissue forms a pale scar **S**, which interrupts the normal pink collagen of the dermis **D** on either side. There are no skin appendages in a skin scar. During the ensuing months and years, the cellularity of the scar diminishes, there is progressive loss of capillary vessels and the scar contracts so that after many years a skin scar may be virtually undetectable macroscopically. Note that healing of skin or mucous membrane involves epithelialisation of the surface by proliferation of epithelium at the edges of the defect (i.e. *epithelial regeneration*).

KELOID

Keloid is the name given to excessive formation of scar tissue. Some individuals, particularly those of African descent, have a tendency to form excessive amounts of collagen. When this occurs but does not extend beyond the bounds of the pre-existing wound, it is called a *hypertrophic scar*. However, when is extends beyond the pre-existing scar it is called keloid and can give rise to a very unsightly appearance. Unfortunately, attempts to remove the excessive scar tissue surgically can give rise to even more keloid formation and an even worse appearance.

KEY TO FIGURES
C capillary   **D** dermis   **F** fibroblasts   **S** scar

Fig. 2.12 Specialised healing in bone (a) LP (b) HP

In most tissues, fibrous scar forms a functionally adequate, albeit unspecialised, replacement for damaged tissues. In bone, the replacement of damaged tissue by fibrous scar is inadequate for restoration of function (e.g. weight bearing) and so in bone healing the processes that form bone during embryonic development are reactivated. This leads to new bone formation, a process of *regeneration* rather than *repair*. As in other forms of wound healing, the process is carefully controlled and orchestrated by an array of mediators, including platelet-derived growth factor (PDGF), transforming growth factor β (TGFβ), fibroblast growth factors (FGF) and bone morphogenetic proteins (BMPs).

Immediately following fracture, there is bleeding in and around the fracture site resulting in a mass of coagulated blood, a *haematoma*. An initial acute inflammatory response is rapidly followed by organisation of the haematoma with formation of granulation tissue as described in Figure 2.9. In the case of bone fracture, this granulation tissue is termed *provisional* or *soft tissue callus* C and forms around the broken ends of the bone B, loosely uniting them; this is seen at low magnification in micrograph (a). Mesenchymal stem cells found in the cambium layer of the periosteum are activated and divide and differentiate into *chondrocytes* and *osteoblasts*, to produce cartilaginous matrix and osteoid, the organic matrix of bone, respectively. This is seen in micrograph (b) where typical granulation tissue G at the top of the field gives way to osteoblasts O, which surround pink-staining, newly formed osteoid Os. Osteoid then becomes mineralised to form the *bony callus* between the two fractured ends. This initial bone is haphazardly arranged (known as *woven bone*) and, over the next few months, undergoes extensive remodelling by osteoclasts and osteoblasts to form lamellar bone with trabecular architecture, best suited to resist local stresses. The end result is normal bony architecture and function.

KEY TO FIGURES

B bone **C** provisional callus **Ca** capillaries **F** fibrin **G** granulation tissue **N** neutrophils **O** osteoblasts
Os osteoid **P** pus

NON-UNION OF FRACTURES
While most fractures heal completely and well with modern management, in some individuals, there is delay in complete healing of a fracture; in others there may be cessation of the healing process without restitution of functional bone, known as **non-union**. A wide range of factors may contribute to delayed or failed healing, the most important of which are poor immobilisation, poor blood supply, poor nutrition (lack of protein, vitamin C, etc.), the presence of infection and foreign bodies or fragments of necrotic bone in the fracture. Old age, drugs such as steroids and non-steroidal anti-inflammatory drugs (NSAIDs), diabetes mellitus, burns and irradiation may also delay or stop healing.

Fig. 2.13 **Abscess formation** **(a)** LP **(b)** HP

An abscess is a localised collection of pus, which usually develops following extensive tissue damage by one of the pyogenic bacteria, such as *Staphylococcus aureus*. Such organisms excite an inflammatory exudate in which neutrophils predominate. In these circumstances, large numbers of neutrophils die, releasing their lysosomal enzymes and undergoing autolysis; the resulting viscous fluid, *pus*, contains dead and dying neutrophils, necrotic tissue debris and the fluid component of the acute inflammatory exudate with a little fibrin. Pyogenic bacteria often remain viable within the abscess cavity and may cause enlargement of the lesion, which is described as an *acute abscess*. At an early stage, expansion of the lesion is limited by the processes of organisation and repair at the margins of the abscess. Thus the abscess may become walled off, isolating the bacteria-containing pus and preventing further spread; an

abscess encapsulated by granulation and fibrous tissue is termed a *chronic abscess*. On the other hand, if the bacteria are highly virulent and present in large numbers, such attempts at organisation and repair may be overwhelmed, and expansion of the abscess ensues with destruction of surrounding tissue. The coexistence of active tissue damage and attempts at repair are typical of *chronic inflammation* (see Ch. 3).

Micrograph (a) shows an abscess in the wall of the colon. The centre consists of a collection of pus **P**. At its margin is a pink-staining zone of fibrin **F**. As yet, there is little evidence of organisation at the margins of the abscess; this therefore represents an acute abscess. Micrograph (b) shows the wall and lumen of a chronic abscess at high power, illustrating the neutrophils **N** and tissue debris in the cavity of the abscess, and the capillaries **Ca** in the inflamed granulation tissue of the wall.

TYPES OF FRACTURE
Fractures are described as **complete** or **incomplete** depending on whether the entire thickness of the bone is fractured. In **closed** fractures the overlying skin is intact, while **compound** fractures include disruption of the overlying skin. A **comminuted** fracture has multiple separate bone fragments. **Pathological fractures** occur in bone with pre-existing disease, such as osteoporosis or metastatic tumour. **Greenstick fracture** is an incomplete fracture where there is initial bending with partial fracture of the side under tension: it typically occurs in children.

Fig. 2.14 Chapter review

Acute inflammation, healing and repair
Key features of acute inflammation
• Oedema due to increased fluid in tissue • Dilated vessels • Infiltration by inflammatory cells – mainly neutrophils in the early stages and macrophages later
Systemic effects of acute inflammation
• Fever • Neutrophilia (increased neutrophils in circulating blood) • Fatigue • Loss of appetite • Increased acute phase proteins in blood
Outcomes of acute inflammation
• Complete resolution with restitution of normal tissue structure and function • Healing by fibrosis – scar formation via the processes of granulation tissue formation and organisation • Abscess formation – acute abscess may persist and become chronic • Progression to chronic inflammation – sometimes with flares of acute inflammation (acute on chronic inflammation) e.g chronic inflammatory bowel disease (see Ch. 13)
Most important mediators in acute inflammation
• Vasodilatation – histamine, prostaglandins and nitric oxide • Increased vascular permeability – serotonin (5-HT), histamine, C5a, C3a and leukotrienes • Leukocyte activation and chemotaxis – C5a, leukotriene B4, various chemokines and bacterial products

3 Chronic inflammation

In developed countries, where the major pyogenic infections have been brought more or less under control, chronic inflammatory conditions result in a huge burden of morbidity and mortality. In less industrialised countries certain infections, such as tuberculosis, typically cause a chronic inflammatory response and are responsible for a large amount of disease. By definition chronic inflammation lasts longer than acute inflammation. Different stimuli may cause variations in the morphological appearances but, overall, in the chronic inflammatory infiltrate lymphocytes, macrophages and plasma cells predominate, in contrast to acute inflammation where the major cell type is the neutrophil. The hallmark features of chronic inflammation are ongoing tissue damage, a chronic inflammatory infiltrate and fibrosis. Chronic inflammation may be subdivided as follows:

- *Non-specific chronic inflammation* – arises following non-resolution of acute inflammation, e.g. chronic peptic ulcer, chronic abscess

- *Specific (primary) chronic inflammation* – arises de novo in response to certain types of injurious agents, e.g. rheumatoid arthritis, idiopathic pulmonary fibrosis

- *Granulomatous inflammation* – is a subset of specific chronic inflammation characterised by the presence of granulomas, e.g. sarcoidosis, tuberculosis (see Ch. 4).

Non-specific chronic inflammation

Chronic inflammation may arise following an episode of acute inflammation (see Ch. 2) where the acute inflammatory response has not been adequate to neutralise or destroy the noxious stimulus. In this situation, tissue damage, acute inflammation, granulation tissue, tissue repair and chronic inflammation coexist. There may be active tissue damage in one area with ongoing acute inflammation, while in adjacent areas fibrosis and a chronic inflammatory infiltrate are seen. The chronic inflammatory infiltrate is dominated by tissue macrophages, lymphocytes and plasma cells (see Fig. 3.2), in contrast to the marked preponderance of neutrophils in the acute inflammatory response. This type of chronic inflammation represents a dynamic balance between tissue destruction and repair. The course of the disease might include repeated acute phases when tissue damage is predominant and intervening chronic phases when chronic inflammation smoulders along with ongoing tissue repair. The outcome of non-specific chronic inflammation depends on whether local and systemic factors favour the injurious agent or the process of healing. Chronic inflammation usually heals by fibrosis.

Fig. 3.1	Factors that affect healing	
Factors that impair resolution and healing	**Factors that aid resolution and healing**
Poor nutrition	Administration of appropriate antibiotics
Immunosuppression	Surgical removal of foreign material
Persisting tissue damage and/or infection	Surgical removal of dead tissue
Retained foreign material	General attempts to improve nutrition
Sequestered dead tissue	Drugs that specifically modify the inflammatory response
Poor blood supply	
Deficiency of intrinsic anti-inflammatory factors	
Diabetes mellitus	

Fig. 3.2 **Cells in chronic inflammation** (HP)

In chronic inflammation the major infiltrating cells types are *macrophages*, *lymphocytes* and *plasma cells* (sometimes collectively called 'mononuclear cells') as well as *eosinophils*, *mast cells* and some *neutrophils*. These cells may be derived from resident tissue populations and/or migrate into the tissue from the circulating blood. As well as killing and disposing of infective organisms, inflammatory cells secrete a wide variety of soluble factors that regulate the inflammatory and healing processes.

In this micrograph, plasma cells **P** are identified by their amphophilic (purple) cytoplasm and eccentric 'clock face' nuclei. Plasma cells are differentiated B lymphocytes that are committed to antibody production. Lymphocytes **L** are seen as dark, rounded nuclei with a thin, almost invisible, rim of basophilic cytoplasm. These are the effector cells of the specific immune response and include both helper and cytotoxic T cells as well as B cells. Macrophages **Ma** are recognised by their oval or kidney-bean-shaped nuclei and pale cytoplasm. Eosinophils **E** have bilobed nuclei and brightly eosinophilic granules in their cytoplasm. When stimulated, eosinophils release their granule contents, including major basic protein, a substance that is effective in killing parasites. Some neutrophils and many active fibroblasts **Fi** are commonly also found in chronic inflammation. Fibroblasts secrete the components of the extracellular matrix including collagen. When the damaging stimulus has been removed and repair is completed, often after weeks or months, these cells progressively disappear from the tissue.

Fig. 3.3 **Chronic peptic ulcer** (a) Entire ulcer (LP) (b) Surface layers of ulcer (MP) (c) Deep layers of ulcer (MP) (*illustrations opposite*)

A common example, which illustrates the principles of non-specific chronic inflammation, is the localised chronic ulceration of the stomach or duodenum, most often in individuals infected by *Helicobacter pylori* (*H. pylori*); such lesions are collectively referred to as chronic peptic ulcers. By definition, an *ulcer* extends through the full thickness of the mucosa; an *erosion* is a lesion involving only the superficial mucosa.

Ulceration is caused by an imbalance between damaging factors (gastric acid and peptic enzymes) and protective factors (gastric mucus secretion, local secretion of alkali).

H. pylori does not invade the tissues but inhabits the protective mucus layer which covers the surface of the mucosa (see Fig. 13.8). It has a unique ability to survive the acid environment of the stomach because of a bacterial enzyme, *urease*. This allows it to produce ammonia by splitting urea, raising pH in the immediate vicinity of the organism. It typically colonises the antrum and, by producing a localised alkaline environment here, *H. pylori* interferes with normal physiological control of gastric acid secretion. The falsely high antral pH stimulates secretion of *gastrin* by the antral G cells, which acts upon the oxyntic cells in the corpus to increase acid production still further. This excess acid production overwhelms normal mucosal defence mechanisms, leading to the formation of an acute ulcer. If the process proceeds unchecked, the ulcer can burrow through the full thickness of the stomach or duodenal wall, leading to perforation and escape of gut contents into the peritoneal cavity (see Fig. 13.8).

Often, the destructive process is arrested by an acute inflammatory response. Tissue repair then begins with the formation of granulation tissue; if conditions are favourable repair may be effective, leaving a fibrous scar. If tissue destruction continues, the concurrent organisation and repair result in chronic inflammation. A chronic peptic ulcer reflects this dynamic balance between tissue destruction and repair. A section through a chronic ulcer is shown in image (a). The ulcerated surface is covered in a slough **Sl**, composed of a pink-staining layer of necrotic debris combined with the fibrin and neutrophils of an acute inflammatory exudate. Beneath the slough is a zone of vascular granulation tissue **V**; these features are seen at a higher magnification in micrograph (b). The next layer is a zone of fibrous granulation tissue **F**, seen in detail in micrograph (c). Deeper still in the ulcer base, is a fibrous scar **Sc**. In this deep ulcer, the muscular wall **M** is completely replaced by the ulcer crater, granulation tissue and scar. If a large blood vessel is present in the ulcer base, erosion into the vessel leads to bleeding into the stomach, giving rise to *haematemesis* (vomiting blood) or *melaena* (black, tar-like faeces composed of altered blood).

The outcome of chronic peptic ulceration depends on whether conditions favour ongoing tissue damage or repair. If healing is favoured, fibrous tissue gradually repairs the ulcer crater and mucosa regenerates from the ulcer margins to cover the epithelial defect and protect the fibrous tissue from further damage. A healed peptic ulcer thus consists of an area of fibrous scarring replacing all or part of the thickness of the stomach wall. Internally, the regenerated mucosa is usually puckered because of contraction of the underlying scarred wall.

KEY TO FIGURES

E eosinophil **F** fibrous granulation tissue **Fi** fibroblast **L** lymphocyte **M** muscular wall **Ma** macrophage **P** plasma cell **Sc** scar **Sl** necrotic slough **V** vascular granulation tissue

Fig. 3.3 **Chronic peptic ulcer** (*caption opposite*)

CLINICAL MANAGEMENT OF PEPTIC ULCER DISEASE

Understanding of the role of *H. pylori* has revolutionised management of peptic ulceration. In the past, peptic ulcers were treated by surgical procedures which aimed to reduce acid production, such as partial gastrectomy (to remove the antral source of gastrin) or vagotomy and pyloroplasty (removing the vagal-driven pathway of acid secretion but requiring release of the pylorus since the vagus also controls gastric emptying). Such operations were associated with considerable morbidity. Conventional medical management of peptic ulcer disease employed a range of drugs, from simple alkalis to neutralise excess acid, through various drugs which interfere with normal physiological control of acid secretion (e.g. adrenergic antagonists and histamine (H2) receptor blockers) to the more recent use of ***proton pump inhibitors (PPIs)*** which effectively block the final common pathway of acid production. Although acid-blocking drugs were usually effective, treatment had to continue life-long. Now, treatment usually requires only a short course of eradication therapy, using a combination of two antibiotics with a proton-pump inhibitor ('triple therapy').

Fig. 3.4 **Bronchiectasis** (LP)

Bronchiectasis is a chronic inflammation of the bronchi associated with destruction of the wall and permanent dilatation. In most cases, repeated episodes of infection and obstruction lead to progressive destruction of the normal elastic and muscular components of the airway wall. Obstruction may be due to foreign bodies in bronchi, tumour, structural abnormalities or stasis of secretions, perhaps related to ciliary malfunction or cystic fibrosis. The elastic and muscular components of the bronchial wall are replaced by granulation tissue and later by fibrous tissue. This process weakens the wall, leading to dilatation of the airway, which in turn

predisposes to stagnation of secretions and further episodes of bacterial infection, creating a vicious cycle.

In this micrograph, two abnormal bronchi are seen, each with the lumen filled with pus **P**. The wall of each affected bronchus is formed of fibrovascular granulation tissue **G**, in which there is a heavy infiltrate of dark-staining cells, just visible at this magnification; these cells are a mixture of plasma cells and lymphocytes. Bronchiectasis exemplifies the concept of coexisting tissue damage and attempts at repair, which are the hallmarks of chronic inflammation.

Fig. 3.5 **Pilonidal sinus** (LP)

A common example of a chronic abscess is the pilonidal sinus. In this condition, a chronic subcutaneous abscess forms, most commonly in the sacrococcygeal area. Hair shafts **H**, derived from locally destroyed follicles and shed body hair, are present in the abscess and act as a focus for chronic inflammation. Successful healing and repair are hindered by the persistence of the hairs which are resistant to phagocytosis. Secondary infection may further complicate the process. As part of the attempt at healing, surface epithelium proliferates and comes to line the tract leading down into the abscess cavity (not seen in this micrograph); such a tract is known as a *sinus*.

In this micrograph, note the subcutaneous abscess cavity **A**, the wall of which is formed by granulation tissue **G**, heavily infiltrated by lymphocytes and plasma cells. There is surrounding fibrosis **F** in the dermis as a result of previous attempts at fibrous repair.

A pilonidal sinus, like any other chronic inflammatory lesion, will only heal if the source of persistent irritation is removed; surgical excision or laying open the complex of sinuses and abscess cavities is usually the only satisfactory method in this situation.

Specific (primary) chronic inflammation

This type of chronic inflammation arises by different mechanisms from non-specific chronic inflammation. Primary chronic inflammation may be either *granulomatous* or *non-granulomatous*. A key feature in chronic inflammation is the activation of macrophages, which orchestrate the chronic inflammatory response. Macrophages may become activated by either immune or non-immune mechanisms. Activated macrophages not only become more efficient at phagocytosis and killing of organisms, but secrete a wide range of factors that control the behaviour of other inflammatory cells (e.g. chemotactic factors, lymphokines) and which induce fibrosis (e.g. fibrogenic cytokines, growth factors). The types of agent which can invoke primary chronic inflammation include:

■ **Immunological**

– Low-toxicity organisms such as *Treponema* sp., the causative organism of syphilis and yaws

– Infective organisms that grow within cells, e.g. viruses, *Mycobacteria*

– Hypersensitivity reactions such as extrinsic allergic alveolitis

– Autoimmune conditions such as systemic lupus erythematosus

– Infections by fungi, protozoa and parasites.

■ **Non-immunological**

– Foreign body reactions

– Inert noxious materials such as silica, talc, asbestos or beryllium.

Primary chronic inflammation of the immune type may be either granulomatous or non-granulomatous. A good example of the non-granulomatous immune type is hepatitis B virus infection (HBV) (see Fig. 14.5). Virus-infected cells in the liver incite a cell-mediated immune response, producing cytotoxic T lymphocytes which kill virus-infected hepatocytes. Some individuals mount an effective immune response and clear the infection, whilst in others there is ongoing infiltration of the liver by lymphocytes over months or years, a condition known as *chronic active hepatitis*. In these people, there is continuing destruction of hepatocytes and fibrosis of the liver that may eventually cause cirrhosis. As in many examples of chronic inflammation, the tissue damage is due to the inflammatory response rather than the virus itself. In non-immune type primary chronic inflammation, the mechanisms are less clear. However, certain materials such as silica can directly activate macrophages to release mediators that induce an inflammatory reaction and fibrosis.

Granulomatous inflammation

The defining feature of granulomatous inflammation is the presence of activated *epithelioid macrophages* and *multinucleate giant cells* derived from macrophages. Epithelioid macrophages are so named because they bear some resemblance histologically to epithelial (squamous) cells. These cells may form well-circumscribed *granulomas* (clusters) which are generally surrounded by lymphocytes, macrophages, fibroblasts and varying degrees of fibrosis. Granulomatous primary chronic inflammation may arise by either immune or non-immune mechanisms. The immune type, known as the *delayed hypersensitivity response*, is epitomised by tuberculosis (see Ch. 4). T lymphocytes responding to mycobacterial antigens are activated and divide and mature to produce helper T cells. The helper T cells in turn secrete lymphokines (e.g. interferon (IFN)-γ) that induce the transformation of macrophages into activated epithelioid macrophages and giant cells.

Non-immune granulomatous inflammation is exemplified by the foreign body reaction, for example in response to suture material after a surgical procedure, or when a rose thorn becomes embedded in the skin. Figure 3.10 is an example of such a reaction and shows plant material (from faeces) embedded in the wall of the bowel in a patient with diverticular disease. In some granulomatous conditions such as Crohn's disease and sarcoidosis, the mechanism is unclear: infective causes have been postulated but never proven.

The term granuloma needs some clarification. In general, granuloma means a cluster of epithelioid macrophages as opposed to granulation tissue as defined in Chapter 2. However, in the past, 'granuloma' was applied to both a granuloma and granulation tissue and a few examples remain in current terminology where the old usage persists. Examples include an *apical granuloma* referring to a mass of granulation tissue at the root of a tooth and a *pyogenic granuloma* (lobular capillary haemangioma), which is a mass of granulation tissue in a healing wound.

KEY TO FIGURES

A abscess cavity   **F** fibrosis   **G** granulation tissue   **H** hair shaft   **P** pus

---

Some granulomas develop necrosis in their central area. The classical form is caseous necrosis, which is almost always found in tuberculosis (see Ch. 4). Caseous necrosis appears creamy macroscopically (caseous = like cream cheese). By light microscopy, caseous necrosis is featureless and eosinophilic, containing few cells. Some other granulomatous conditions, such as atypical mycobacterial infection, also develop central necrosis but the necrosis is suppurative with plentiful neutrophils, often called *'suppurating'* or *'necrotising granulomas'*. Some common types of granulomatous inflammation are characterised by their lack of necrosis; good examples of this type are Crohn's disease and sarcoidosis.

Fig. 3.6 **Pulmonary fibrosis (idiopathic)** **(a)** LP **(b)** HP

Idiopathic pulmonary fibrosis (or *cryptogenic fibrosing alveolitis*) is a good example of a chronic inflammatory condition which in its earliest phases has a chronic inflammatory infiltrate. At this early stage, it may be called *interstitial pneumonitis* (or *usual interstitial pneumonia*), where an unknown damaging agent repeatedly triggers the inflammation of the alveolar walls leading to extensive fibrosis as part of the healing process. Idiopathic pulmonary fibrosis is one of a group of disorders known as interstitial pneumonias.

The later stages of this process are well illustrated in these micrographs where the alveolar walls are thickened because of the deposition of dense fibrous tissue **F**. The thickened alveolar walls are distorted and less permeable to gases. In the final stages, there may be great distortion of alveoli, giving rise to greatly enlarged alveolar spaces **A**, known as *honeycomb lung* (see Fig. 12.11). In addition, there is

damage to the alveolar lining cells and these are replaced by hyperplastic or regenerating type II pneumocytes. In micrograph (b), the inflammatory infiltrate of lymphocytes and plasma cells is readily seen, as well as type 2 pneumocyte hyperplasia **P**.

The usual presentation of cryptogenic fibrosing alveolitis is of insidious onset of breathlessness associated with finger clubbing. However, a histologically identical picture may arise as an end stage of *diffuse alveolar damage* owing to oxygen toxicity in premature infants, i.e. *hyaline membrane disease* (see Fig. 12.10) and acute viral pneumonitis. The condition may also follow a range of other conditions such as extrinsic allergic alveolitis, drug toxicity, miliary tuberculosis, connective tissue disorders and sarcoidosis. Some of these disorders are associated with granulomatous inflammation in the early stages and this may still be apparent at the end stage.

CHRONIC FIBROSIS

Chronic fibrosis, whatever the cause, can be a cause of great morbidity and sometimes mortality. Fibrosis and scar formation are normal parts of tissue healing after significant damage. However, in some individuals, in association with some insults there is tendency to develop excess fibrosis such that the fibrous tissue impairs the function of the organ. Idiopathic pulmonary fibrosis as described above is one example; others include keloid scars, idiopathic retroperitoneal fibrosis, intra-abdominal adhesions that may arise and persist after abdominal surgery and Reidel's thyroiditis.

The mechanisms and pathogenesis of these uncommon diseases are still a mystery and various theories have been proposed including persistent infective organisms, other persistent antigens and autoimmune mechanisms. The end result seems to be abnormal regulation of the healing process such that there is exuberant and inappropriate fibrosis. Macrophages become activated in such a way that they produce pro-fibrotic cytokines (e.g. interleukin-10, TGFβ) leading to activation and proliferation of fibroblasts and myofibroblasts and excessive production of extracellular matrix. Other instances of excessive fibrosis result from known causes (e.g. infections such as tuberculosis (see Ch. 4) and fibrosis of a transplanted kidney in chronic rejection (see Fig. 3.7)).

Fig. 3.7 **Transplant rejection: kidney** (LP)

Organ transplantation introduces non-self antigens into the recipient. Specifically, the HLA antigens (human leukocyte antigens) of the donor are very rarely identical to those of the recipient, except in the case of transplantation of organs between identical twins. The HLA antigens of the donor excite both *antibody-* and *cell-mediated immune responses* in the recipient in an attempt to rid the body of the foreign material by killing donor cells. This is, of course, a gross simplification of the many and complex faces of transplant rejection, which are dealt with in more detail in Chapter 15. This micrograph illustrates a cell-mediated immune response to a transplanted kidney. There is an infiltrate of lymphocytes, most of which are T cells, in the interstitium **I** of the kidney. The tubules are atrophic and widely separated. Lymphocytes **L** can be seen within the tubular basement membrane between the tubular epithelial cells (*tubulitis*). These lymphocytes are attacking the tubular epithelial cells, causing tubular damage and eventual loss of tubules. Loss of any part of the nephron leads to loss of the entire nephron so that the transplanted kidney is unable to function. As in many cases of chronic inflammation, tissue damage is caused primarily by the inflammatory infiltrate. The transplanted kidney makes no attack on the recipient and, if left alone by the immune system, does nothing but good. Various combinations of immunosuppressant drugs are used to suppress the cell-mediated immune response to the transplanted kidney to allow it to function, thus freeing the recipient from a life of dialysis.

Fig. 3.8 **Giant cells** **(a)** Foreign body giant cell (HP) **(b)** Langhans' giant cell (HP)

As described in the introduction, multinucleate giant cells are formed by the fusion of epithelioid macrophages and are a highly characteristic, though not universal, feature of chronic granulomatous inflammation. These micrographs illustrate typical appearances of giant cells. Micrograph (a) is a good example of a *foreign body-type giant cell*, which is characterised by a central group of nuclei similar to those seen in adjacent epithelioid macrophages **E**. These cells may be found in association with implanted foreign material, for example a remnant of a surgical suture or a rose thorn in the skin (see Fig. 3.10). These cells are usually found in association with epithelioid macrophages, although they may not form the discrete granulomas seen in other types of granulomatous inflammation.

The second important form of giant cell is the *Langhans' giant cell*, said to be characteristic of tuberculosis. As shown in micrograph (b), the multiple nuclei of Langhans' giant cells are arranged in a horseshoe formation around the periphery. Again, epithelioid macrophages **E** are seen in the surrounding tissues.

Both epithelioid macrophages and giant cells are specialised secretory cells, rather than phagocytic cells. The plentiful eosinophilic cytoplasm seen in both cell types is indicative of abundant rough endoplasmic reticulum, as opposed to the pale foamy cytoplasm of phagocytic macrophages. Although Langhans' giant cells and foreign body cells are said to be more or less specific for different types of granulomatous inflammation, in practice this is not so.

KEY TO FIGURES

A enlarged alveolar space **E** epithelioid macrophage **F** fibrous tissue **I** interstitium **L** lymphocytes
P type 2 pneumocyte hyperplasia

Fig. 3.9 **Sarcoidosis** **(a)** Sarcoidosis in a lymph node (MP) **(b)** Sarcoid granulomas (HP)

Sarcoidosis is a chronic granulomatous disease of unknown aetiology, characterised by the formation of multiple discrete granulomas in many tissues. In marked distinction to classical tuberculous granulomas (see Ch. 4), those of sarcoidosis do not typically undergo central caseous necrosis, although small foci of necrosis may be seen in large granulomas.

Sarcoidosis may occur in any organ or tissue, notably the spleen, liver, skin and lymph nodes, but frequently also involves the lungs which may be peppered with numerous granulomas. In most cases of pulmonary sarcoidosis, the hilar lymph nodes are also grossly enlarged by masses of granulomas; such massive nodes are a useful diagnostic feature when visible on chest imaging.

Micrograph (a) illustrates part of a typical lymph node. Note the scattered non-caseating granulomas **G**. Since there is no central mass of caseation, the sarcoid granuloma differs from the tuberculous granuloma by having a much broader zone of epithelioid macrophages. As in tuberculosis, sarcoid granulomas are surrounded by a zone of lymphocytes, although this feature is much less obvious in sarcoid

lesions. In tissues other than lymph nodes, the granulomas are described as being 'naked', i.e. lacking a rim of lymphocytes and fibroblasts.

Micrograph (b) shows a typical sarcoid granuloma at high magnification. Note the epithelioid macrophages **M**. Multinucleate giant cells are a feature of most of the granulomas. The cytoplasm of sarcoid giant cells may contain inclusion bodies of two types: eosinophilic star-shaped *asteroid bodies* **A** or small, laminated calcified concretions called *Schaumann bodies* **S**. In practice, these inclusion bodies are rare. Although characteristic of sarcoid giant cells, such inclusion bodies are not pathognomonic of sarcoidosis (i.e. not exclusive to sarcoidosis) and are occasionally found in other chronic inflammatory granulomas.

Sarcoidosis has many possible clinical presentations, including no clinical symptoms; in persistent cases, the granulomas undergo progressive fibrosis, although some giant cells still remain. In the lungs, this may culminate in pulmonary fibrosis and honeycomb lung (see Fig. 3.6) and may lead to chronic respiratory failure.

KEY TO FIGURES

A asteroid body   **F** foreign body giant cells   **G** non-caseating granuloma   **L** lipogranuloma   **M** epithelioid macrophages   **P** plant material   **S** Schaumann body

Fig. 3.10 **Foreign body reaction** (a) Foreign body granuloma (LP) (b) Giant cell with inclusion (HP)

The presence of certain non-soluble foreign materials in tissues may excite a chronic granulomatous inflammatory response, with or without discrete granuloma formation. Common examples of such *foreign body reactions* are those produced by suture material, wood or other vegetable matter, metal or glass splinters, and inorganic materials such as silica and beryllium, inhaled deep into the lungs during industrial dust exposure. Inhaled materials are of particular clinical importance because of their tendency to produce progressive pulmonary fibrosis, similar to that which may occur in idiopathic pulmonary fibrosis. Many of these foreign bodies are refractile when viewed with polarised light and can thus be identified within the granulomas or giant cells.

At low magnification, micrograph (a) shows plant material **P**, derived from faeces, that has become embedded in the wall of the colon in a patient with *diverticulitis*. Diverticular disease is a condition where the mucosa of the bowel herniates through the muscular wall, forming a pouch or diverticulum in which faecal material may become impacted, leading to inflammation and sometimes perforation (see Ch. 13). The pale, incompletely digested plant material is surrounded by aggregates of foreign body giant cells **F** and epithelioid macrophages **M** as well as other inflammatory cells. At high power in micrograph (b), a fragment of plant material **P** can be easily seen within the cytoplasm of a Langhans' type giant cell.

Fig. 3.11 **Xanthogranulomatous inflammation and lipogranuloma** (a) Xanthogranulomatous cholecystitis (MP) (b) Lipogranuloma in fat necrosis (HP)

Xanthogranulomatous inflammation is a rare condition most often seen in the kidney or the gallbladder. Although rare, these are important lesions as they may form a mass that can be mistaken for a malignant tumour. Micrograph (a) shows xanthogranulomatous inflammation in the gallbladder at medium power. The lesion consists of sheets of macrophages whose cytoplasm is loaded with droplets of lipid, thus giving it a foamy appearance. The lipid in the macrophage gives the lesion an orange-yellow appearance macroscopically. Interspersed among the foamy macrophages are lymphocytes, plasma cells, eosinophils and, sometimes, a few neutrophils. Older lesions are often very fibrotic and the gallbladder may

become shrunken and thick walled. Xanthogranulomatous pyelonephritis tends to occur in patients with *Proteus* urinary tract infection and has similar histological appearances.

Another much more common appearance is the accumulation of lipid-laden macrophages in areas where fat is released from adipocytes, often in areas of fat necrosis. Micrograph (b) shows such an area where necrotic fat cells are easily identified by their lack of nuclei. Interspersed among the fat cells are sheets of foamy macrophages, often with very few other inflammatory cells. Occasional lipogranulomas **L** may be seen, consisting of a droplet of lipid surrounded by foamy macrophages.

BASIC PATHOLOGICAL PROCESSES ■ CHRONIC INFLAMMATION

Fig. 3.12 Chapter review

Type of chronic inflammation	Histological features	Some examples	Figure
Non-specific – follows on from unresolved acute inflammation	Mixed inflammatory response with lymphocytes, plasma cells, eosinophils, neutrophils. Characterised by mixture of acute inflammation, chronic inflammation and attempts at healing (granulation tissue, fibrosis)	Chronic peptic ulcer Bronchiectasis Pilonidal sinus Ulcerative colitis	3.3 3.4 3.5 13.19
Specific chronic inflammation (non-granulomatous)	The inflammatory infiltrate consists predominantly of lymphocytes, plasma cells and macrophages Sometimes there are variable numbers of eosinophils and mast cells	Viral infections Usual interstitial pneumonitis/ idiopathic pulmonary fibrosis Cellular rejection of transplanted kidney Lichen planus	4.12–4.14 3.6 3.7 21.7
Specific chronic inflammation (granulomatous)	This type of inflammation is characterised by the formation of granulomas – aggregates of epithelioid macrophages, with or without giant cells	Sarcoidosis Foreign body giant cell reaction Tuberculosis Leprosy Crohn's disease	3.9 3.10 4.3–4.7 4.9 13.13

4 Infections of histological importance

Introduction

A number of infections may be diagnosed from the characteristic appearances seen in biopsy specimens. In some cases, the diagnosis may first be suspected when a biopsy is examined by light microscopy. In other cases, the clinician suspects an infective agent and seeks confirmation by biopsy as well as by other means. Although histological appearances are often characteristic, it is usually necessary to confirm the presence of the infective agent by other techniques such as microbiological cultures or serology. In addition, the pathologist may employ a wide variety of techniques such as electron microscopy, immunohistochemical staining with specific monoclonal antibodies and a wide range of special stains to confirm the diagnosis.

Many infections which are otherwise difficult to diagnose arise in immunosuppressed patients, for example AIDS patients and organ transplant recipients and, as the number of such patients increases, so the role of histopathology in diagnosis of infection expands. This chapter aims to give an overview of infections which are important in routine diagnostic pathological practice, to illustrate the appearances of these organisms in the tissues and to consider the patterns of tissue damage they cause. As prion disease specifically affects the central nervous system, this is discussed in Chapter 23.

Bacterial infections

Most bacteria cause disease by exciting an acute exudative inflammatory response (*pyogenic bacteria*). This inflammatory exudate is responsible for many of the clinical features of the disease (e.g. lobar pneumonia, Fig. 2.3; bronchopneumonia, Fig. 12.5). The pattern of tissue damage is similar irrespective of the pyogenic bacteria causing it and the organism can only be identified by microbiological methods. More complex mechanisms are involved in the tissue damage caused by infection with bacteria such as *Helicobacter pylori*, which cause inflammation by interfering with the normal physiological regulation of gastric acid secretion (see Fig. 3.3, Fig. 13.8). Other bacteria cause disease as a direct result of producing toxins which induce necrosis of cells and tissues (e.g. *Clostridium difficile* toxins destroy the surface epithelium of the colon, see Fig. 4.1), and some bacteria initiate a type IV hypersensitivity reaction (e.g. *Mycobacteria* and some *Treponema* organisms) and so produce characteristic histological changes.

Fig. 4.1 Pseudomembranous colitis

In pseudomembranous colitis, there is focal necrosis of the surface epithelium of the colon. This necrotic epithelium is replaced by an area of 'membrane' which is composed of a predominantly fibrinous acute inflammatory exudate. Typically, it occurs in older people following treatment with certain antibiotics. The antibiotic destroys the natural bacterial flora, allowing uncontrolled multiplication of *Clostridium difficile*. This bacterium produces a toxin which causes extensive, patchy colonic epithelial necrosis, which may be fatal.

The pattern of superficial necrosis of the mucosa is characteristic. There are multiple focal lesions of necrosis with tufts of exudate **E** which have been likened to an erupting volcano. The deep components of the mucosa remain largely intact, but the superficial parts of the colonic crypts **C** appear acutely inflamed and atrophic.

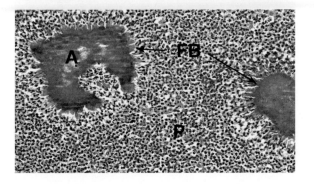

Fig. 4.2 *Actinomyces* organisms

These are filamentous bacteria which grow in characteristic fungal-like colonies, appearing macroscopically as yellow *sulphur granules* and causing chronic abscesses and *fistulation*. Typical sites of infection include oral cavity, lung, GI tract and female genital tract (usually linked to use of intrauterine contraceptive devices).

Histologically, the *Actinomyces* **A** lie within a pool of pus **P** and appear encrusted by eosinophilic proteinaceous material (the *Splendori–Hoeppli phenomenon*). The filamentous shape of the bacteria **FB** can be seen at the edges of these colonies.

KEY TO FIGURES

A *Actinomyces*   **C** colonic crypts   **E** inflammatory exudate   **FB** filamentous bacteria   **P** pus

Mycobacterial infections

Infections caused by various *Mycobacteria* can frequently be diagnosed histologically because of the tissue reaction to their presence. The organisms are difficult and slow to grow in microbiological culture and so biopsy often plays an important role in early diagnosis. *Mycobacterium tuberculosis* causes **tuberculosis**, a disease which is increasing in incidence because of the emergence of drug-resistant strains. *Mycobacterium leprae* is the cause of **leprosy** (Fig. 4.9). There are other pathogenic *Mycobacteria* (called atypical *Mycobacteria*) which cause a range of disorders.

Important points to note about the histology of mycobacterial infections are:

■ Most show a **granulomatous** pattern of chronic inflammation (see Ch. 3) due to a delayed type hypersensitivity reaction.

■ **Caseous necrosis** (see Fig. 4.3) is particularly associated with *M. tuberculosis* infection.

■ Suppurating granulomas (with neutrophils in the central necrotic area of the granuloma) may occur in infections by atypical *Mycobacteria* (Fig. 4.8). These organisms are also referred to as **Mycobacteria other than tuberculosis (MOTT)** or **non-tuberculous Mycobacteria (NTM)**.

■ The causative organism can sometimes be identified in histological sections by the use of special stains (Ziehl–Neelsen, Wade–Fite).

Fig. 4.3 **Early pulmonary tuberculosis** (*caption opposite*)

KEY TO FIGURES

CN caseous necrosis　**F** fibroblast　**L** Langhans' giant cell　**M** epithelioid macrophages　**W** fibrous wall

Fig. 4.3 **Early pulmonary tuberculosis** **(a)** Early tubercle (MP) **(b)** Early tubercle (HP) **(c)** Later tubercle (MP) **(d)** Later tubercle (HP) *(illustrations opposite)*

PART I

CHAPTER

4

BASIC PATHOLOGICAL PROCESSES ■ INFECTIONS OF HISTOLOGICAL IMPORTANCE

The characteristic histological lesion in tuberculosis is the granuloma, which in this case is known as a *tubercle*.

When *Mycobacteria* gain access to the lungs by inhalation, they tend to localise in the periphery of the lung where they excite a transient neutrophil response. The organisms survive neutrophil enzyme activity, probably because of their thick and resistant glycolipid cell wall. They are then ingested by macrophages where they may initially continue to divide within macrophage cytoplasm. The macrophages present mycobacterial antigen to T lymphocytes, which become activated and initiate a cell-mediated (type IV hypersensitivity) response. The sensitised lymphocytes produce various soluble factors (*cytokines*), which attract and activate the macrophages, enhancing their ability to secrete substances that kill *Mycobacteria*. Such activated macrophages become large and develop granular, eosinophilic cytoplasm. As a result of their supposed resemblance to epithelial cells, they are known as *epithelioid macrophages* (see Ch. 3). These cells form a major component of all granulomas, including tubercles.

Micrograph (a) shows an entire tubercle at an early stage, and (b) illustrates a sector of the same tubercle at higher magnification. At the centre of the tubercle is an area of caseous necrosis **CN** containing *Mycobacteria*. These can only be demonstrated by specific staining methods for acid-fast bacilli (Fig. 4.10). The caseous area is surrounded by a zone of epithelioid macrophages **M** with abundant eosinophilic cytoplasm. Some of the macrophages fuse to produce multinucleate giant cells called *Langhans' giant cells* **L**; a typical Langhans' giant cell is shown in more detail in Figure 3.8. Peripheral to the macrophages, there is a rim of lymphocytes.

Progressive, central, caseous necrosis results in enlargement of the tubercle and the zone of peripheral macrophages and lymphocytes becomes relatively thinner. These changes can be observed by comparing micrograph (a) with micrograph (c), which shows a more advanced tubercle. With further development, spindle-shaped fibroblasts **F** appear in the peripheral lymphocytic zone of the tubercle, where they are stimulated by factors produced by epithelioid macrophages to lay down collagen in the extracellular tissue; this process is evident in micrograph (c) and at higher magnification in (d).

At this stage, further changes in the tubercle can occur in one of two ways. If the organisms are virulent and present in large numbers, and particularly if the body's resistance is low (as, for example, in a debilitated or immunosuppressed patient), then the tubercle rapidly enlarges owing to increasing caseous necrosis. The macrophage–lymphocyte–fibroblast defensive reaction is overwhelmed, failing to confine the infection. This can result in tuberculous bronchopneumonia (Fig. 4.6). On the other hand, if the balance of resistance and attack is reversed, the macrophage–lymphocyte fibroblast barrier resists enlargement of the tubercle, and proliferation of fibroblasts produces a firm shell confining the infection. Production of collagen by these fibroblasts further strengthens this capsule, imprisoning the necrotic tissue and its contained *Mycobacteria* and isolating the organisms from other susceptible tissue (see Fig. 4.4). Calcium salts may become deposited in the collagenous shell and necrotic centre. In the lung, carbon is also taken up by the macrophages of the granuloma.

In primary tuberculous infection, the initial tubercle in the lung is known as a *Ghon focus* and is usually situated in the subpleural area in the mid zone of the lung. This lesion rarely attains a large size and undergoes the process of fibrosis described above. Before the lung lesion is walled off, however, *Mycobacteria* pass via lymphatics to regional lymph nodes in the lung hilum, where tubercles develop in a manner identical to the Ghon focus in the lung. The outcome of the infection depends on what happens to this tuberculous infection of the hilar lymph nodes; possible outcomes are discussed in Figures 4.4 to 4.7.

Fig. 4.4 Fibrocaseous tuberculous nodule (LP)

In most cases of primary tuberculosis, the Ghon focus heals by fibrosis leaving a small fibrous nodule which is often calcified. Some individuals are unable to contain the initial infection and develop *post-primary tuberculosis*. Others contain the initial infection but later, because of relatively suppressed immunity, further active infection occurs due to reactivation. In either case, a variety of lesions may result, including a localised lesion at the apex of the lung known as an *Assmann focus*. This may progress to further spread of infection or may be contained by chemotherapy, giving rise to a *fibrocaseous nodule*. A thick fibrous wall **W** completely encircles a mass of caseous necrotic material **CN**. In this case, there is little calcification.

Fig. 4.5 Tuberculous lymph node (LP)

With the formation of a Ghon focus in a child's lung, tubercle bacilli pass via lung lymphatics to regional lymph nodes where they initiate caseous necrosis and tubercle formation similar to that in the lung. The combination of a Ghon focus in the lung and tuberculous regional (peribronchial) lymph nodes is called a **primary complex** or **Ghon complex**. The outcome of infection depends on the fate of the lymph node lesion. If defences are strong, healing of the tubercles occurs by fibrosis, leaving only small fibrocalcific nodules in the lung periphery and regional lymph nodes. If defence mechanisms are inadequate, the lymph node tubercle enlarges due to extensive caseous necrosis, tending to overwhelm the surrounding macrophage–lymphocyte–fibroblast reaction. The lymph node enlarges until its capsule is breached then ruptures, discharging many tubercle bacilli into the surrounding tissues. The enlarging node may ulcerate into nearby bronchi, causing tuberculous bronchopneumonia (see Fig. 4.6), or into blood vessels (see Fig. 4.7), leading to extensive systemic spread of the organisms. Here, the tubercle has greatly enlarged so that the lymph node has almost been destroyed by caseous necrosis **C** and the zone of cellular reaction around it is very thin. Necrosis has almost reached the lymph node capsule and rupture is imminent.

Fig. 4.6 Tuberculous bronchopneumonia (MP)

When the wall of a bronchus is eroded by an enlarging tuberculous node or an apical Assmann focus, tubercle bacilli pass into the bronchial lumen from which they may be spread in various ways. If coughed up in sputum, the infection may be transmitted to other susceptible persons by droplet infection, sometimes infecting the patient's larynx (**tuberculous laryngitis**) on the way. Infected sputum may be swallowed and subsequently produce **tuberculous oesophagitis** or **ileitis**. Infected sputum may also gravitate to lower areas of the same or opposite lung where, by destruction of a bronchiolar wall, the organism may invade peribronchial lung tissue to form further caseating tubercles. This is called **tuberculous bronchopneumonia**.

In this example of an early lesion in tuberculous bronchopneumonia, note a bronchiole containing infected material. The walls of the bronchiole are indicated by the arrows marked **B**. A segment of the bronchiolar wall has been destroyed **D**, permitting access of bacilli which have initiated a caseating tubercle **T** in the nearby lung parenchyma. Large numbers of such lesions may form, merging with one another to produce a wide area of rapidly enlarging caseation, usually in the lower lobes of the lungs. This is the pathogenesis of the once dreaded '**galloping consumption**'.

SOME OTHER ASPECTS OF TUBERCULOSIS

In all cases of suspected tuberculosis, material should be submitted for culture. Culture of *Mycobacterium tuberculosis* is difficult and time consuming and may take 6 or more weeks. When the organisms have been cultured successfully, this allows assessment of antimicrobial resistance and sensitivity. It is often necessary to begin treatment empirically whilst awaiting microbiological confirmation and so initial histological findings supportive of this diagnosis can be very valuable. Histological identification of the organisms using special staining techniques is dependent upon the nature of the mycobacterial cell wall. This lipid-rich coating allows the organisms to retain certain dyes, even upon heating with acid and alcohol solutions, and so mycobacteria are often termed '**acid and alcohol fast bacilli**' (see Fig. 4.10). Another name for *Mycobacterium tuberculosis* which is sometimes used in clinical practice is the eponymous designation **Koch's bacillus**.

KEY TO FIGURES

B bronchiole **Bo** bony trabeculae **C** caseous necrosis **D** destroyed wall **G** granuloma **L** Langhans' giant cell
T tubercle

Fig. 4.7 **Disseminated tuberculosis** **(a)** Liver (MP) **(b)** Kidney (MP) **(c)** Bone (MP) **(d)** Tuberculous meningitis (MP)

If a ruptured tuberculous lymph node (or a rapidly enlarging focus of post-primary tuberculosis) erodes a blood vessel wall, masses of *Mycobacteria* are discharged into the circulation and lodge in the microvasculature. When the eroded vessel is a branch of the pulmonary artery, the organisms pass to other areas of the lung, but when a pulmonary venous tributary is involved, they are spread in the systemic circulation to many organs, notably the liver, kidney and spleen. In this way, vast numbers of new tubercles may be produced throughout the body. Such multiple lesions rarely attain any great size because this occurrence usually produces rapid clinical deterioration and death. Because the gross appearance of individual lesions resembles millet seeds, this condition is known as *miliary tuberculosis*.

Micrograph (a) shows several miliary tubercles **T** in the liver. One of the tubercles exhibits Langhans' giant cells **L** and the larger tubercle shows early central caseous necrosis.

It seems that a relatively small number of organisms can be disseminated by the bloodstream to various organs without causing overt disease, only to become reactivated at a later date when the host's immune status is impaired. These organisms remain viable but quiescent and active tuberculosis may then reappear in tissues remote from the original lesion many years later. This phenomenon is known as *metastatic* or *isolated organ tuberculosis* and most commonly involves the kidneys, adrenals, meninges, bone, Fallopian tubes, endometrium and epididymis.

Micrograph (b) illustrates renal involvement with the formation of small tubercles **T** in the renal cortex. Continuation of this process results in destruction of much of the renal cortex and medulla, with eventual rupture of large confluent tubercles into the pelvicalyceal system which becomes distended with caseous material. This condition is known as *tuberculous pyonephrosis*. In more advanced cases, infection spreads to involve the ureter and bladder. Renal tuberculosis is frequently bilateral and may result in renal failure.

Bone tuberculosis (*tuberculous osteomyelitis*) most frequently affects the long bones, associated joints and the vertebrae (*Pott's disease*). In long bones, infection may produce a localised, painful swelling which may drain to the skin to form a chronic sinus. Joint involvement (*tuberculous arthritis*) is most common in children and often affects the hips or joints associated with the vertebrae (*tuberculous spondylitis*) as part of Pott's disease of the spine. As in other tissues, image (c) shows the characteristic caseating granulomas **G** which cause progressive destruction of the bony trabeculae **Bo**. The infection tends to spread extensively in the cancellous medullary bone, leading to necrosis of surrounding cortical bone.

Tuberculous meningitis is an uncommon but frequently fatal complication of tuberculosis. Most often, it affects the meninges around the base of the brain and the spinal cord. As shown in (d), tuberculous granulomas **G**, with characteristic central areas of caseation, develop in the leptomeninges and adjacent brain tissue where they may damage cranial and spinal nerves. The presence of numerous lymphocytes in CSF obtained from lumbar puncture is useful in distinguishing tuberculous meningitis from purulent (bacterial) meningitis. In the latter, neutrophils are the major cell type present.

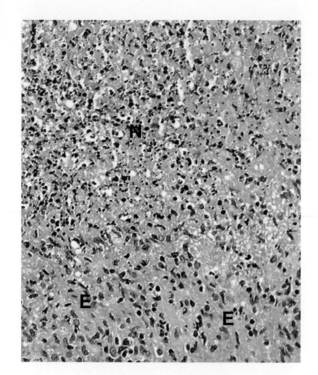

Fig. 4.8 **Atypical mycobacterial infection involving lymph node** (MP)

Infection with non-tuberculous *Mycobacteria* (also known as atypical *Mycobacteria* or *Mycobacteria* other than tuberculosis, MOTT) is not uncommon in the cervical lymph nodes of young children. Another group at risk from these organisms is AIDS patients who, because of severe immunosuppression, commonly develop widespread infections involving the liver, lymph nodes and spleen. In these patients, there is usually a deficient immune response and the histological appearance may simply be of aggregates of epithelioid cells or even foamy macrophages in the tissue with no lymphocytic component.

This micrograph shows a lymph node from an otherwise healthy child with MOTT infection. The lymphoid tissue is replaced with a granulomatous inflammatory response, consisting of confluent sheets of epithelioid macrophages **E**. In contrast to *M. tuberculosis*, the granulomas in MOTT infection show suppurative necrosis with aggregates of neutrophils **N**, rather than caseous necrosis. As in this example, giant cells may be sparse.

Fig. 4.9 **Leprosy (a)** Dermal infiltration (LP) **(b)** Nerve involvement (HP)

Leprosy is a disease caused by infection with *Mycobacterium leprae*. The tissue reaction to the bacillus depends on the immune response of the infected person. In the **tuberculoid** form of the disease, there is an active cell-mediated immune response and granulomas are formed which are similar to those seen in tuberculosis, but without evidence of caseation. In the **lepromatous** form, there is no effective cell-mediated immune response and tissues are infiltrated with macrophages colonised by large numbers of bacteria. Intermediate forms of leprosy exist with both tuberculoid and lepromatous features.

Clinically, people with the lepromatous form of the disease have nodular dermal and subcutaneous deposits of macrophages filled with bacteria and lipid. The disease affects the face, ears, arms, knees and buttocks, as the leprosy bacilli require cooler areas of the body for proliferation. In contrast, the tuberculoid form of the disease gives rise to macular or plaque-like skin lesions and, in addition, causes extensive inflammatory destruction of peripheral nerves. This typically gives rise to anaesthesia (loss of sensation) in the limbs, which then become prone to damage through repeated non-perceived injury.

Micrograph (a) is from the skin of a person with tuberculoid leprosy. Histiocytic granulomas **G** with a heavy surrounding lymphocytic infiltrate are present at all layers throughout the dermis, but particularly in relation to small nerves. This is illustrated at higher magnification in micrograph (b). Here, a small dermal nerve **DN** is shown which is surrounded by a cuff of lymphocytes. There is an associated granuloma **G** adjacent to the nerve.

KEY TO FIGURES

C carbon pigment   **DN** dermal nerve   **E** epithelioid macrophages   **G** granuloma   **N** neutrophils

Fig. 4.10 **Special staining for** *Mycobacteria* **(a)** Ziehl–Neelsen stain in tuberculosis (HP) **(b)** Wade–Fite stain in lepromatous leprosy (HP)

Mycobacterium tuberculosis and atypical *Mycobacteria* are not visible on routine H&E stains. To demonstrate the presence of *Mycobacteria* in tissue, the Ziehl–Neelsen (ZN) staining method is employed. The stain is taken up by the cell walls of the *Mycobacteria* and remains despite treatment with acid and alcohol. This is the origin of the term *acid and alcohol fast bacilli*, which is used in describing *Mycobacteria*. In this very high-power micrograph (a), scattered magenta-coloured, rod-shaped organisms can be seen in the lung of an immunocompromised patient. Some carbon pigment C can be identified within alveolar macrophages. In an immunocompetent individual, these organisms may be very sparse and difficult to find, but even a single organism in the appropriate background of a caseating granuloma is diagnostic. In immunosuppressed individuals (as shown here) and also in MOTT infection, the organisms are often much more numerous.

Micrograph (b) of lepromatous leprosy shows the Wade–Fite stain, which is a modified version of the ZN stain. Again, it stains the organisms red. The similarity in appearance between *M. tuberculosis* and *M. leprae* can be readily appreciated.

Spirochaete infections

The major form of spirochaete infection worldwide is *syphilis*, due to *Treponema pallidum*. *Yaws* and *pinta* are further important treponemal infections, but these are rare except in specific tropical regions. Although now relatively uncommon, late-stage syphilis is still regarded as one of the classical examples of specific chronic inflammation. The infecting organism, the spiral-shaped spirochaete *Treponema pallidum*, resists usual tissue defences and excites a progression of fascinating pathological and clinical phenomena which represent typical chronic inflammatory responses with superimposed hypersensitivity reactions mounted by the immune system. Classically, the condition proceeds through three stages extending over a long period.

In brief, the organism usually gains access to the body by penetrating the genital mucosa where it produces a single, small primary lesion known as a *chancre*. The chancre is a raised, reddened nodule caused by an intense local accumulation of plasma cells and lymphocytes in the subepithelial connective tissue. The chancre may ulcerate at this stage, but it is often painless and may easily pass unnoticed. By the time the chancre has developed, the organism has multiplied extensively and has been disseminated to regional lymph nodes and thence into the bloodstream, causing a generalised bacteraemia. The chancre and concomitant bacteraemia (*primary syphilis*) are followed some weeks or months later by a transient *secondary stage*. This is characterised by a widespread, variable skin rash, often with moist, warty, genital lesions and ulceration of the oral mucosa. These various mucosal lesions are histologically similar to the primary chancre and are full of treponemal organisms. The disease is now at its most contagious, yet the patient usually feels well and the only other evidence of a generalised infection is a widespread lymphadenopathy and positive serological findings.

In most untreated cases, the infection is effectively resolved by body defences and, in many of these patients, even serological evidence of previous infection disappears. Unfortunately, a proportion of untreated cases proceed from the secondary stage to develop *tertiary syphilis*, after a variable interval of from one to many years. The lesions of tertiary syphilis may be either focal or diffuse and it is the focal lesion of tertiary syphilis, known as the *gumma*, which exhibits many of the features of a granulomatous inflammation. Tertiary lesions may occur in almost any organ or tissue and the clinical consequences vary enormously. The diffuse form of tertiary syphilis most notably involves the cardiovascular system, particularly the ascending aorta and, less commonly, the central nervous system; the well-known *tabes dorsalis* and *general paresis of the insane (GPI)* are two of the manifestations of neurosyphilis. In the focal form of tertiary syphilis, gummas may develop in the liver, bone, testes and other sites. The clinical outcome depends upon the nature and extent of local tissue destruction.

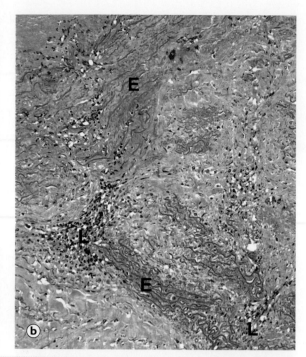

Fig. 4.11 **Syphilis** **(a)** Syphilitic gumma of the liver (LP) **(b)** Syphilitic aortitis (MP)

Micrograph (a) illustrates the classical appearance of a gumma with central, homogeneous, coagulative necrosis **N** surrounded by a zone of epithelioid macrophages, lymphocytes, plasma cells and plump fibroblasts. Fibrous healing of liver gummas may produce a pattern of coarse, deep scars dividing the liver surface into numerous irregular lobules. This condition is known as **hepar lobatum**.

Micrograph (b) illustrates **syphilitic aortitis**, the most common form of diffuse tertiary syphilitic lesion. The characteristic feature of syphilis is a low-grade, chronic vasculitis of small vessels with thickening of the wall, particularly the endothelium, and a perivascular cuff of lymphocytes and plasma

cells (**endarteritis obliterans**). In the aorta, the vasculitis affects the vasa vasorum of the tunica adventitia and their smaller branches which extend into the tunica media. The blue-stained areas in the tunica media represent lymphocytic cuffing **L** around numerous small vessels. The smooth muscle and elastic fibres of the media degenerate, probably because of ischaemia, and the aortic wall is replaced by collagen. Residual elastin **E** is stained deep pink. The loss of elasticity and contractility in the aortic wall allows progressive stretching with the formation of an **aneurysm** (see Chs 8 and 11), usually affecting the ascending aorta or aortic arch.

Viral infections

Viruses cause disease in three main ways:

■ By causing death of the cell they infect, either by a direct effect or by modifying the genome such that the host cell is recognised as foreign and is destroyed by the host immune system.

■ By causing excessive proliferation of the infected cell line, which may result in the development of malignant tumours. Human papilloma virus (HPV) is particularly important in this respect.

■ By integrating themselves in the cell nucleus where they produce latent infection.

Although viral culture and the demonstration of rising titres of antibodies against the virus remain the mainstays of diagnosis, some viral infections can be diagnosed by characteristic histological appearances. Individual viruses are too small to be seen by light microscopy, but when congregating together in enormous numbers within the host cell, they are visible as **viral inclusion bodies** and may be either intranuclear, intracytoplasmic, or both. Inclusion bodies provide a histological clue to the causative virus and this can be confirmed by electron microscopy and immunohistochemistry.

One viral infection of particular importance is the **Human immunodeficiency virus (HIV)** which is the cause of the **acquired immune deficiency syndrome (AIDS)**. As well as producing certain characteristic histological changes, particularly affecting lymph nodes, HIV compromises the host immune system and so a range of other unusual infections may result. HIV-1 is a lymphotropic virus which gains access to cells by way of the CD4 surface protein, normally found on T helper cells as well as on most monocytes and other macrophages. Infection with HIV-1 is associated with several clinical and pathological syndromes. Some patients develop fever, weight loss, diarrhoea and generalised lymph node enlargement (lymphadenopathy) in which there is generalised follicular hyperplasia. In patients with the full-blown immunodeficiency state of AIDS, lymph nodes show loss of follicles, lymphocyte depletion, vascular proliferation and fibrosis.

KEY TO FIGURES
E elastin   **I** inclusion body   **L** lymphocytes around vessels   **N** necrosis   **S** syncytial cells   **V** vesicle

The two main consequences of the immunodeficiency state seen in AIDS are:

■ Predisposition to opportunistic infections, particularly

– *Pneumocystis* pneumonia (Fig. 4.17)

– Cytomegalovirus infection (Fig. 4.13)

– Mycobacterial infections, tuberculosis as well as atypical *Mycobacteria* (Fig. 4.8)

– Mucocutaneous and other fungal infections (Fig. 4.15) including *Cryptococcus* (Fig. 4.18)

– Toxoplasmosis

■ Predisposition to certain tumours, particularly

– Kaposi's sarcoma (Fig. 11.12)

– Non-Hodgkin's lymphoma, especially diffuse large B-cell lymphoma (see Ch. 16).

CLINICAL FEATURES OF HERPES VIRUS INFECTION

Herpes simplex virus types 1 and 2 (HSV-1 and HSV-2) cause the common skin eruptions known as '**cold sores**' and genital herpes, whilst the chicken pox virus (Herpes zoster) is responsible for '**shingles**'. In immunocompetent individuals, Herpes viruses may remain latent in nerve cells with intermittent episodes of reactivation when the virus replicates within and destroys either epidermal cells or the epithelial cells of mucous membranes. Clinically, this gives rise to the typical appearance of groups of vesicles on an erythematous background. Most lesions heal spontaneously although the latent viral DNA remains in the nerve cells and can emerge in subsequent clinical episodes. In immunosuppressed patients, such as those with AIDS or those on immunosuppressive treatment, herpetic infection may result in widespread skin or visceral infections, rather than the self-limiting rash seen in the immunocompetent.

Fig. 4.12 **Herpes virus infection** **(a)** Skin (LP) **(b)** Oesophagus (HP)

Micrograph (a) shows a biopsy from a patient with HSV-2 infection. At low power, there is **vesiculation V** due to hydropic degeneration and necrosis of epithelial cells.

Micrograph (b) shows a high-power image of an oesophageal biopsy from a patient undergoing chemotherapy for gastric carcinoma. There is severe inflammation of the squamous mucosa and numerous intranuclear eosinophilic **inclusion bodies I** can be seen within the nuclei, pushing the hyperchromatic host chromatin to the periphery. These consist of masses of virus particles. Another characteristic feature is fusion of epithelial cells to form multinucleate **syncytia S**. These nuclei contain inclusions and typically mould together within the cells.

Neonates can become infected during passage through the birth canal if there is active infection and may succumb to a severe, generalised infection of the lymph nodes, spleen, lungs, liver, adrenals and central nervous system.

Fig. 4.13 Cytomegalovirus infection (HP)

Cytomegalovirus (CMV), another of the Herpes virus group, causes a mild, non-specific infection in immunocompetent individuals. Most adults will have been exposed to this virus by late middle age and will have specific serum antibodies. CMV infects white blood cells and may remain latent in leukocytes for many years. If the individual then becomes immunosuppressed for any reason, widespread systemic infection may result. Common sites of infection include the lungs, brain, retina, gastrointestinal tract and kidney.

CMV pneumonitis is shown in this micrograph. The characteristic feature is markedly enlarged cells with large, dark-staining, intranuclear inclusion bodies **I**. These are surrounded by a clear halo. Cytoplasmic inclusions may be seen, but are not illustrated in this micrograph. Sometimes, there is focal necrosis but there is usually minimal, if any, inflammation. Cytomegalic inclusions are usually seen in epithelial cells, endothelial cells and in macrophages and, as is the case in other Herpes virus infections, these inclusions may be sparse.

Fig. 4.14 Human papilloma virus (HP)

Human papilloma virus (HPV) is the causative agent of the common viral skin warts and genital warts. It has also been shown to be very closely associated with cervical intraepithelial neoplasia (CIN) and with invasive squamous cell carcinoma of the cervix, vagina, vulva and other sites.

HPV infects squamous epithelial cells and causes characteristic morphological changes. The epithelium is usually thickened (acanthotic) or may have the papillary appearance of an exophytic wart (*condyloma acuminatum*). Infection of cells in the upper layers of the epithelium produces enlargement of the nuclei which are hyperchromatic and have a folded appearance. A prominent cytoplasmic halo is also seen. These cells are called *koilocytes* **K**. In addition, the epithelium contains binucleate cells **B** and *dyskeratotic cells* **D** (i.e. individual cell keratinisation).

Such changes are usually seen in association with low-grade CIN, as in this specimen from a woman with CIN I. In high-grade CIN, these changes are usually less apparent, being overshadowed by more advanced dysplastic changes. HPV infection can be demonstrated by molecular techniques in almost all high-grade CIN lesions (see also Figs 17.5 and 17.6).

Fungal infections

Fungal infections range from minor localised skin infections to life-threatening systemic diseases in immunosuppressed patients. The inflammatory reaction in fungal infections may have one of three patterns. The classical appearance is of a granulomatous inflammation which may exhibit central suppurative necrosis. A second pattern is of acute inflammation with an infiltrate consisting primarily of neutrophils. This pattern is seen in *Candida* infection of the oesophagus. The third is a very minimal inflammatory response, as in superficial infections of the skin by dermatophytic fungi.

Fungi are not usually obvious on routine H&E staining, but the thick cell walls are highlighted by special stains such as PAS or silver stains. Some fungi are easily recognised histologically because of the characteristic shape and structure of the hyphae and the pattern of budding of the yeast forms. Despite this, culture techniques are preferable for definitive identification of fungal species. An important diagnostic point is that the presence of fungal yeast forms, such as *Candida* at a mucosal surface or on the skin, does not necessarily indicate active infection, as these agents are common commensals. Evidence of active invasion must be demonstrated and, in most cases, there is an appropriate inflammatory response.

SOME CLINICAL ASPECTS OF FUNGAL INFECTION

Many superficial forms of fungal infection are very indolent and slow growing and, as a result, treatment with antifungal drugs may need to extend over a prolonged period. It may be important to identify the precise type of fungus which is causing infection in order to ensure that the organism is sensitive to the form of treatment chosen. As fungi tend to have different growth requirements from bacteria, the microbiology laboratory must be informed if fungal infection is suspected so that appropriate cultures can be undertaken.

Fig. 4.15 **Candidiasis** **(a)** Oral candidiasis (PAS) (HP) **(b)** Oesophageal candidiasis (PAS) (HP) **(c)** Myocardial candidiasis (PAS) (HP)

Candida albicans is a ubiquitous commensal fungus on the epithelial surfaces of the skin, mouth and genital tract. It exists in both a hyphal/mycelial form and as rounded yeasts. Although usually commensal, it can become pathogenic, usually producing reddening and soreness of the affected epithelium, often with a whitish surface membrane comprising excess keratin production and fungal hyphae.

The common sites for this are the mouth (oral candidiasis or thrush) and the vulvo-vaginal region (candidal vulvo-vaginitis). Both may be precipitated by debilitation or as a complication of systemic antibiotic therapy destroying the normal bacterial flora and allowing overgrowth of the fungus.

More severe infections can occur in patients who are immunosuppressed. Surface epithelial infections are more extensive and symptomatic, with large numbers of organisms in both hyphal and yeast forms (see micrograph (b)). Organisms may also gain access to the bloodstream and in immunosuppressed patients

may produce disseminated candidiasis, with organisms in many organs.

Micrograph (a) shows candidal infection, mainly in hyphal forms **H**, on the surface of the buccal epithelium from a case of oral thrush in a patient taking antibiotics.

Micrograph (b) shows abundant candidal infection, both in hyphal **H** and yeast **Y** forms, in the oesophagus of an elderly man debilitated by terminal cancer. There is also abundant necrotic debris **ND** forming a thick surface membrane. The infection had started as severe oropharyngeal thrush, but had spread down his oesophagus.

Micrograph (c) shows *Candida* yeast forms **Y** in giant cells **G** in the myocardium, forming a small granuloma. Often, bloodstream spread of *Candida* produces small abscesses filled with neutrophils (pus), but this patient was severely immunosuppressed and was unable to mount an acute inflammatory reaction.

KEY TO FIGURES

B binucleate cell **D** dyskeratotic cell **G** giant cell **H** hyphae **I** inclusion body **K** koilocyte **ND** necrotic debris **Y** yeast forms

Fig. 4.16 *Aspergillus* (*caption opposite*)

KEY TO FIGURES
A *Aspergillus* hyphae   **E** exudate   **F** fruiting bodies   **H** hyphae   **I** inflammatory cells   **L** lymphocytes
N necrotic tissue   **S** septa

Fig. 4.16 *Aspergillus* (a) MP (b) HP (c) HP (d) Silver stain (HP) (e) *Aspergillus niger* (MP) (*illustrations opposite*)

Aspergillus is a ubiquitous fungus which may cause an allergic pulmonary response in otherwise healthy individuals. This is known colloquially as brewer's lung and belongs to the group of diseases known by the term *extrinsic allergic alveolitis*. In this case, the *Aspergillus* does not colonise or invade the lung.

Asthmatic individuals may have their bronchial tree colonised by *Aspergillus* without invasion. They are then likely to suffer from an exacerbation of their asthma as a result of *allergic bronchopulmonary aspergillosis*. This is a hypersensitivity response to *Aspergillus* antigens to which they are constantly exposed.

Aspergillus may also colonise pre-existing abscess cavities, classically old tuberculous cavities, where it may form a fungus ball (*aspergilloma*). Invasive *Aspergillus* infections occur in individuals who are immunosuppressed.

Micrograph (a) shows a medium-power view of invasive *Aspergillus* infection in the lung. A mass of *Aspergillus* hyphae **A** is surrounded by an inflammatory infiltrate **I** consisting mainly of neutrophils. Adjacent to this, there is a zone of necrotic lung tissue **N**. At high power, micrograph (b) shows the mass of *Aspergillus* hyphae. These characteristically branch at an acute angle as is shown in micrograph (c). The hyphae are also *septate*, i.e. the hyphae have divisions or septa **S** which divide them into segments. The typical appearance of *Aspergillus* on a silver stain is shown in micrograph (d), which shows the fungal hyphae clearly.

Micrograph (e) shows a mass of hyphae of *Aspergillus niger* **H** and inflammatory cells **I** from the external ear canal of a patient with chronic otitis externa. In the centre of the field there are two characteristic *fruiting bodies* **F** or *conidia*. These are similar to the fruiting bodies of other *Aspergillus* species except that they are pigmented. The brownish-black pigment is visible around the periphery of the fruiting body and gives rise to the name *Aspergillus niger*. This is a common cause of chronic otitis externa, an infection of the outer ear, mainly the auditory canal.

OTHER FUNGAL INFECTIONS – ZYGOMYCOSIS

Zygomycosis (also termed *mucormycosis*) is a form of opportunistic fungal infection caused by one of a range of environmental fungi of the class *Zygomycetes*. These organisms pose no threat to immunocompetent individuals, but can cause very serious and often life-threatening infections in those who are immunocompromised, particularly in diabetic patients in whom the organisms may infect the nose and paranasal sinuses, invading from this site to involve the orbits and cerebrum (*rhinocerebral mucormycosis*). The hyphae in cases of mucormycosis are broad and irregular, branching at near right angles (in contrast to the acute angles seen in *Aspergillus* infection). Also, the hyphae typically appear open and non-septate in routine preparations. Often, the fungi invade into artery walls and may then give rise to thrombosis and tissue necrosis.

Fig. 4.17 *Pneumocystis* in lung (a) H&E (MP) (b) Silver stain (HP)

The organism *Pneumocystis jirovecii* (formerly known as *Pneumocystis carinii*) was previously classified as a protozoan, but more recently it has become clear that it is a member of the fungal family. It is a ubiquitous organism and can be demonstrated in the lungs of most normal individuals where it causes no disease. *Pneumocystis* has, however, been brought into the spotlight by AIDS, although it may infect patients with immunosuppression from other causes. In AIDS patients, *Pneumocystis* causes a diffuse patchy pneumonia which may be the presenting feature of full-blown AIDS and is often fatal. Diagnosis may be difficult and transbronchial lung biopsy is often required. With routine H&E staining, as in micrograph (a), the organisms may not be apparent.

The alveoli are often filled by a foamy, acellular exudate **E** with an interstitial infiltrate of lymphocytes **L** in the alveolar wall. The inflammatory infiltrate may be minimal or more severe, showing features of diffuse alveolar damage (see Fig. 12.10) with hyaline membranes, capillary dilatation and exudation of red cells. Demonstration of the organisms requires a silver stain as shown in micrograph (b). The organisms are cup-shaped and measure 4–6 μm. Giemsa and toluidine blue stains may also be employed. The above stains may also be carried out on sputum samples and bronchial washings. AIDS patients frequently have concurrent infections with other organisms such as Cytomegalovirus (see Fig. 4.13).

Fig. 4.18 *Cryptococcus* **(a)** Brain H&E (MP) **(b)** Alcian blue stain (HP) **(c)** Mucicarmine stain (HP)

Cryptococcus neoformans is another yeast which causes serious infections in many tissues, mainly in immunosuppressed individuals such as patients with AIDS, haematological malignancy and transplant recipients. Occasionally, however, it may cause meningitis, meningoencephalitis or lung infection in an otherwise well individual.

Micrograph (a) shows the typical appearance of *Cryptococcus* in the brain. The organisms are seen forming a cyst in a Virchow–Robin perivascular space. These lesions are known as 'soap bubble' lesions. The *Cryptococci* **C** have a thick surrounding capsule which appears as a clear space. This capsule is an important virulence factor as it inhibits phagocytosis of the organisms and reduces normal leukocyte migration. Typically, there is a minimal inflammatory response which may be due to the immunosuppressed state of the patient. However, in chronic infections in non-immunosuppressed individuals, the organisms may incite a granulomatous response.

Techniques employed in demonstrating *Cryptococci* are highly dependent upon the thick capsule of the organisms. One simple method uses India ink to create a negative image, showing the organism with a clear capsular halo against a dark background. Micrographs (b) and (c) show other special staining techniques which are useful in highlighting *Cryptococci*. The organism's thick polysaccharide capsule **Cap** can be stained using Alcian blue as illustrated in image (b). Here, the nuclei of surrounding cells are counter-stained red. Image (c) shows brain tissue stained using the mucicarmine method. The *Cryptococci* **C** organisms are surrounded by a thick, magenta-coloured capsule **Cap**.

In the lung, *Cryptococcus* may cause a diffuse infection or it may form a solitary mass lesion in previously healthy individuals. Focal lesions such as this may lead to suspicion of other pathologies, such as bronchial carcinoma. In this case, the lesion is actually a large granuloma with a jelly-like centre, formed by a mass of organisms surrounded by a thick layer of macrophages, lymphocytes and giant cells.

Protozoa and helminths

Of the wide range of ***protozoa*** which are of pathological importance, only a few are usually diagnosed histologically. Many of these organisms are major causes of morbidity and mortality in particular geographic regions in the developing world. Increasingly, such infections may be seen elsewhere as a result of more widespread travel and migration. Protozoa are unicellular organisms which may reproduce asexually or sexually. Many have a complex life cycle involving one or more animal hosts. ***Giardia lamblia*** is a common protozoan infecting the small intestine in communities worldwide (Fig. 4.19). ***Trichomonas vaginalis*** is another protozoan parasite which is a common cause of female genital tract infection (Fig. 4.20). This organism is frequently encountered in cervical cytology screening. ***Malaria*** and ***amoebiasis*** are also described in this chapter (Figs 4.21 and 4.22). A wide variety of ***helminths*** infect humans, many primarily infecting the gut, although they may pass through other anatomical sites en route. Some helminths, such as the nematodes ***Enterobius vermicularis*** and ***Toxocara canis***, are found worldwide, while others, such as ***Wuchereria bancrofti***, have a more limited tropical distribution. ***Enterobiasis*** is fairly commonly seen in routine practice (Fig. 4.24) and ***Schistosomiasis*** is of particular histological importance (Fig. 4.23). These infections are illustrated here.

Fig. 4.19 Giardiasis (HP)

Giardia lamblia is a common protozoan parasite which causes diarrhoea. The organism is spread via contaminated water and is more common in institutionalised and immunocompromised patients. Diagnosis is commonly made by biopsy of the small intestine. The organisms **G** are seen on the surface of the villi **V**. A few erythrocytes **E** are also seen. The mucosa may appear normal or may be inflamed, sometimes resembling coeliac disease (see Fig. 13.15).

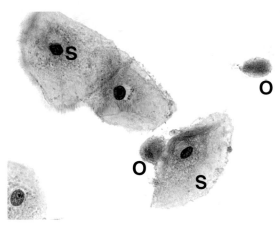

Fig. 4.20 *Trichomonas vaginalis* (Papanicolaou stain) (HP)

This flagellated protozoan parasite commonly infects the female genital tract, presenting with itching and a frothy greenish vaginal discharge. The organism is motile and can be demonstrated in wet preparations, but is most commonly noted at the time of examination of a routine cervical smear test ('Pap' test). The organisms **O** are pear-shaped or ovoid and are somewhat smaller than the surrounding squamous epithelial cells **S**. The organisms stain a smudgy grey-green colour. Indistinct nuclei and red cytoplasmic granules may be seen. Flagellae are not usually identifiable on routine preparations. The surrounding epithelial cells may show reactive changes and scattered neutrophil polymorphs may be present.

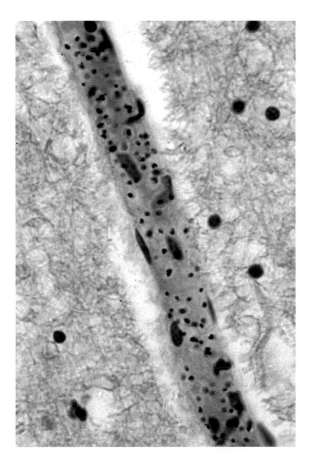

Fig. 4.21 Cerebral malaria (HP)

Malaria, which is caused by four species of the protozoan *Plasmodium*, is common in the tropics and subtropics and is a major cause of mortality. After entering the blood via the proboscis of a mosquito, the merozoites enter erythrocytes. Further cycles of division occur within the erythrocytes which rupture, allowing further cycles of infection. The sexual phase of the life cycle occurs within the mosquito. *Plasmodium falciparum* is the most virulent form of malaria, with cerebral involvement being a major cause of death. The cerebral tissue is characteristically congested, as shown in this micrograph, where a dilated small blood vessel is packed with erythrocytes within which the malarial parasites can be seen as dark brown dots. Falciparum malaria has the property of causing erythrocytes to adhere to endothelium, thus obstructing blood flow. The congested vessels often rupture to cause 'ring haemorrhages' (not shown here). Without specific treatment, cerebral malaria is almost always fatal and the increasing incidence of drug resistance makes it difficult to treat. Malarial parasites can be seen within erythrocytes in any other tissues and the diagnosis is usually made by examination of a blood smear. The different species can be identified by their characteristic appearance. The other species that cause malaria, namely *P. vivax, P. ovale* and *P. malariae*, cause a much milder illness which may be recurrent. *P. falciparum* may cause severe anaemia, pulmonary oedema, renal failure, shock, hypoglycaemia and cerebral disease.

KEY TO FIGURES

C *Cryptococcus*   **Cap** capsule   **E** erythrocytes   **G** *Giardia*   **O** *Trichomonas* organisms   **S** squamous cells   **V** villi

Fig. 4.22 Amoebiasis (HP)

Infections with *Entamoeba histolytica* occur worldwide. The organism is restricted to man and it is estimated that about 10% of the world's population may carry the organism in the colon. The most common form of infection is ***amoebic dysentery***, where the *Entamoebae* invade the mucosa of the colon and rectum, causing painful, bloody diarrhoea. Pathologically, the mucosa is extensively undermined, producing typical flask-shaped ulcers which may perforate. This micrograph shows organisms **A** adherent to colonic mucosa **M**. The *Entamoebae* are slightly larger than a macrophage and characteristically phagocytose erythrocytes (visible within the organisms). The organisms may invade and obstruct colonic arteries, causing superimposed ischaemic necrosis. The organism may spread to the liver, causing an ***amoebic abscess***, and thence to the lung or pleural, peritoneal or pericardial cavities. Venereal infections of the cervix and penis also occasionally occur.

Fig. 4.23 Schistosomiasis (a) MP (b) HP

Schistosomiasis is a systemic parasitic infection caused by the organism *Schistosoma*, a genus of ***trematode worms (flukes)***. Three species are of pathological importance. Their life cycle includes water snails (the intermediate host), with man (the definitive host) becoming infected by bathing or working in water containing the larvae or ***cercaria*** released from snails. The cercaria penetrate the skin, in the process converting to ***schistosomules***, and then migrate via the venous system to the pulmonary vessels where they mature for 4 weeks before entering the systemic circulation. From here, they migrate to the hepatic branches of the portal vein (*S. mansoni* and *S. japonicum*) or the pelvic veins (*S. haematobium*) where they mature and may persist for several years or even more. In their chosen location, the adult worms mate with the females, producing up to 3000 eggs per day. Some eggs leave the body in urine or faeces and, on reaching still or gently flowing fresh water, hatch into a ciliated form called ***miracidia*** and thus reach their intermediate snail hosts. Other eggs lodge in the tissues (*S. mansoni* and *S. japonicum* in the small and large intestine and thence to the liver; *S. haematobium* in the bladder and rectum), exciting a florid granulomatous reaction progressing to extensive fibrosis. In the liver, there is severe fibrosis of the portal tracts where the eggs lodge. Schistosomiasis is the major cause of portal hypertension worldwide. *S. haematobium* causes a similar reaction in the bladder, with a number of manifestations including papillomas, ulcers and bladder contractures. Chronic inflammation predisposes to dysplasia and malignancy. Eggs may also be found at many other sites such as the lungs and CNS.

Micrograph (a) shows a low-power view of schistosome eggs **SE** in the small intestine. Unusually, part of the adult worm **W** is seen. Micrograph (b) shows two schistosome eggs **SE** at high power. The groups of eggs are surrounded by epithelioid cells **E**, giant cells **G** and eosinophils. The eggs of each species can be identified by their size and the position of the spine, which in this case is terminally located and therefore likely to come from *S. haematobium*.

KEY TO FIGURES

A amoebae   **AP** alar projection   **C** cuticle   **E** epithelioid cells   **G** giant cell   **M** mucosa   **N** neutrophils
SE schistosome eggs   **W** adult worm

Fig. 4.24 *Enterobius vermicularis* (HP)

Enterobius vermicularis is also known as pinworm or threadworm. The organism is spread by the faecal–oral route and is commonly present within the lumen of the bowel, particularly in children. The organisms do not invade into the tissues. The female worm lays eggs in the perianal area and symptoms, if any, tend to be of perineal irritation. The adult worms inhabit the ileocaecal area and are most commonly identified in the appendix. This micrograph shows a transverse section through an adult worm within the lumen of the appendix. There is no invasion of the mucosa **M**. The thick cuticle **C** of the worm has a typical alar projection **AP** on each side and the oesophagus and other internal structures of the worm can also be seen.

Fig. 4.25 Chapter review

Disorder	Main features	Figure
Bacterial infections		
Clostridium difficile	Pseudomembranous colitis with focal epithelial necrosis due to toxin. 'Volcano' pattern with inflammatory exudate	4.1
Actinomyces	Filamentous bacteria forming 'sulphur granule' colonies with encrusted proteinaceous material	4.2
Mycobacterium tuberculosis	Granulomatous inflammation with caseation and Langhans' giant cells. Ghon complex. May progress to miliary disease if immunosuppressed	4.3–4.7, 4.10(a)
Atypical Mycobacteria (MOTT, NTM)	Often in immunocompromised patients. Suppurative granulomas	4.8
Mycobacterium leprae	Pattern depends upon immune status (tuberculoid/lepromatous). Granulomatous inflammation of skin and dermal nerves	4.9, 4.10(b)
Treponema pallidum	Primary, secondary and tertiary syphilis. Chancre, gumma, endarteritis obliterans	4.11
Viral infections		
Herpes simplex virus	Types 1 & 2. Oral and genital herpes. Disseminated in immunosuppressed. Vesiculation with syncytial giant cells and intranuclear inclusions	4.12
Varicella zoster virus	Cause of chickenpox and shingles. Morphology similar to HSV	Like 4.12
Cytomegalovirus	Non-specific symptoms normally. Disseminated in immunosuppressed. Very large cells with intranuclear and intracytoplasmic inclusions	4.13
Human papilloma virus	Many types, causes common wart. Oncogenic forms cause cervical cancer. Koilocytosis, binucleation, dyskeratosis and dysplasia (CIN)	4.14, 17.5, 17.6
Fungal infections		
Candida	Common, often affects mucous membranes. Typically neutrophil response. Yeast forms and branching pseudohyphae	4.15
Aspergillus	Mostly lung disease. Allergic, colonising and invasive forms. Narrowing septate hyphae with branching at acute angles	4.16
Zygomyces	Mucormycosis. Typically sinonasal disease in diabetic patients. Invades vessels. Broad and non-septate hyphae with right-angle branching	
Pneumocystis	Environmental fungus, pathogenic in immunocompromised, e.g. AIDS. Foamy exudate in alveoli, cup-shaped organisms on silver stains	4.17
Cryptococcus	Mostly in immunocompromised patients. Can cause lung disease in normal people. Yeasts with thick outer capsule	4.18
Protozoa and helminths		
Giardia lamblia	Cause of infective diarrhoea. Protozoan parasite infecting small intestine. Small sickle-shaped organisms on mucosal surface	4.19
Trichomonas vaginalis	Common cause of vaginal discharge and irritation, often seen in cervical smear tests. Pear-shaped protozoan parasites with flagellae	4.20
Plasmodium sp.	Cause of malaria. Intracellular parasites with complex life cycle, spread by mosquito. Pigmented organisms in erythrocytes, vascular complications	4.21
Entamoeba histolytica	Very common cause of dysentery world wide. Invades colorectal mucosa. Flask-shaped ulcers and organisms larger than macrophages, PAS positive	4.22
Schistosoma sp.	Important worldwide. Complex lifecycle involving snail. Eggs lodge in various tissues and cause granulomatous inflammation	4.23
Enterobius vermicularis	Threadworm or pinworm. Common, colonises ileocolic area. Worms do not invade. Eggs cause perianal irritation. Often seen in appendix	4.24

5 Amyloidosis

Introduction

Amyloidosis is a condition which is characterised by the extracellular deposition of abnormal fibrillar proteins known as *amyloid*. These may be deposited in many tissues and organs (*systemic amyloidosis*) or in a single organ (*localised amyloidosis*). Amyloid is defined by its staining characteristics with certain stains such as *Congo red* and by its ultrastructural appearance, forming rigid non-branching fibrils 7–12 nm in diameter.

Amyloid is formed from one of a range of peptide molecules (forming 90–95% of the deposited material), in combination with a small amount of *amyloid P component*, a glycoprotein molecule synthesised by the liver. This shows structural similarity to C reactive protein (CRP) but unlike CRP, amyloid P component is not an acute-phase reactant. These molecules are deposited as fibrils in the extracellular space where they form a *β-pleated sheet* configuration, a structure which is highly resistant to proteolysis.

Amyloidosis has traditionally been classified as primary or secondary, according to whether or not there was a pre-existing disease which was known to be associated with amyloid. This classification has been superseded as the peptide structure of amyloid has now been elucidated and classification according to peptide structure is more clinically useful. More than 25 distinct amyloidogenic peptides have now been described in humans. These peptides are derived from normal body proteins and some of the main forms are outlined in Figure 5.2. The most common subtypes are *AL amyloidosis* and *AA amyloidosis*. There are also various inherited forms of amyloidosis caused by polymorphisms in genes encoding a range of proteins.

CLINICAL ASPECTS OF AMYLOIDOSIS

AA amyloid is produced from a normal serum acute-phase protein (serum amyloid A). Conventionally, AA amyloidosis was termed **secondary amyloidosis**, because it occurred as a complication of certain underlying chronic inflammatory conditions. In the past, the most common predisposing conditions were tuberculosis, bronchiectasis and chronic osteomyelitis. With improved antibiotic therapy, these disorders are now comparatively rare and most cases of AA amyloidosis now arise secondary to connective tissue diseases such as rheumatoid arthritis and chronic inflammatory bowel disease.

AL amyloid protein consists of the variable segment of immunoglobulin light chains. Rather confusingly, this was traditionally termed **primary amyloidosis** because, in most cases, no underlying disorder could be identified. In reality, these light chains are produced in abnormal quantities by abnormal plasma cells and a proportion of patients so affected have overt evidence of **multiple myeloma**, a malignant proliferation of plasma cells (see Fig. 16.16). More commonly, there is no clinical evidence of a malignant plasma cell neoplasm but molecular testing confirms the presence of monoclonal immunoglobulins.

Fig. 5.1 | Amyloid ultrastructure (EM)

Electron microscopy is a useful method for the detection of amyloid in tissues, particularly when it is present in small quantities and does not show up with special stains. This electron micrograph shows amyloid deposited in renal glomeruli and resulting in *proteinuria* (excess protein leaking into the urine). A renal biopsy was performed and light microscopy revealed thickening of the glomerular basement membrane.

Ultrastructural examination of a portion of the thickened basement membrane revealed the deposition of amyloid. The amyloid is seen to have a fibrillar ultrastructure, each fibril being composed of the precursor peptide arranged as finer filaments of a β-pleated sheet. In this instance, the amyloid was deposited as a result of long-standing rheumatoid disease and was presumably of the serum amyloid A protein type (see Fig. 5.2).

Fig. 5.2 Overview of classification based on amyloid fibril protein

Pattern of deposition	Precursor protein	Clinical features
Systemic amyloidosis	Immunoglobulin light chain (AL)	Primary or myeloma-associated
	Immunoglobulin heavy chain (AH)	Primary or myeloma-associated
	Serum amyloid A protein (AA)	Secondary to chronic inflammation
	Serum amyloid A protein (AA)	Familial Mediterranean fever
	β_2-Microglobulin	Dialysis-associated
	Transthyretin (prealbumin)	Familial neuropathy
	Transthyretin (prealbumin)	Senile systemic amyloidosis
Localised amyloidosis	Atrial natriuretic factor	Senile cardiac amyloidosis
	Pro-calcitonin	Medullary thyroid carcinoma
	Islet amyloid polypeptide (amylin)	Islets of Langerhans, NIDDM, insulinoma
	Prolactin	Ageing pituitary, prolactinoma
	Aβ protein precursor (APP)	Alzheimer's disease, Down's syndrome
	Aβ protein precursor (APP)	Cerebral amyloid angiopathy
	Prion protein	Spongiform encephalopathies

Distribution and classification of amyloid

Amyloid is deposited in the extracellular compartment of tissues and, in H&E preparations, it is seen as uniformly *eosinophilic* (pink-staining) material. It can be highlighted in histological sections by use of special stains such as *Congo red* and *Sirius red*. Congo red staining is commonly used for diagnostic purposes, amyloid staining orange-red in colour and exhibiting a characteristic green appearance when viewed with polarised light.

Amyloidosis may involve many tissues in the body but most commonly affects the kidneys, liver, spleen, adrenals and heart (Fig. 5.3 to Fig. 5.6). It has a particular predilection for deposition in blood vessel walls (Fig. 5.7) and basement membranes. The progressive accumulation of amyloid leads to cellular dysfunction, either by preventing normal diffusion through extracellular tissues or by physical compression of functioning parenchymal cells.

Amyloid associated with monoclonal proliferation of plasma cells or B lymphocytes is usually made up of the variable segment of immunoglobulin light chains (AL protein). All patients so affected have a monoclonal gammopathy (circulating immunoglobulins produced by a single clone of plasma cells) but only a small proportion have overt evidence of malignant disease such as multiple myeloma or other B-cell lymphomas.

AA type amyloid occurs in a minority of cases of chronic inflammatory disease. The end result is deposition of amyloid derived from serum amyloid A protein (AA), an acute-phase protein which is produced by the liver in response to inflammation and circulates in the serum. It is not clear why some individuals have deposition of amyloid in this situation and others do not.

Certain familial types of amyloid involve the deposition of *transthyretin*-derived amyloid (transthyretin is so named because it transports thyroxine and retinol in plasma; this was formerly termed pre-albumin). In the familial types, transthyretin amyloid is associated with amino acid substitutions in the protein which predisposes to the formation of the β-pleated sheet amyloid structure.

Tumours of peptide-secreting endocrine cells may form amyloid from an abnormal form of the hormone peptide. A well-known example is the localised deposition of calcitonin-derived amyloid in medullary carcinoma of the thyroid (Fig. 5.8).

The central nervous system provides one of the most common examples of localised amyloid deposition in Alzheimer's disease (Fig. 23.3). Here, it is due to deposition of a peptide termed *amyloid β protein*. This is derived from a normal neuronal protein termed β-amyloid precursor protein (APP), the gene for which is found on chromosome 21. This may be related to deposition of the same protein in Down's syndrome (trisomy 21).

Fig. 5.3 **Renal amyloidosis** **(a)** H&E (HP) **(b)** Sirius red (HP)

The kidneys are the organs most commonly involved by systemic amyloidosis and renal failure is one of the most serious clinical complications, accounting for the majority of deaths from the disease. These sections from the same glomerulus are from an autopsy specimen, taken from a 58-year-old woman with a 20-year history of rheumatoid arthritis. The sections have been stained with contrasting histological methods to illustrate the principal features.

Amyloid deposition usually begins in the glomerular mesangium and around capillary basement membranes, leading to progressive obliteration of capillary lumina, destruction of glomerular endothelial, mesangial and podocyte cells, and eventually complete replacement of the glomerulus by a confluent mass of amyloid. Concurrently, the walls of renal arterioles and arteries may become infiltrated by amyloid, causing impairment of the blood supply to the glomerulus. Interstitial spaces between renal tubules may also become infiltrated, further compromising tubular function. With H&E staining, amyloid appears as a homogeneous eosinophilic (pink) material, difficult to distinguish from collagen or hyaline deposition. Staining methods such as Congo red or Sirius red, as in micrograph (b), readily distinguish amyloid which stands out as red-stained material. In this case, amyloid is present in the glomerulus and in the wall of an affected afferent arteriole **AA**.

Amyloid of the kidney usually presents with proteinuria, often severe enough to produce the *nephrotic syndrome*. Increasing amyloid deposition leads to glomerular ischaemia and tubular atrophy, and chronic renal failure supervenes.

Fig. 5.4 **Hepatic amyloidosis** (HP)

In the liver, amyloid is deposited in the space of Disse, between the sinusoidal lining cells and the hepatocytes. With progressive deposition, hepatocytes become compressed by sheets of amyloid and undergo atrophy.

Amyloid is visible as ribbon-like, pink-staining deposits **A** within hepatic sinusoids. The plates of hepatocytes **H** have become compressed and are atrophic.

Clinically, hepatic amyloidosis may be a cause of *hepatomegaly* (enlargement of the liver) and upon autopsy examination of patients with systemic amyloidosis, there is commonly evidence of hepatic involvement. Despite this, even when liver involvement is severe, it is rare to find evidence of clinically significant functional impairment in amyloidosis.

KEY TO FIGURES
A amyloid   **AA** afferent arteriole   **Ep** epithelium   **H** hepatocytes   **P** white pulp   **V** vessel

Fig. 5.5 **Splenic amyloidosis** **(a)** Diffuse type (LP) **(b)** Nodular type (LP)

There are two patterns of amyloid deposition seen in the spleen, described as either *diffuse* or *nodular*.

Micrograph (a) shows the more common diffuse pattern. Splenic amyloidosis most commonly begins with deposition in the walls of splenic sinuses, progressing until the deposits coalesce to form large diffuse masses **A**. Little red pulp and lymphoid tissue (white pulp **P**) remains. This form is sometimes termed '*lardaceous*' because of the waxy firmness of the spleen when the specimen is cut.

Less commonly, amyloid deposition results in the formation of the so-called '*sago*' spleen, illustrated in micrograph (b). In this pattern, the amyloid **A** becomes deposited in the periarteriolar lymphoid sheaths (white pulp), giving the appearance of discrete deposits on the cut surface of the gross specimen. Note the small vessels in the centre of the pink-staining nodular amyloid deposits. Amyloid deposition in the spleen can give rise to clinically palpable *splenomegaly* (splenic enlargement).

Fig. 5.6 **Cardiac amyloidosis** (MP)

Amyloid involvement of the heart may be an incidental finding at autopsy in the elderly. It may be a manifestation of localised senile cardiac amyloid (derived from atrial natriuretic peptide) or of systemic senile amyloidosis (derived from transthyretin). The most severe form of cardiac amyloid is seen in systemic heredo-familial amyloidosis, derived from serum amyloid A protein, as in familial Mediterranean fever. Cardiac involvement may also occur in cases of systemic AA amyloidosis.

Myocardial amyloidosis leads to intractable cardiac failure with enlargement of the heart. Subendocardial deposition of amyloid may interfere with the conducting system resulting in cardiac arrhythmias. In the case illustrated here, amyloid has accumulated in the walls of myocardial vessels V and is extending to form masses within the myocardium.

Fig. 5.7 **Vascular amyloid in rectal biopsy** (HP)

The diagnosis of systemic amyloidosis can be confirmed by tissue biopsy. The rectum is the commonest site of biopsy. In rectal biopsies, amyloid can be detected in the submucosal vessels in 60–70% of cases of generalised amyloidosis. This photomicrograph, taken at very high magnification, shows rectal glandular epithelium **Ep** with a small blood vessel in the adjacent lamina propria. The vessel wall is thickened by homogeneous, pink-staining amyloid **A**. Amyloid in small vessels such as this may be subtle and it is usual to confirm the diagnosis using a special stain such as Congo red.

Fig. 5.8 Amyloid in medullary carcinoma of the thyroid (HP)

An example of localised amyloidosis is seen in tumours derived from the calcitonin-secreting cells of the thyroid, namely medullary carcinomas. Large islands of pink-stained amyloid **A** are present between zones of tumour cells **T**. The amyloid is derived from pro-calcitonin secreted by the tumour. Amyloid is present only within the tumour and is not deposited in other tissues. Another example of localised amyloid is seen in *insulinomas*, tumours arising from the islets of Langerhans' in the pancreas. In this case, it appears that the amyloid is formed from a protein similar to calcitonin, termed *islet amyloid polypeptide* or *amylin*.

Fig. 5.9 Chapter review

Amyloid	Main features	Figure
Definition	Indigestible extracellular fibrillary protein	
	Defined by physicochemical properties	
	β-pleated sheet structure	
	7–12 nm diameter non-branching fibrils on EM	5.1
	Stains orange-red with Congo and Sirius red	5.3
	Apple green birefringence with polarised light	
Component peptides	Many different precursor peptides	5.2
	Common types AA and AL	
	All types include amyloid P component (glycoprotein synthesised by liver)	
AA amyloidosis	Derived from serum amyloid A protein	
	Traditionally termed 'secondary'	
	Associated with systemic chronic inflammatory diseases such as rheumatoid arthritis	
AL amyloidosis	Derived from immunoglobulin light chains	
	Traditionally termed 'primary'	
	Abnormal immunoglobulins produced by clone of abnormal plasma cell	
	Often no overt clinical evidence of plasma cell tumour	
	Some associated with myeloma or lymphoma	16.16
Other features	Localised or systemic deposition	
	Localised forms often associated with endocrine peptides and tumours	5.8
	Familial types due to subtle alterations in normal peptides, predisposing to fibril formation	
	CNS deposition occurs in various settings, including Alzheimer's disease	23.3
	Diagnosis confirmed by biopsy – amyloid often seen in walls of rectal blood vessels	5.7

KEY TO FIGURES
A amyloid **T** tumour cells

6 Disorders of growth

Introduction

Cells exist in, and must adapt to, an environment which is continually changing, reflecting not only physiological processes but also external influences such as drugs or toxins. As briefly discussed in Chapter 1, if the stimulus is overwhelming, the cells undergo degeneration or cell death. However, many less noxious stimuli cause cells to adapt by altering their pattern of growth. This may occur in three main ways:

■ alteration in the size of cells

    – *hypertrophy* – increase in size of existing cells

    – *atrophy* – decrease in size of existing cells

■ increase in the number of cells (*hyperplasia*)

■ change in the differentiation of cells (*metaplasia*).

In an organ composed of different types of cell, only one of the cell types may be affected, leading to a marked change in tissue appearance and function.

In all tissues, there is a population of undifferentiated cells (*stem cells*) which differ from mature cells throughout the body in three ways:

■ they are capable of dividing and renewing themselves (self-renewal)

■ they are unspecialised

■ they can give rise to specialised cell types.

Extrinsic to the cell, factors such as blood supply, innervation, hormonal stimulation, physical stress or biochemical alterations will determine the normal pattern of cell growth in an organ or tissue. Depending on the intrinsic characteristics of a particular cell type, a change in environment may result in a change in the growth pattern. Such responses are now recognised as being under the control of various growth factors which act upon specific cell surface receptors. Alterations in the concentrations of growth factors or the expression of growth factor receptors will result in altered cell growth.

STEM CELL THERAPY

Harnessing the therapeutic potential of stem cells, with their capacity for self-renewal and ability to differentiate into a variety of specialised cell types, represents one of the major challenges facing modern medicine. Stem cell therapy, in the form of stem cell transplants, is now common in treating some leukaemias. However, ongoing research into the potential regenerative/reparative capacity of stem cells in the treatment of conditions such as myocardial infarction, spinal cord injuries and degenerative conditions such as Parkinson's disease reflect the hopes for stem cell therapy in medicine.

In stem cell therapy for leukaemia the recipient's bone marrow must first be cleared of cells through a process known as *myeloablation* using a combination of chemotherapy and radiotherapy. This process removes any remaining, diseased marrow and reduces the likelihood of transplant rejection. Transplanted stem cells can then be introduced through an intravenous infusion. These cells are referred to as either *autologous* or *allogeneic*. In an autologous transplant the patient's own stem cells are used. These are collected at a time when the leukaemia is under control (in *remission*), though occasional tumour cells may still be present and can be removed through a process called *purging*. Allogeneic transplants use stem cells collected from a donor with a tissue type which closely matches that of the recipient, often a family member.

Increased cell mass

Organs may respond to environmental stimulation by an increase in functional cell mass through hyperplasia and/or hypertrophy. Hyperplasia occurs where cells are capable of dividing to generate an increased number of cells. In contrast, hypertrophy is typified by increase in cell size without an increase in cell number. An important feature of these forms of increased cell mass is that, following removal of the environmental stimulus, the altered pattern of growth ceases and the tissue may revert to its former state. Hypertrophy and hyperplasia can, in many circumstances, be regarded as normal physiological adaptations, as exemplified by exercise-induced skeletal muscle hypertrophy and the hyperplasia and hypertrophy of the myometrium during pregnancy.

Many pathological stimuli invoke the responses of hypertrophy and hyperplasia, and it appears these responses occur in many cases by the same mechanism which induces the normal physiological response. Thus, in the first part of the menstrual cycle, the endometrium proliferates with elongation of glands and increased numbers of epithelial cells. When an excessive concentration of oestrogen acts on the endometrium, such as at the menopause or owing to injudicious hormone replacement therapy, similar but more pronounced changes occur, leading to crowding of endometrial glands. Removing the stimulus to this excess growth can result in a regression. This contrasts with the abnormal, uncontrolled proliferation of cells associated with the development of cancers, referred to as *neoplasia* (see Ch. 7) where growth is independent of any external stimuli. Therefore, hyperplastic tissue is not of itself neoplastic, but may carry with it an increased risk of neoplastic change. Thus, hyperplastic endometrium is more likely than normal endometrium to progress to cancer. This risk is increased further when the hyperplasia is combined with cytologic atypia (termed *atypical hyperplasia*).

For poorly understood reasons, the process of hyperplasia may not be uniform throughout an organ or tissue and, in these instances, nodules of excessive cell growth arise in between areas of unaltered cell growth. This phenomenon, known as *nodular hyperplasia*, is seen in the thyroid gland (Fig. 20.5), the adrenal gland (Fig. 20.9) and the prostate gland (Fig. 19.9).

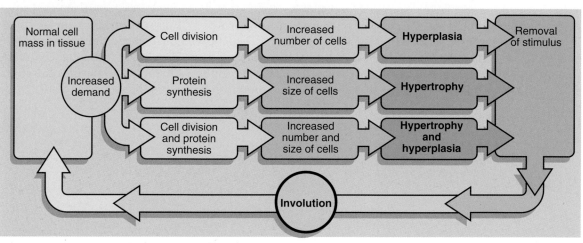

Fig. 6.1 **Increased functional cell mass**

Fig. 6.2 **Hypertrophy** **(a)** Normal myocardium (MP) **(b)** Hypertrophic myocardium (MP)

Pure hypertrophy, without coexisting hyperplasia, is virtually only seen in muscle, where the stimulus is an increased demand for work. An example is adult myocardium, the cells of which are incapable of division and are therefore unable to undergo hyperplasia. As such, myocardium becomes hypertrophic when it is subjected to an increased haemodynamic load over a period of time, such as in systemic hypertension or valvular stenosis.

Micrograph (a) shows normal myocardium **M** while micrograph (b), which is at the same

magnification, shows enlargement of myocardial cells **M** and their nuclei **N**. This enlargement is due to increased synthesis of proteins and filaments, permitting an increased workload; thus the size and weight of the heart are increased.

Other examples of muscular hypertrophy include bowel wall smooth muscle in chronic obstruction of the bowel by tumour, bladder detrusor muscle in chronic obstruction due to prostatic hyperplasia and in regularly exercised skeletal muscles.

Fig. 6.3 **Hyperplasia** **(a)** Normal proliferative phase endometrium (HP) **(b)** Hyperplasia of endometrium (HP)

Endometrial hyperplasia occurs when there is abnormal oestrogenic stimulation. Micrograph (a) shows normal proliferative-phase endometrium responding to normal ovarian oestrogenic stimulation. In contrast, in micrograph (b), the endometrial glands are markedly hyperplastic, and continued increase in the number of cells in each gland has resulted in some glands **G** showing cystic dilatation. In addition, there is irregularity and crowding of the glands as well as crowding of the epithelial cells lining the glands. This example is from

a woman on hormone replacement therapy where the effects of oestrogen were not counterbalanced by progestogens, resulting in persisting growth of the endometrium. Similar changes may also be seen in the endometrium of women with oestrogen-secreting ovarian tumours. Thus, hyperplasia results from exaggeration of a normal physiologic mechanism.

In such examples, removal of the abnormal oestrogenic stimulation restores the normal pattern of endometrial growth.

KEY TO FIGURES
G gland   **M** myocardial cells   **N** nuclei

BASIC PATHOLOGICAL PROCESSES ■ DISORDERS OF GROWTH

Reduction in functional cell mass

When the functional cell mass in a tissue is reduced, the tissue is said to have undergone *atrophy*. The mechanisms of atrophy may involve reduction in cell volume and/or in cell number, both leading to a reduction in functional capacity. Macroscopically, the appearance of the tissue depends on whether the functional cells lost are replaced by other tissue. Commonly, when atrophy occurs, the lost cells are replaced by either adipose or fibrous tissue, often maintaining the overall size of the organ. When adipose or fibrous replacement does not occur, the overall size of the organ is reduced. Examples are the testis in the elderly (Fig. 6.4) and the adrenal gland when suppressed by exogenous steroid administration (Fig. 20.9). Atrophy may occur as a physiological event (termed *involution*), such as in embryologic development or the normal involution of the thymus during adolescence.

A variety of causes of atrophy is recognised, in general conditions opposite to those causing hypertrophy or hyperplasia. Thus, disuse of skeletal muscle will result in a loss of cell mass (*disuse atrophy*). Removal of endocrine stimulation causes atrophy in target organs. Reduction in blood supply to a tissue may result in loss of functional cells (*ischaemic atrophy*), a situation commonly encountered in the kidney.

Atrophy must be distinguished from *hypoplasia*, a condition where there is incomplete growth of an organ, and *agenesis*, where there is complete failure of growth of an organ during embryological development.

In many atrophic tissues a granular, brown pigment (*lipofuscin*), which is composed of degenerate lipid material in lysosomal granules, may accumulate within the shrunken cells. It is most readily identified in atrophic myocardial fibres of the hearts of elderly people, giving rise to the term *brown atrophy*.

Hyaline is a term used to describe replacement of tissue by an amorphous pink-staining material similar to basement membrane matrix. It is a common end result of atrophy or cell damage, being frequently accompanied by fibrosis.

Fig. 6.4 Atrophy (a) Normal testis (HP) **(b)** Atrophic testis (HP)

Atrophy of a tissue occurs by shrinkage of cells, with reduction of cytoplasmic components such as organelles and enzyme proteins, and also by loss of cells by apoptosis.

Micrograph (b) illustrates atrophy of the testis in a 94-year-old man. Compared with the normal testis in micrograph (a), the seminiferous tubules of the atrophic testis show almost no spermatogenic activity; however the Sertoli cells **Se** are still easily identified. The basement membranes of the tubules are thickened and pink-stained (*hyalinised*). The interstitial tissue shows an increased deposition of fibrous tissue **F**.

Change in cell differentiation

Under certain circumstances, cells may undergo a change in differentiation to another, mature, differentiated cell type (*metaplasia*). This is thought to be an adaptive response which produces cells better equipped to withstand an environmental change (usually pathological). For example, in the bronchi the specialised columnar respiratory epithelium may be replaced by squamous epithelium under the influence of chronic irritation by cigarette smoke (*squamous metaplasia*). Similarly, in response to environmental changes during the reproductive cycle, the normal columnar endocervical epithelium is replaced by a stratified squamous epithelium (Fig. 6.5(a)).

In the lower oesophagus, the normal stratified squamous epithelium may, in response to acid reflux from the stomach, be replaced by gastric (*gastric metaplasia*) or small intestinal (*intestinal metaplasia*) mucosa (Fig. 6.5(b)). In common with metaplasia at other sites, the basic alteration appears to occur in the stem cells of the tissue such that, rather than differentiating into a squamous cell, they mature instead into a mucus-producing columnar cell which is better able to protect itself from an acid environment. When the stimulus is removed, the stem cells may revert to producing differentiated cells of the original type.

Metaplasia most commonly occurs in epithelial tissues but may also be seen in mesodermal tissues; for example, areas of fibrous tissue exposed to chronic trauma may form bone (*osseous metaplasia*). Metaplasia may coexist with hyperplasia and, more importantly, *dysplasia* (see Ch. 7).

Fig. 6.5 **Metaplasia** **(a)** Squamous metaplasia of cervix (MP) **(b)** Gastric metaplasia of lower oesophagus (MP)

Squamous metaplasia of the cervix is so common it may almost be regarded as physiologically normal. During a woman's reproductive life, the shape of the cervix changes cyclically, exposing the endocervical columnar epithelium to the environment of the vagina. This *ectropion*, often incorrectly referred to as an 'erosion', is apparent macroscopically as an area of velvety pink epithelium at the external os.

In response to this change of environment, the endocervical epithelium is replaced by stratified squamous epithelium as shown in micrograph (a). At the top, the surface is covered by mature stratified squamous epithelium **S** which overlies endocervical glands lined by the normal mucus-secreting columnar epithelium **C**, which is also present at the surface at the bottom. In time, the metaplastic squamous epithelium may extend into the glands. Inflammation of the cervix accelerates this process.

In micrograph (b), the reverse change is occurring in the lower oesophagus where normal native squamous epithelium **S** at the top and bottom is being replaced by gastric-type columnar epithelium **C**, which is able to produce mucus to protect the epithelium from acid reflux. This is known as *Barrett's oesophagus*.

KEY TO FIGURES
C columnar epithelium   **F** fibrous tissue   **S** squamous epithelium   **Se** Sertoli cells

	Main features	**Examples**	**Figure**
Hypertrophy	Increase in size of existing cells	Myocardium in hypertension	6.2
		Skeletal muscle with exercise	
Hyperplasia	Increase in number of cells	Endometrium under oestrogenic stimulation	6.3
Atrophy	Reduction in cell size and/or number	Ischaemic atrophy of kidney	
		'Brown atrophy' of myocardium	
		Testicular atrophy	6.4
Metaplasia	Change of differentiation in a cell	Squamous metaplasia of cervix	6.6(a)
		Gastric/intestinal metaplasia of lower oesophagus	6.6(b)

Fig. 6.6 Chapter review

7 Dysplasia and neoplasia

Cellular atypia and dysplasia

In the previous chapter we considered cellular adaptations to a variety of stimuli resulting in alterations in their pattern of growth, whilst still achieving full differentiation/maturation. Occasionally, cells have an increased rate of division such that they do not have time to reach complete maturation (with full development of cytoplasmic specialisation) before another cycle of cell division supervenes. This leads to a population of cells which are structurally abnormal, having a high nuclear to cytoplasmic ratio with large nuclei containing abundant, dark-staining chromatin and prominent, occasionally multiple, nucleoli. These nuclear changes are associated with evidence of incomplete maturation of the cytoplasm, which may be lacking in the specialised structures normally seen in that cell type, such as mucin vacuoles or surface cilia. This is called *failure of differentiation* and the cells are said to show *atypia*.

Cellular atypia may be a consequence of rapid multiplication of cells as a response to cell destruction due to a persistent damaging stimulus. In this case, atypia is a result of the high turnover of cells attempting to regenerate damaged epithelium. When the damaging stimulus is removed, these abnormalities should revert to normal with full differentiation of the cells returning. However, sometimes the atypia is persistent and is not simply the result of regeneration. In these cases the population of atypical cells may eventually be the focus from which invasive cancer develops. This type of persistent cellular atypia is called *dysplasia* (Fig. 7.1). The problem for the pathologist is in distinguishing between cellular atypia, representing a reactive, regenerative response to tissue damage, and dysplasia, which is indicative of early pre-cancer. There is no simple answer.

Dysplasia often arises in metaplastic tissues and it is likely that the stimuli which cause dysplasia are also responsible for metaplastic change. Thus metaplastic epithelium in the cervix and Barrett's oesophagus is at risk of dysplasia and subsequent neoplasia. In dysplastic cells, molecular biological techniques have demonstrated some of the genetic abnormalities found in invasive neoplasms. Because of the sinister association of dysplasia with the subsequent development of neoplasia, treatment of dysplastic conditions is undertaken to minimise the risk of subsequent development of a malignancy. Recognition of dysplastic changes by cytological examination of cervical smears forms the basis of screening for cancer of the cervix (see Fig. 17.5).

MOLECULAR ORIGINS OF CANCER 1: INTRODUCTION

Our knowledge of the molecular origins of cancer grows at an exponential rate, such that any account of the field is destined only to be a snapshot in time of our understanding. Nevertheless, the basic principles underlying the cellular events in the development of cancers remain. In essence, all cancers arise as a consequence of non-lethal damage to DNA (i.e. the cell survives the damage). Typically, the genes damaged are in one of three classes regulating the cell cycle:

■ **Proto-oncogenes** which code for proteins regulating cell growth and differentiation. Activation by either genetic damage (*mutation*) or increased expression results in the development of *oncogenes*.

■ **Tumour suppressor genes** which code for proteins involved in regulating the cell cycle, repairing damaged DNA or, if the DNA is damaged beyond repair, inducing programmed cell death (*apoptosis*)

■ **MicroRNAs (miRNA)** which, unlike the other genes involved in the development of cancer, do not code for proteins, but are single-stranded RNA molecules with a role in regulation of the cell cycle.

Such non-lethal damage frees the cell from the normal restraints and controls on growth and maturation leading to uncontrolled, *clonal* expansion of the cell.

Fig. 7.1 **Dysplasia** **(a)** Normal cervix (HP) **(b)** Dysplasia in the cervix (HP) **(c)** Normal skin (HP) **(d)** Dysplastic skin (HP)

Dysplasia is a morphological feature characterised by increased cellular proliferation with incomplete maturation of cells. It occurs most commonly at the uterine cervix and in the skin.

Micrograph (a) illustrates normal stratified squamous epithelium from the cervix. Cellular proliferation is confined to the basal layer **B** where the cells are small, uniform and darkly stained. As the cells mature towards the surface, their cytoplasm expands and becomes more eosinophilic. Near the surface, the cells become progressively flattened. The ratio of nucleus to cytoplasm diminishes as the cells pass from the basal to surface layers.

In contrast, micrograph (b) shows dysplastic cervical epithelium where there is disruption of the normal orderly maturation sequence. Cells in all layers now exhibit larger than normal nuclei, some with prominent nucleoli. Mitotic figures **M** may be seen well above the basal layer. The nuclei of the cells are more variable in shape and size than normal

(*pleomorphism*) and the nuclear to cytoplasmic ratio is greater than normal. It is the presence of such surface cells with large nuclei which alerts the cytologist to underlying dysplasia in a cervical smear (see Fig. 17.5).

Micrographs (c) and (d) demonstrate similar features in normal and dysplastic skin, respectively. Note how the normal cellular stratification is disrupted in the dysplastic specimen by cells with large, darkly staining nuclei and multinucleated cells **N** extending into the middle strata. In addition, a disturbed pattern of maturation is reflected in the development of a thick layer of keratin which contains purple-stained nuclear remnants (*parakeratosis*). It is this keratin layer which becomes clinically evident as thickening and scaling of the skin. Mitotic figures **M** are also apparent above the basal layers.

Both of these conditions have a greatly increased tendency to develop into invasive carcinoma.

KEY TO FIGURES
B basal layer   **M** mitotic figures   **N** multinucleated cells

In a neoplasm, cellular proliferation and growth occur in the absence of any continuing external stimulus. Therefore, the term *neoplasia* (from the Greek for 'new growth') describes a state of autonomous cell division and the abnormal mass of cells that results is termed a *neoplasm*. The state of neoplastic growth contrasts with *hyperplasia*, discussed in the preceding chapter, where, although there is abnormal proliferation of cells, this ceases with removal of the causative stimulus.

As well as abnormal cell proliferation, neoplasia is characterised by abnormal maturation of cells. A feature of normal tissue growth is the maturation of constituent cells into a form adapted to a specific function. Such adaptation may involve the acquisition of specialised structures such as mucin vacuoles, neurosecretory granules, microvilli or cilia. This process of structural and functional maturation is termed *differentiation*. A fully mature cell of any particular cell line is said to be *highly differentiated*, whereas its primitive precursor cells are described as being *undifferentiated*. In any given tissue, the normal cells have a characteristic state of differentiation. In contrast, neoplastic cells exhibit variable states of differentiation and commonly fail to achieve a highly differentiated state. Neoplasms are divided clinically into two main groups (Fig. 7.3):

- *benign neoplasms* grow slowly and remain localised to the site of origin

- *malignant neoplasms* grow rapidly and may spread widely,

There is a broad correlation between histological appearances and biological behaviour, allowing prediction of the likely prognosis. In general, the cells of benign neoplasms are well differentiated. In the case of malignant neoplasms, there is a variable degree of differentiation. At one end of the spectrum the constituent cells may closely resemble the tissue of origin, in which case the tumour is described as being a *well differentiated malignancy*. Alternatively, the constituent cells may bear little resemblance to the tissue of origin, in which case the neoplasm is described as being *poorly differentiated*. At the extreme end of the spectrum, neoplasms which exhibit no evidence of differentiation are termed *anaplastic* and, in many cases, it may not be possible to identify the cell of origin on morphological grounds alone. Generally, the degree of differentiation of a neoplasm is related to its behaviour. A poorly differentiated neoplasm tends to be more invasive and more aggressive than a well-differentiated neoplasm.

BASIC PATHOLOGICAL PROCESSES ■ DYSPLASIA AND NEOPLASIA

MOLECULAR ORIGINS OF CANCER 2: CARCINOGENESIS

Transformation from normally functioning and growing cells to cancer, termed **carcinogenesis**, is regarded as a multistep process. For example, the consequences of a mutation in a single oncogene invariably would be overcome by otherwise normally functioning tumour suppressor genes. This concept is summarised by the **Knudson hypothesis** which states that multiple mutations, or 'hits', are required for cancer to develop. In the typical example of familial cancer syndromes, the first hit is in inheriting the abnormal DNA which is balanced by normally functioning genes until the second hit, where these too are damaged and cancer develops.

In addition to a growing list of inherited cancer syndromes a considerable number of environmental agents associated with the development of cancer are now recognised including chemical agents, radiation and viruses. Examples are given below.

Inherited cancer syndromes		Chemical agents		Viruses	
Gene	**Association**	**Agent**	**Association**	**Virus**	**Association**
NF1, NF2	Neurofibromatosis types 1 and 2	Asbestos	Mesothelioma, lung, GI tract	HPV	Cervical carcinoma
APC	Familial adenomatous polyposis, colon cancer	Nitrosamines	Gastric carcinoma	EBV	Burkitt, Hodgkin lymphomas
BRCA1/ BRCA2	Breast and ovarian cancers	Benzene	Leukaemia, Hodgkin lymphoma	Hep B/C	Hepatocellular carcinoma
RB	Retinoblastoma	Nickel	Lung cancer	HHV8	Kaposi's sarcoma

The term *carcinoma in situ* is used when an epithelial tissue shows the cytological and histological features of carcinoma (architectural and cytological abnormalities such as cell crowding, pleomorphism, increased and abnormal mitotic activity), but there is no evidence that the basement membrane bounding the abnormal epithelial tissue has been breached and there is no encroachment of atypical cells into the underlying stroma. The process whereby tumour cells breach the basement membrane and extend into the surrounding tissues is described as *invasion*. Thus, with carcinoma in situ the epithelial cells show the cytological, but not the behavioural, characteristics of malignancy. However, many forms of carcinoma in situ will become invasive if left untreated.

Certain benign epithelial tumours may progress to form an invasive malignant tumour by development and selective persistence of mutations in key oncogenes. A sequence from benign neoplasm through increasing dysplasia to carcinoma in situ and on to invasive carcinoma is well recognised in certain sites (e.g. the colon).

Carcinoma in situ occurs particularly in skin (see Fig. 21.14), cervix (cervical intraepithelial neoplasia; see Fig. 17.6), vulva (vulval intraepithelial neoplasia, VIN) and other sites. It also occurs in solid glandular organs, most notably the breast (ductal and lobular carcinoma in situ; see Fig. 18.9).

Fig. 7.2 Carcinoma in situ

Diagram (a) shows the regular architecture of a normal stratified squamous epithelium. The layered epithelium is formed by mitotic replication of the basal layer, producing layers of regular cells which differentiate and flatten as they approach the surface (stratification). The cells are regular in shape and size, as are the nuclei, and mitotic activity is confined to the basal layer.

Diagram (b) shows an epithelium in which there is dysplasia in the lower layers. The cells and their nuclei are irregular in shape and size and the nuclei occupy more of the cell. Mitoses are present in layers other than the basal layer. The cells still differentiate and eventually mature near the surface.

Diagram (c) shows fully developed carcinoma in situ. The dysplastic epithelial cells now occupy the full thickness of the epithelium and stratification and differentiation are largely lost. Mitoses can be present

in any of the layers, even in surface cells. Although all the cells in this epithelium show cytological characteristics of malignancy (cellular and nuclear pleomorphism, high nuclear to cytoplasmic ratio, nuclear hyperchromasia and increased abnormal mitotic activity), the epithelial cells as yet show no tendency to invade across the basement membrane into the stroma.

The changes shown in (b) are regarded as an early stage in the development of carcinoma in situ. In certain locations, this is acknowledged by applying a numerical value. Hence, in the squamous epithelium of the uterine cervix, the changes in (c) would be called CIN 3 (cervical intra-epithelial neoplasia 3), whereas those in (b) would be called CIN 2. A similar scheme exists in the nomenclature of dysplastic/in situ neoplastic changes in the vulva (VIN) and vagina (VAIN).

As mentioned before, the property whereby a malignant tumour can grow into the surrounding tissue is termed invasion. A further property of malignant neoplasms is distant spread of neoplastic cells away from the main neoplasm (termed the *primary tumour*) to form subpopulations of neoplastic cells which are not in continuity with the primary tumour. The property of distant spread of a tumour is termed *metastasis*; the *secondary tumours* which result are often termed *metastases*.

In general terms, a benign tumour will behave in a relatively innocuous manner and a malignant tumour will have deleterious effects, often leading to death. There are, however, exceptions to these generalisations and factors other than the biological growth pattern of a tumour may be important in influencing the outcome. Of these, the most notable is the location of the tumour. For example, a benign tumour of the brain stem may lead to rapid death, whereas a malignant tumour of the skin may progress slowly over many years.

Systemic symptoms such as weight loss, loss of appetite, fever and general malaise frequently accompany malignant tumours. In most cases, the pathophysiology is poorly understood, but includes effects of secreted cytokines such as *tumour necrosis factor*. Some tumours, benign and malignant, retain the function of their organ of origin. If this happens to be an endocrine function, then the tumour may exert harmful effects by secretion of excess hormone. Other tumours secrete hormones not usually secreted by that tissue, for example the secretion of parathyroid hormone by lung carcinomas. This is known as *ectopic hormone secretion* and the clinical manifestations are described as *paraneoplastic syndromes* (see below).

Fig. 7.3 Summary of features of neoplasms

		Benign	Malignant
Behaviour		Expansile growth only; grows locally	Expansile and invasive growth; may mestastasise
		Often encapsulated	Not encapsulated
Histology		Resembles cell of origin (well differentiated)	May show failure of cellular differentiation
		Few mitoses	Many mitoses, some of which are abnormal forms
		Normal or slight increase in ratio of nucleus to cytoplasm	High nuclear to cytoplasmic ratio
		Cells are uniform throughout the tumour	Cells vary in shape and size (cellular pleomorphism) and/or nuclei vary in shape and size (nuclear pleomorphism)

PARANEOPLASTIC SYNDROMES

In addition to direct, local invasion and metastatic spread, cancers may give rise to distant symptoms and/or signs through two main mechanisms:

■ **an immune response** to the malignancy producing antibodies to tumour cells which cross-react with normal cells. In many cases the antibodies may target normal neurons producing well-characterised, complex neurological presentations.

■ **release of cytokines/ hormones** by malignant cells, such as ectopic adrenocorticotrophic hormone (ACTH; see Ch. 20) which may be released by a variety of cancers, including pulmonary carcinomas.

The associated clinical syndromes may precede, follow or present at the same time as the primary malignancy.

Histological assessment of neoplasms

Histological assessment of a tumour provides a useful guide to its behaviour, i.e. whether the tumour is benign or malignant, and provides a rational basis for treatment. Histological assessment should establish the following features:

■ **The type of tumour**. This is based on the presumed tissue of origin and/or differentiation of the tumour.

■ **The degree of differentiation**. This is known as *grading* and takes into account some or all of the following features:

  – the similarity of the tumour to the supposed tissue of origin both architecturally and cytologically (*differentiation*)

  – the degree of variability of cellular shape and size (*pleomorphism*)

  – the proportion of mitotic figures (dividing cells).

■ **The extent of spread of tumour (*staging*)** is partly assessed histologically, particularly:

  – size of the primary tumour

  – histological assessment of local, vascular, lymphatic and perineural invasion

  – the presence of metastatic tumour deposits, for example in lymph nodes and bones.

■ **The presence or absence of other prognostic factors**. For instance, the presence of oestrogen receptors in breast carcinoma cells confers an improved prognosis. The expression of certain oncogenes is increasingly being related to prognosis in some tumours.

Tumour nomenclature and classification

The classification and nomenclature of neoplasms have developed from gross morphological, histological and behavioural observation. Ideally, the name given to a tumour should convey information about the cell of origin and the likely behaviour (either benign or malignant). While this is so for the majority of tumours of epithelial and connective tissues, there are many tumours which are given eponymous or semi-descriptive names out of either poor understanding of pathogenesis or long-established tradition. Some tumours have several different names which are synonymous, but derive from different classifications.

Tumours of epithelial origin

■ Benign neoplasms of surface epithelia, for example skin, are termed *papillomas*. This term is preceded by the cell of origin, for example squamous papilloma of skin, squamous papilloma of larynx.

■ Benign neoplasms of both solid and surface glandular epithelia are termed *adenomas*. This is prefixed by the tissue of origin, for example thyroid adenoma, salivary gland adenoma. Frequently, a benign tumour of surface glandular epithelium (almost always in the large bowel) assumes a papillary growth pattern when it is termed a *villous adenoma*.

■ A malignant tumour of any epithelial origin is termed a *carcinoma*. Tumours of glandular epithelium (including that lining the gut) are termed *adenocarcinomas*. Tumours of other epithelia are preceded by the cell type of origin, for example *squamous cell carcinoma*, *transitional cell carcinoma*. To classify a carcinoma further, the tissue of origin is added, for example adenocarcinoma of prostate, adenocarcinoma of breast, squamous cell carcinoma of larynx.

The nomenclature of epithelial tumours is summarised in Figure 7.4.

Fig. 7.4 Nomenclature of epithelial tumours

Tissue of origin	Benign	Malignant
Surface epithelium	Papilloma/adenoma	Carcinoma
Examples:		
Squamous	Squamous cell papilloma	Squamous cell carcinoma
Glandular (columnar)	Adenoma (villous or tubular)	Adenocarcinoma
Transitional	Transitional cell papilloma	Transitional cell carcinoma
Solid glandular epithelium	Adenoma	Adenocarcinoma
Examples:		
Thyroid	Thyroid adenoma	Thyroid adenocarcinoma
Kidney	Renal adenoma	Renal cell carcinoma
Liver	Hepatic adenoma	Hepatocellular carcinoma

Tumours of connective tissue origin

In connective tissues, there is a simpler and more descriptive classification of neoplasms. First, the tissue of origin is designated, with the addition of the suffix *-oma* for a benign tumour or *-sarcoma* for a malignant tumour. As an example, a benign tumour of adipose tissue is termed a lipoma, whilst a malignant tumour of the same origin is termed a liposarcoma. A summary of other connective tissue tumours is shown in Figure 7.5.

Fig. 7.5 Nomenclature of connective tissue tumours

Tissue of origin	Benign	Malignant
Fibrous tissue	Fibroma	Fibrosarcoma
Bone	Osteoma	Osteosarcoma
Cartilage	Chondroma	Chondrosarcoma
Adipose tissue	Lipoma	Liposarcoma
Smooth muscle	Leiomyoma	Leiomyosarcoma
Skeletal muscle	Rhabdomyoma	Rhabdomyosarcoma
Blood vessel	Haemangioma	Haemangiosarcoma

Nomenclature of other tumours

There are other neoplasms which do not fit into either the epithelial or the connective tissue category described above and these are grouped according to their tissue of origin. The main categories are as follows:

- **Melanoma**: tumours of melanocytes (Fig. 7.11 and Ch. 21)

- **Lymphomas**: tumours of solid lymphoid tissue (Fig. 7.10 and Ch. 16)

- **Leukaemias**: tumours derived from haemopoietic elements which circulate in the blood and only rarely form tumour masses (Ch. 16)

- **Gliomas**: tumours derived from the non-neural support tissues of the brain (Ch. 23)

- **Germ cell tumours**: tumours derived from germ cells in the gonads (Fig. 7.12, Ch. 17 and Ch. 19)

- **Neuroendocrine tumours**: tumours derived from cells of the neuroendocrine system. Examples include phaeochromocytoma (Fig. 20.11), carcinoid tumour (Fig. 13.13) and medullary carcinoma (Fig. 5.8).

Finally, there is a group of tumour-like lesions known as **hamartomas** which represent non-neoplastic overgrowths of tissues indigenous to the site of their occurrence. These are thought to be developmental abnormalities. A common example is the 'port-wine stain' of the skin composed of blood vessels and known as a **haemangioma**. An example of a haemangioma in the liver is shown in Figure 11.9.

Fig. 7.6 **Squamous cell carcinoma** **(a)** Well differentiated (HP) **(b)** Poorly differentiated (HP)

Squamous cell carcinomas may arise in any site of native stratified squamous epithelium, for example skin, oesophagus or tongue. They may also arise in stratified squamous epithelium which has formed by the process of metaplasia, for example in bronchus or urinary bladder.

The degree of differentiation varies widely. Well-differentiated tumours, as seen in micrograph (a), have cytological features similar to the prickle cell layer of normal stratified squamous epithelium. The cells are large and slightly fusiform in shape and the nuclei exhibit a moderate degree of pleomorphism. Mitotic figures are infrequent. The cells are commonly arranged in broad sheets and large nests **N**. At very high magnification, intercellular bridges (typical of normal prickle cells) may be visible. The most characteristic feature of well-differentiated squamous carcinomas is the formation of keratin, which may be seen within individual cells (known as *dyskeratosis* **D**), but which more often forms lamellated, pink-stained masses known as *keratin pearls* **KP**.

In contrast, poorly differentiated squamous carcinomas, as in micrograph (b), lose most of their resemblance to normal prickle cells and have a high nuclear to cytoplasmic ratio. Keratin pearl formation is not seen, although individual dyskeratotic cells **D** may be present. In the most anaplastic squamous carcinomas, the only evidence of the cell of origin may be intercellular bridges, which are only visible at high magnification after a careful search, or the detection of certain types of cytokeratin by immunocytochemistry.

Fig. 7.7 Transitional cell (urothelial) carcinoma (a) Well differentiated (papillary) (LP) (b) Poorly differentiated (HP)

These tumours arise almost exclusively from native transitional epithelium in the urinary tract.

Well-differentiated lesions usually adopt a papillary growth pattern (see Fig. 15.21) and the cytological features may be almost indistinguishable from those of normal transitional epithelium. Micrograph (a) shows a typical papillary tumour resembling normal urothelium, but with slight nuclear pleomorphism and minimal evidence of mitotic activity.

As transitional cell carcinomas become less differentiated, the growth pattern becomes more solid and nuclear pleomorphism becomes more marked. In anaplastic tumours, it may not be possible to determine the tissue of origin except by knowing that the tumour has arisen in the urinary tract. Micrograph (b) shows a poorly differentiated solid tumour from the bladder wall. Note the nests of highly pleomorphic tumour cells T invading between bundles of smooth muscle M.

BASIC PATHOLOGICAL PROCESSES ■ DYSPLASIA AND NEOPLASIA

KEY TO FIGURES
D dyskeratotic cells   **KP** keratin pearl   **M** smooth muscle   **N** cell nest   **T** tumour cell

MOLECULAR ORIGINS OF CANCER 3: MORE DETAIL ON ONCOGENES

As noted above, **oncogenes** encode proteins controlling proliferation, programmed cell death (*apoptosis*) or both. Activation of these genes, with resultant abnormal production of their protein products (**oncoproteins**), can take place in a number of ways:

■ **Point mutation**: resulting in a permanently active gene, such as in the **RAS oncogene**, which encodes a signal transduction protein. Mutations in this gene are very common, occurring in around 20% of all human cancers.

■ **Translocation**: This is a common molecular abnormality in cancer cells. The result is that either the oncogene comes to lie adjacent to a gene which is constitutively expressed, or relocation of the gene results in its fusion with a second gene, so producing a new protein with increased activity. The former is a common event in haematological malignancies such as in **Burkitt lymphoma**, where the **c-Myc** oncogene on chromosome 8 becomes relocated adjacent to the **immunoglobulin heavy chain gene** on chromosome 14, which is constitutively expressed in mature B lymphocytes. In 95% of cases of **chronic myeloid leukaemia**, translocation results in the **ABL gene** on chromosome 9 fusing with the **BCR gene** on chromosome 22, the outcome being the '**BCR-ABL**' gene, also known as the **Philadelphia chromosome**. The protein product of this fused gene is constitutively active and has a role in activating proteins controlling the cell cycle.

■ **Amplification**: Here, multiple copies of a gene are formed, resulting in increased production of the oncoprotein. This is of particular note in tumour progression and hence correlates with poor prognosis. One such example is the **ERBB2 (HER2/neu**; human epidermal growth factor receptor 2) gene in breast carcinoma, where amplification of the gene correlates with poorer prognosis.

> **Fig. 7.8** **Colonic adenocarcinomas (*illustrations opposite*) (a)** Well differentiated (MP) **(b)** Poorly differentiated (HP) **(c)** Signet ring (HP) **(d)** Mucinous (MP)

Carcinomas which derive from surface glandular epithelium, such as colon and stomach, tend to exhibit a glandular pattern of growth and are known as *adenocarcinomas*. The same is true of carcinomas arising in solid glandular tissues, such as kidney, breast and prostate, and of tumours of the liver (which in embryological terms develops as an outgrowth of primitive gut epithelium).

Micrograph (a) illustrates a typical well differentiated colonic adenocarcinoma. Although it is a carcinoma, it still exhibits a glandular pattern **G** reminiscent of normal colon. The cell nuclei are, however, hyperchromatic, with a high nuclear to cytoplasmic ratio and numerous mitoses **M** are seen. Unlike the normal colon, the glandular pattern is irregular and there is little evidence of mucin secretion.

Poorly differentiated adenocarcinomas, as shown in micrograph (b), display a minimal tendency to form a glandular pattern and the cells are extremely pleomorphic. The only evidence of glandular origin is the presence of occasional cells with secretory vacuoles **V** containing mucin.

Two other patterns of adenocarcinoma, seen much more commonly in other tissues than in colon, are *signet ring cell* and *mucinous* forms. In signet ring cell carcinoma, as shown in micrograph (c), the tendency to produce mucin-filled cytoplasmic vacuoles is greatly exaggerated such that the majority of cells have their nuclei **N** pushed to one side by a mucin-filled vacuole **V**. This pattern is much more common in the stomach (see Fig. 13.12) than in the colon, although focal areas of this pattern may be seen in adenocarcinomas from a wide variety of tissues. In contrast, in a mucinous carcinoma, as shown in micrograph (d), excessive secretion of mucin **Mu** results in so-called 'mucin lakes' in which small nests of tumour cells **T** are found. This pattern of adenocarcinoma is not uncommon in the colon and is also well recognised in the breast (see Fig. 18.10).

KEY TO FIGURES
G glandular pattern   **M** mitoses   **Mu** mucin   **N** nucleus   **T** nests of tumour cells   **V** mucin vacuoles

Fig. 7.8 **Colonic adenocarcinomas** (*caption opposite*)

Fig. 7.9 **Sarcomas** **(a)** Leiomyosarcoma (HP) **(b)** Ewing's sarcoma (HP)

Sarcomas are malignant tumours derived from connective tissues including adipose tissue, bone, cartilage and smooth muscle. Many sarcomas resemble the tissue of origin either cytologically, structurally or by producing characteristic extracellular materials such as collagen and ground substance. For example, liposarcomas have intracellular lipid vacuoles and chondrosarcomas produce cartilaginous ground substance.

Micrograph (a) shows an example of a uterine *leiomyosarcoma*, a sarcoma derived from smooth muscle. The tumour cells are spindle-shaped and resemble normal smooth muscle cells. However, they have large pleomorphic nuclei with evident mitoses including an abnormal, ring-form mitotic figure **MF**.

Micrograph (b) shows a typical *Ewing's sarcoma*. This malignant tumour typically arises in the medullary cavity of long or flat bones in children, though the cell of origin is unknown. As here, the tumours consist of sheets of small round cells with a glycogen-rich cytoplasm (clear on standard H&E staining). Given the appearance of these tumours in H&E they are often described, with other primitive, poorly differentiated tumours, as *small round blue cell tumours*. Ewing's tumours are aggressive and may metastasise early. Treatment with combinations of surgery, chemotherapy and radiotherapy can improve the outcome.

Fig. 7.10 **Lymphoma** (HP)

Lymphomas are solid tumours derived from cells of the lymphoid system. The majority arise in lymphoid organs such as lymph nodes, spleen and bone marrow, but may spread to other tissues, particularly the skin, liver and CNS. Primary lymphomas may also arise at extranodal sites, often in tissues where a longstanding chronic inflammatory or autoimmune response is present such as the small intestine in coeliac disease or the thyroid in Hashimoto's thyroiditis.

Histologically, lymphomas consist of sheets of lymphoid cells arranged either diffusely or in a follicular pattern. Lymphomas are discussed in detail in Chapter 16.

This micrograph illustrates a primary lymphoma of the brain composed of large lymphoid cells arranged around a central vessel **V**. Atypical mitotic figures **MF** are readily identified. Such tumours may have a rapidly progressive clinical course.

Fig. 7.11 Melanoma (HP)

Melanomas are malignant tumours of melanocytes, most often arising in sun-exposed skin, though examples arising in sites not traditionally associated with sun exposure do occur, such as bowel and dura. Clinically, melanomas appear as irregular, variably pigmented, raised or flat lesions which may be prone to bleeding.

In the example shown here the tumour cells are large, irregularly shaped and have abundant cytoplasmic melanin pigment. Unfortunately, this 'typical' appearance may not always be apparent, particularly in metastatic tumour, for example in a lymph node specimen where the primary may be unknown. For this reason melanomas are often regarded as the classical 'mimic metastases', in that they can assume the morphological features of almost any other malignancy. Under such circumstances a careful and thorough search for melanin pigment, combined with the judicious use of immunocytochemistry stains, can be helpful in achieving a diagnosis.

Fig. 7.12 Teratoma (MP)

Teratomas are tumours derived from germ cells and most commonly arise in the testis or ovary. The tumours contain neoplastic tissues derived from all of the three germ cell layers, i.e. endoderm, mesoderm and ectoderm (including neuroectoderm), and thus can contain tissues as diverse as skin, teeth, thyroid, brain and muscle. The tumours range from benign to highly malignant.

A benign teratoma of the ovary is shown in this micrograph. Epidermis-type epithelium, including hair follicles H and sebaceous glands G, has formed a cystic space C. Connective tissue elements including fat F are also seen. Neural tissue N is present in the form of well-differentiated clusters of ganglion cells. Teratomas arising in the ovary are usually benign, whereas those in the testis are usually malignant and contain more primitive, immature tissue such as primitive mesenchyme.

KEY TO FIGURES
C cystic space   F fat   G sebaceous glands   H hair follicles   MF abnormal mitotic figure   N Neural tissue
V vessel

Fig. 7.13 **Degrees of tumour differentiation: colon** **(a)** Normal mucosa (HP) **(b)** Benign neoplasm (HP) **(c)** Well differentiated malignant neoplasm (HP) **(d)** Poorly differentiated neoplasm (HP)

This series of micrographs demonstrates the variable degree of differentiation which may be seen in tumours arising from the same cell of origin.

Note the similarity between normal colonic mucosa in micrograph (a) and a benign neoplasm (*tubular adenoma*) in micrograph (b). In both cases, the epithelial cells **E** are tall, columnar and regular in form. The main points of difference are that the cells of the benign neoplasm contain less mucin **Mu** and their nuclei are larger and more crowded.

The cells of the well differentiated malignant neoplasm shown in micrograph (c) are also tall and columnar, but the nuclei are more irregular in shape and arrangement with no mucin secretion, most of each cell being occupied by the nucleus. The nuclei are crowded and are no longer arranged along the basal parts of the cells. The nucleoli are also large and irregular in size and shape. In contrast, in the poorly differentiated colonic neoplasm in micrograph (d), the cells bear little resemblance to the tissue of origin and are arranged haphazardly. The cells show a great variability in size and nuclear shape, mitoses **M** are seen and there is little evidence of mucin secretion.

Modes of spread of malignant neoplasms

There are four main modes of tumour spread:

■ **Local invasion.** Invasive tumours tend to spread into surrounding tissues by the most direct route. Examples include carcinoma of the breast invading overlying skin or deeply into underlying muscle and carcinoma of the cervix invading rectum or bladder.

■ **Lymphatic spread.** Tumours may spread via lymphatic vessels draining the site of the primary tumour. Neoplastic cells are conducted to local lymph nodes where they may form secondary tumours, e.g. breast cancer spreading to lymph nodes in the axilla or carcinoma of the tongue spreading to lymph nodes in the neck.

■ **Vascular spread.** Tumours can spread via the veins draining the primary site. Gut tumours tend to spread via the portal vein to the liver where secondary tumours are very common. In the systemic circulation, neoplastic cells may be trapped in the lung to form pulmonary metastases.

■ **Transcoelomic spread.** Certain tumours can spread directly across coelomic spaces, for example across the peritoneal or pleural cavities. Carcinoma of the ovary may spread transcoelomically to produce large numbers of metastatic deposits on the peritoneal surfaces.

Fig. 7.14 Growth characteristics of surface neoplasms: colon (a) Benign neoplasm: villous adenoma (LP) **(b)** Malignant neoplasm: adenocarcinoma (LP)

Benign neoplasms of surface epithelia usually grow in the form of warty, papillary or nodular outgrowths and show no tendency to infiltrate downward into the submucosa. Micrograph (a) shows one form of benign colonic neoplasm. This *villous adenoma* has grown into the lumen in the form of papillary fronds **F** with a stromal core covered by moderately dysplastic epithelial cells. The underlying muscularis mucosae **MM** is intact and there is no downward tumour spread.

Malignant neoplasms not only form a mass in the lumen, but also spread across the epithelial basement membrane into subepithelial tissues. In micrograph (b) of a colonic *adenocarcinoma*, the tumour cells have grown in complex, abnormal gland formations **G** within the mucosa. Malignant glands are also seen invading into the submucosa **SM**, having breached the muscularis mucosae **MM**, and have spread beneath the adjacent normal mucosa **Muc**. Even at low power, it is obvious that the malignant cells are disorganised, crowded together and less differentiated than are the cells of the benign adenoma. Note the nuclear hyperchromasia of both benign and malignant lesions in comparison to the normal.

BASIC PATHOLOGICAL PROCESSES ■ DYSPLASIA AND NEOPLASIA

79

KEY TO FIGURES

E epithelial cells   **F** papillary fronds   **G** abnormal glands   **M** mitotic figure   **MM** muscularis mucosae
Mu mucin   **Muc** normal mucosa   **SM** submucosa

Fig. 7.15 **Local invasion** **(a)** Benign neoplasm of myometrium (LP) **(b)** Margin of lesion in (a) (MP) **(c)** Malignant neoplasm of breast (LP) **(d)** Margin of lesion in (c) (MP)

These micrographs compare the local growth patterns of benign and malignant neoplasms within solid organs. Micrograph (a) shows a benign neoplasm of the uterine smooth muscle, a *leiomyoma* L, surrounded by normal myometrium M. The tumour margin is shown at higher magnification in micrograph (b). Note that the neoplasm is well circumscribed and shows no evidence of local invasion. This neoplasm has expanded symmetrically and compressed the supporting stroma of the myometrium to form a *pseudocapsule* C.

Micrograph (c) illustrates a breast carcinoma. Note the neoplasm has an irregular outline with tongues of neoplastic cells invading the fatty tissue **Fa** and collagenous stroma **St** of the breast. There is no tendency to form a capsule. The ill-defined tumour margin is illustrated in micrograph (d) in which hyperchromatic malignant cells can be seen infiltrating the surrounding adipose tissue.

KEY TO FIGURES
C pseudocapsule   **Fa** fatty tissue   **L** leiomyoma   **Ly** lymphatic   **M** myometrium   **MS** medullary sinus
S subcapsular sinus   **St** stroma   **T** tumour cells

Fig. 7.16 **Lymphatic spread** **(a)** Tumour in lymphatic vessel (HP) **(b)** Metastasis in a lymph node (MP)

Malignant tumours may invade through the walls of lymphatics and spread either by growth of solid cores along the lumina or by fragments breaking off the intralymphatic tumour mass to form emboli, which pass to regional lymph nodes.

Micrograph (a) illustrates a large, valved lymphatic **Ly** containing an embolic clump of malignant tumour cells **T** en route to a lymph node. Tumour spread via lymphatics to regional lymph nodes is a very common mode of spread for carcinomas.

Micrograph (b) shows a lymph node draining a primary breast carcinoma. Tumour cells, which arrive via afferent lymphatics, lodge and proliferate in the subcapsular sinus **S**. From here, the malignant cells may then infiltrate down the medullary sinuses **MS** and go on to form solid masses in the parenchyma of the node (not illustrated here).

Fig. 7.17 **Haematogenous spread of malignant neoplasms** **(a)** Malignant colonic neoplasm (MP)
(b) Malignant breast neoplasm (MP)

The thin-walled vessels of the venous system provide a ready means of spread for many types of malignant tumour. In contrast, invasion of arterial vessels is rare and tends to result in haemorrhage or infarction, rather than tumour spread. Malignant cells may grow along veins in solid cores from which fragments may break off to form tumour emboli, which tend to lodge in the first capillary bed encountered. The lungs and liver are frequent sites of metastatic deposition. From here, tumour cells may pass through the heart to the arterial system and spread throughout the body. Hence, brain and bone marrow are other common sites for metastatic deposits.

Micrograph (a) shows a large serosal vein from a colon in which there was an extensive malignant neoplasm. A solid mass of tumour is growing along the vessel lumen. The site of invasion of the vessel wall was proximal to this section and, therefore, cannot be seen.

Venous invasion by carcinoma of the breast is seen in micrograph (b). Solid masses of tumour cells **T** infiltrate the fatty tissue of the breast. Tumour emboli are seen within three small venules **V** and also two small lymphatics **L**, adjacent to a nerve **N**. The arterioles **A** close by are not affected. Vascular and lymphatic invasion by tumour is an important factor in the prognosis of many types of tumour.

Fig. 7.18 **Transcoelomic spread of malignant neoplasms** (HP)

Malignant tumours may spread into coelomic spaces by direct extension from adjacent organs. Tumour emboli may then break free from the tumour to float in the small amount of fluid normally present in these spaces and spread to other areas of the mesothelial surface. Thus, breast and lung tumours commonly involve the pleural space. Ovarian and gastric tumours are usually responsible for peritoneal involvement.

In response to tumour growth in these serous spaces, there is commonly an inflammatory response in the lining with accumulation of protein-rich fluid and inflammatory cells, proliferation of mesothelial cells and often haemorrhage to form a *malignant pleural effusion* or *malignant ascites*.

This example is a smear of ascitic fluid from a patient with metastatic breast carcinoma. The tumour had spread through the pleural space and reached the peritoneum, probably via the diaphragm. Aspiration of the fluid serves to relieve symptoms and to confirm the diagnosis cytologically (*diagnostic paracentesis*). Tumour cells **T** are present as single cells and small aggregates. They are pleomorphic with large, hyperchromatic nuclei and prominent nucleoli. Reactive mesothelial cells **Me** are also present and, in contrast to the tumour cells, are smaller with bland nuclear features. In this example, inflammatory cells are sparse.

Fig. 7.19 **Metastatic tumour deposits in solid organs** **(a)** Liver (MP) **(b)** Lung (LP)

As noted above, metastatic deposits of tumour are frequently encountered in liver, lung, bone marrow and brain as a result of haematogenous spread. Other tissues are less common sites for deposition of metastatic tumour (e.g. heart and skeletal muscle). However, metastases can occur in any tissue or organ. Certain types of tumour have characteristic patterns of spread. For example, malignant tumours of the prostate gland have a propensity to spread to bone. It is thought that the malignant cells and the target organ must express mutually compatible receptors and cell-surface adhesion molecules which facilitate cellular anchorage and subsequent growth.

Micrographs (a) and (b) show examples of hepatic and pulmonary blood-borne metastases **M**,

respectively. Hepatic metastases often arise from organs drained by the portal system; the lesion in micrograph (a) is from a moderately differentiated adenocarcinoma of the colon. Lung metastases, on the other hand, arise from tumour emboli from the systemic venous circulation, and micrograph (b) is an example of secondary spread from a primary breast carcinoma. Note that both tumours have induced a stromal reaction in the form of fibrous connective tissue containing blood vessels and inflammatory cells. Without this ability to induce the formation of a vascular supply (***angiogenesis***), the growth of metastases would not be possible.

Fig. 7.20 **Perineural spread** (HP)

Spread along the course of nerve bundles is a common feature of some tumours, such as adenocarcinoma of the prostate, but may also be seen in other tumour types. This micrograph shows perineural invasion by a well-differentiated prostatic adenocarcinoma. Tumour cells **T** in a glandular conformation are seen infiltrating around and between bundles of nerve fibres **N**.

KEY TO FIGURES
A arteriole   **L** lymphatic   **M** metastases   **Me** mesothelial cells   **N** nerve fibres   **T** tumour cells   **V** venule

Staging of malignant tumours

The extent of local, regional and distant tumour spread is an important determinant of tumour management and prognosis. Several systems have been devised for defining these characteristics in a standardised fashion; this is known as *staging* of a tumour. The *TNM system* is the most widely used method and involves scoring the extent of local Tumour spread, regional lymph Node involvement and the presence of distant Metastases. Despite advances in diagnostic techniques, the stage of a tumour is still a very good indicator of likely prognosis. Tumour stage assessment is also important in planning therapy. Tumours at an advanced stage (extensive spread) may require aggressive treatment, while early-stage tumours (localised) can be treatable by more conservative measures such as surgical excision alone. Staging is usually performed by a combination of histopathology, radiology and clinical assessments.

By way of example, the TNM method for renal cancer staging is illustrated in Figure 7.21.

Fig. 7.21 TNM staging of renal carcinoma

T0	No evidence of primary tumour in kidney	N0	No nodes involved	M0	No distant metastases
T1	Tumour no greater than 7 cm diameter and within renal capsule	N1	Spread to one node	M1	Distant metastases
T2	Tumour greater than 7 cm diameter, but within renal capsule	N2	Spread to more than one node		
T3	Spread to local tissues				
T4	Spread beyond local tissues				

MOLECULAR ORIGINS OF CANCER 4: THERAPY TARGETED AT ONCOGENES

Knowledge of the molecular origins of cancer, with an awareness of the genes and their protein products which drive cancerous cells, has provided researchers with targets for intervention in cancer treatment. This offers clinicians the opportunity to deliver treatment to patients based on the particular molecular signature of their specific tumour, so-called *individualised therapy*. Thus, molecular assessment of many cancers has become part of the routine pathology work-up in a growing number of cancers. Throughout this book many examples of diagnostic molecular pathology providing insight into tumour behaviour and/or directing therapy are given. Here we discuss the principles of these therapies using two common examples.

Those protein products which are expressed on the cell surface, in theory, provide a target for attack by appropriately designed monoclonal antibodies. This principle forms the basis of many targeted therapies in cancer. We have already mentioned the ERBB2 (HER2/neu; human epidermal growth factor receptor 2) gene in breast carcinoma which, when amplified, is associated with a poorer prognosis. This protein has also provided an opportunity for development of targeted therapy through production of a monoclonal antibody to HER2/neu (trastuzamab; trade name *Herceptin*) which has proved successful in treatment of some patients with breast carcinoma, specifically those tumours shown to over-express the HER2/neu receptor. Thus, assessment of 'HER2 status' is now commonplace in the evaluation of breast carcinoma.

In addition to monoclonal antibodies targeting cancer-associated proteins, a number of small molecules have been developed which can interfere with the function of oncoproteins. *Tyrosine kinases* are enzymes which phosphorylate proteins and have key roles in cell growth and differentiation (among other functions). One example where tyrosine kinase activity is increased in cancers is in relation to the BCR-ABL gene in chronic myelogenous leukaemia (CML) where the protein product of the gene has tyrosine kinase activity. To counter this, inhibitors of tyrosine kinase have been developed and are now used in routine practice with considerable success, not only in treatment of CML, but also in other cancers where tyrosine kinase activity is implicated in the development of the tumour such as gastrointestinal stromal tumours.

Fig. 7.22 **Chapter review**

	Definition/main features	Examples	Figure
Dysplasia	Increased cell proliferation with failure of maturation	Uterine cervix	7.1
		Skin	7.1
Carcinoma in situ	Features of carcinoma in an epithelium, but no invasion		7.2
		Uterine cervix	17.6
		Skin	21.14
		Breast	18.9
Epithelial tumours	Benign tumours either *papillomas* or *adenomas*		7.4
	Malignant tumours termed *carcinomas*		7.4
		Squamous cell carcinoma	7.6
		Transitional cell carcinoma	7.7
		Colonic adenocarcinoma	7.8
Connective tissue tumours	Benign tumours named after tissue of origin with suffix *-oma*		7.5
	Malignant tumours named after tissue of origin with suffix *-sarcoma*		7.5
		Leiomyosarcoma	7.9
Lymphoma	Solid tumours derived from cells of lymphoreticular system	Primary CNS lymphoma	7.10
Melanoma	Tumour derived from melanocytes		7.11
Teratoma	Tumour derived from germ cells		7.12
Invasion	Spread of tumour to surrounding tissues	Breast carcinoma	7.14
		Colonic adenocarcinoma	7.15
		Perineural invasion	7.20
Metastasis	Distant spread of tumour by one of several mechanisms	Lymphatic spread	7.16
		Haematogenous	7.17
		Transcoelomic	7.18

8 Atherosclerosis

Introduction

The walls of arterial vessels are composed of smooth muscle, elastin and collagen, which together make up a resilient system for maintaining vascular tone. Alterations in the relative amounts of these specialised elements occur with age and lead to hardening, thickening and loss of elasticity of vessel walls and are a major cause of illness and death, particularly in affluent societies. The term *arteriosclerosis* (from the Greek *arteria-* artery, *skleros-* hardening) is often used as a general descriptive term for such diseases.

Atheroma (from the Greek word for porridge or gruel) affects large and medium-sized arteries and is the commonest type of arteriosclerosis, referred to as *atherosclerosis*. Other forms of arteriosclerosis occur, such as thickening of the walls of arterioles in association with hypertension (arteriolosclerosis; see Figs 11.1 and 11.2). However, from a histopathological and clinical point of view, atherosclerosis is the condition of overwhelming importance, contributing to around half of all deaths in the Western world.

To some extent, atherosclerotic changes can be demonstrated in large and medium-sized arteries in almost all adults; however, clinical consequences mainly occur in association with severe atherosclerosis. The factors predisposing to severe lesions with a high incidence of complications can be divided into *non-modifiable* (factors we have no control over) and *modifiable* (factors we can influence/control); these are summarised in Figure 8.1.

Fig. 8.1 | **Risk factors in atherosclerosis**

Non-modifiable risk factors	
Age	Incidence of severe disease rises with each decade after age 55
Sex	Higher risk in men and postmenopausal women
Genetic	Increased risk if a first-degree relative has had stroke/coronary artery disease before age 55 (male relative) or 65 (female relative)
Ethnicity	People with African or Asian ancestry are at increased risk
Modifiable risk factors	
Hypertension	Most important risk factor for stroke and one of most important for cardiac disease
Hyperlipidaemia	High total cholesterol, high triglycerides, high levels of low-density lipoprotein or low levels of high-density lipoprotein cholesterol increase the risk of atheromatous disease
Tobacco use	Risk increased if started smoking when young, smoke heavily or female
Physical inactivity	Increases risk by up to 50%
Obesity	Major risk for cardiovascular disease and predisposes to diabetes
Diabetes	Doubles the likelihood for developing cardiovascular disease
Psychosocial	Chronic stress, anxiety and depression increase the risk of atheromatous disease

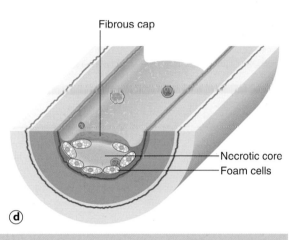

Fig. 8.2 **Stages in atheroma formation**

(a) *Normal elastic artery* with a distinct internal elastic lamina. The artery is lined internally by a smooth, flat endothelium lying on a delicate, fibroelastic, loose connective tissue which contains occasional multifunctional myointimal cells (tunica intima). Beneath the intima is a strong internal elastic lamina followed by a layer of smooth muscle containing some elastic fibres (tunica media). On the outer surface is the loose tunica adventitia.

(b) *Endothelial dysfunction*. At certain locations in the arterial system, such as vessel branch points, turbulent flow and shear stress are associated with expression of cell adhesion factors by the endothelium, which result in the accumulation and migration of monocytes and T lymphocytes. In parallel, the endothelium may become permeable to lipoproteins.

(c) *Fatty streak*. Continued endothelial dysfunction, with associated permeability to lipoproteins and monocyte and T-lymphocyte

migration, produces an intimal collection of lipid-laden macrophages (foam cells) and inflammatory cells. This is followed by migration of smooth muscle from the media producing the early atheromatous fatty streak lesion

(d) *Advanced/complicated atheroma*. Further progression of the early atheromatous fatty streak sees the formation of a fibrous cap between the vessel lumen and the accumulating constituents of the mature plaque, including lipid-laden macrophages, free lipid, inflammatory cells and debris. This fibrous cap forms from modified smooth muscle cells. Over time, the plaque continues to evolve, re-model and, frequently, undergoes calcification. Complications may arise from these advanced plaques through rupture (thereby exposing the highly thrombotic plaque contents), thrombosis associated with rupture, aneurysmal dilatation of the vessel or haemorrhage into the plaque, in turn leading to rupture.

STATINS

The statins are a group of drugs which act by inhibiting an enzyme involved in the production of low-density lipoprotein (LDL) cholesterol, which transports cholesterol to arteries where it can be incorporated as atheroma. Blocking the enzyme results in increased LDL receptor expression in the liver and, as a consequence, an increased clearance of LDL from the blood with associated decrease in blood cholesterol levels.

As a result of their success in lowering blood cholesterol levels and, with this, reducing the risk of atheromatous disease, these drugs are now widely used in adults where there is clinical evidence of cardiovascular disease and as one factor in the primary prevention strategy for adults at high risk of developing cardiovascular disease.

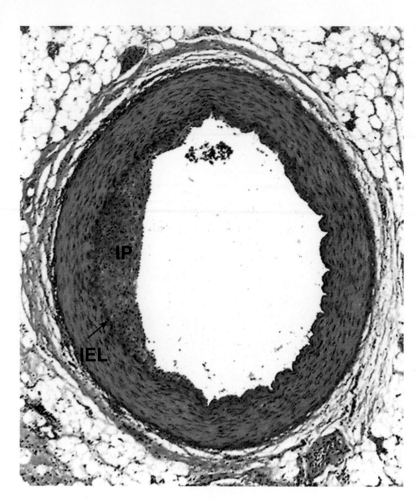

Fig. 8.3 **Arteriosclerosis**

Intimal thickening of arteries and arterioles is extremely common with increasing age. This may form part of the spectrum of atherosclerotic disease or may simply represent a physiological adaptation which occurs with age.

This micrograph shows a small artery exhibiting eccentric intimal proliferation **IP**. The thickened intima, clearly defined by the internal elastic lamina **IEL**, can be seen to consist of multiple cell layers and involves approximately half the circumference of the vessel.

Fig. 8.4 **Atheromatous plaque development** **(a)** Early atheromatous plaque (LP) **(b)** Foam cells and lipid (HP) **(c)** Fibrofatty plaque (LP) **(d)** Fibrous plaque (LP) (*illustrations opposite*)

Stages in development of a mature, fibrous atheromatous plaque are illustrated in these four images. Image (a) shows a pale-staining area of thickening of the intima **In** composed of aggregated myointimal cells containing lipid and some intimal fibrous tissue. Macroscopically, these lesions appear as slightly raised, flat areas termed ***atheromatous plaques***. Note that the medial layer of the vessel **M** is uniform and appears normal at this stage. Early atheroma is a disease confined to the intima.

Image (b) reveals detail of the intimal thickening at higher power. Foam cells **FC** filled with lipid appear as large, pale-staining cells with vacuolated cytoplasm. These cells may be derived from either myointimal cells or macrophages. As the lesion progresses, some of the foam cells break down and liberate free lipid into the intima which appears as non-staining, angular clefts **C** (***cholesterol clefts***).

Early intimal atheromatous lesions enlarge by further accumulation of lipid both in foam cells and free within extracellular intimal tissue. This is associated with a more marked fibrotic response in the intima, leading to increased thickening of the lesion to produce a ***fibrofatty plaque*** **P** as shown in image (c). Note the areas of non-staining lipid **L** surrounded by pink-staining fibrous tissue **F** making up the thickened intima. A zone of denser, more intensely stained fibrous tissue, sometimes termed a ***fibrous cap*** **Cap**, runs between the endothelial surface and the underlying fibrofatty aggregate.

With progression of the lesion, the fibrous cap thickens and the intimal lesion becomes larger and more raised. Image (d) shows such a plaque **P**, which is mostly composed of fibrous tissue. Note that in both images (c) and (d) there is early thinning of the tunica media **M** beneath the plaque compared to the adjacent normal vessel wall. This is the result of loss of supporting elastic tissue, atrophy of smooth muscle cells and progressive medial fibrosis. With time, the medial fibrous tissue stretches owing to loss of elastic recoil in the vessel wall and the vessel dilates. This dilatation is the basis of the formation of an atheromatous aneurysm.

KEY TO FIGURES

C cholesterol clefts **Cap** fibrous cap **F** fibrous tissue **FC** foam cells **IEL** internal elastic lamina
In intima **IP** intimal proliferation **L** lipid **M** media **P** fibrofatty plaque

Fig. 8.4 Atheromatous plaque development (*caption opposite*)

Consequences of atheroma

Atherosclerosis may affect all arterial vessels, but the aorta, coronary, cerebral, carotid, renal and ilio-femoral arteries tend to be most severely affected and are the most common sites of significant clinical disease.

The most important pathological and clinical sequelae of atherosclerosis are as follows:

■ **Occlusion**: narrowing of the arterial lumen produces partial or complete obstruction to blood flow; this may result in ischaemia and *infarction* of the tissue supplied by the atheromatous vessel (see Ch. 10).

■ **Thrombosis**: endothelial ulceration stimulates formation of an overlying thrombus. This may occlude the vessel at the site of thrombosis, or fragments of thrombus may become detached to form *emboli* which block one or more smaller vessels distally (see Ch. 9).

■ **Aneurysm**: loss of muscle and elastin from the media causes weakening of the vessel wall, predisposing to a localised area of dilatation; such a dilatation is known as an *aneurysm*. Rupture of the weakened and dilated artery wall leading to fatal haemorrhage is a further serious complication and is most common in the abdominal aorta. Aneurysms may also lead to thrombus formation (see Ch. 9) because of areas of stasis in the aneurysm cavity.

The main histopathological complications are shown in Fig. 8.5 to Fig. 8.8.

Fig. 8.5 **Complicated atheroma** (MP)

As an atheromatous plaque enlarges, it may become very thick relative to the normal thickness of the vessel wall, and, in addition to lipid, foam cells and fibrous tissue, calcium may be deposited in the lesion. With thickening and fibrosis the lesion may undergo rupture or surface ulceration. This is then described as a *complicated atheromatous plaque*. The normal smooth endothelial lining having gone, the highly thrombogenic plaque contents are exposed directly to the blood flow. The coagulation sequence is thus activated and thrombus is formed on the vessel wall at the site of ulcerated atheroma (see Ch. 9).

This image shows the top of an atheromatous plaque with foam cells **F** and free lipid **L**. The surface has ulcerated and is encrusted with thrombus **T** composed of fibrin, platelets and entrapped blood cells. In a small vessel, for example a coronary artery, such a thrombus can occlude the lumen.

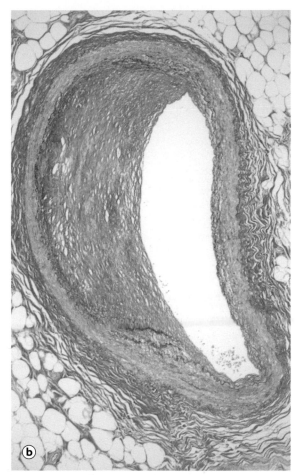

Fig. 8.6 **Arterial narrowing by atheroma** (LP) **(a)** H&E **(b)** EVG

The formation of a plaque of atheroma **A** in the intima of a small or medium-sized artery, such as this branch of a coronary artery, can greatly reduce the size of the lumen **Lu**. The consequent reduction in blood flow leads to ischaemia of the tissues supplied. Note that the media **M** underlying the atheroma is thinned. Such partly occlusive atheroma is frequent in the coronary arteries of cigarette-smoking males, particularly in the region of the bifurcation of the left coronary artery. Image (b) is stained by a special method to demonstrate elastin and illustrates the disruption of the internal elastic lamina.

A common symptom of this arterial narrowing is known as **angina pectoris**, a gripping pain in the chest particularly experienced on exertion and settling with rest. This pain is a manifestation of ischaemia of the myocardium and patients with longstanding angina often show replacement of small areas of myocardium by fibrous scar tissue

Similar luminal narrowing by atheroma occurs in many other arteries. In the leg arteries, such changes can produce severe calf pain on walking (**intermittent claudication**) and may eventually lead to the development of gangrene of the lower leg. In the vertebrobasilar arterial system, which supplies the cerebellum and brain stem, severe atheroma can produce transient ischaemia manifest clinically as dizziness, loss of balance and, occasionally, unconsciousness (**vertebrobasilar syndrome**).

ANGIOPLASTY AND STENTING

Where a vessel is narrowed by atheroma, typically a coronary artery, it is possible to widen the narrowed segment by a process known as **angioplasty**. Here an elongated, deflated balloon attached to the end of a catheter is passed along the systemic arterial system from a peripheral vessel (such as the femoral artery) to the diseased coronary artery. Once at the site of narrowing, the balloon can be inflated, so compressing the lipid-laden atheroma and improving the diameter of the vessel lumen.

In many cases following this angioplasty, a metal mesh tube known as a **stent** is deployed at the site to act as a scaffold holding the vessel open to limit the re-formation of atheromatous plaque.

KEY TO FIGURES
A atheroma   **F** foam cells   **L** lipid   **Lu** lumen   **M** tunica media   **T** thrombus

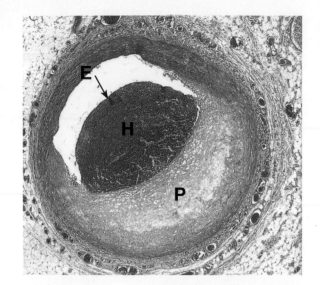

Fig. 8.7 Haemorrhage into atheromatous plaque (LP)

There are two possible mechanisms for the development of haemorrhage in an atheromatous plaque. First, the rigid fibrotic plaque may split under the constant trauma of pulsatile movements and allow blood from the vessel lumen to greatly expand the plaque lesion; such a process is termed *plaque fissuring*. Alternatively, small capillary vessels which develop in established plaques may rupture and lead to haemorrhage. Whatever the mechanism, because of the confined space in which such apparently trivial haemorrhage occurs, the consequences can be disproportionately devastating. In this micrograph, a small haemorrhage **H** has occurred in the superficial area of a fibrofatty atheromatous plaque **P**. The accumulated blood has tracked beneath the non-ulcerated endothelium **E**, causing it to bulge markedly into the artery. This has led to even greater narrowing of a lumen already reduced to about half its normal size by the pre-existing atheromatous plaque. Such an abrupt reduction in arterial flow leads to acute ischaemia in the supplied tissues.

In this patient, the lesion was situated in the anterior descending branch of the left coronary artery and resulted in acute ischaemia of a substantial area of the anterior wall of the left ventricle and the anterior half of the interventricular septum. Necrosis of heart muscle ensued, a process known as *myocardial infarction*, resulting in this patient's death (see Fig. 10.2).

CORONARY ARTERY BYPASS SURGERY

Where atheroma in a coronary vessel is such that symptoms from the reduced flow through the stenotic segment cannot be controlled through medication and/or the region of diseased vessel is not suitable for an angioplasty or stent procedure, it is possible to perform surgery to bypass the blocked segment of vessel. This is achieved by utilising a nearby vessel (e.g. internal thoracic artery) or inserting a length of vessel from elsewhere in the body (e.g. a vein from the leg) between the aorta and the diseased vessel beyond the point of stenosis. This length of vessel is sometimes referred to as the *graft*. Hence, the procedure is commonly referred to as a *coronary artery bypass graft* or, more often, by its acronym as a *CABG* (pronounced 'cabbage').

Whilst angioplasty and stenting may be favoured for disease in a single coronary vessel, bypass surgery is preferred where more than one vessel is diseased. Hence, the number of vessels bypassed may be referred to when discussing the procedure (e.g. *double bypass, triple bypass*).

Together, the procedures of angioplasty, stenting and bypass surgery are referred to as *revascularisation* procedures. Although these procedures have transformed outcomes in patients with coronary artery atheromatous disease, it should be borne in mind that while they may overcome the diseased arterial segment, they do not prevent further atheroma from developing. As such, following revascularisation it is advised that patients do all they can to tackle the modifiable risk factors that may have contributed to the development of their atheromatous disease.

KEY TO FIGURES
C clot **E** endothelium **H** haemorrhage **P** plaque **T** thrombus

Fig. 8.8 **Thrombus formation on atheroma** (LP)

The most important complication of atheroma in small and medium-sized arteries is the development of a *thrombus* on the surface of an atheromatous plaque. The process of thrombus formation is discussed in detail in Chapter 9. Thrombus, which consists of a mass of platelets and insoluble fibrin, tends, in the arterial system, to form on any intimal surface which is denuded to expose the underlying tissues. Endothelial ulceration over an atheromatous plaque is the commonest cause of thrombosis in the arterial system, although plaque fissuring, as discussed in Figure 8.7, can also initiate thrombosis.

This micrograph of a coronary artery shows an ulcerated atheromatous plaque **P** which has already significantly constricted the arterial lumen. A thrombus **T** has then developed on the ulcerated surface, largely obliterating the remaining lumen. The thrombus is deep pink in colour and is composed of fibrin and platelets with entrapped red blood cells.

The residual lumen is occupied by bright red post-mortem blood clot **C** composed entirely of tightly packed red blood cells. The naked cyc distinction between genuine ante-mortem thrombus and post-mortem clot is important. Thrombus is pinkish red, granular and firm, whereas clot is predominantly dark red, shiny and jelly-like.

When thrombus formation occurs on an atheromatous lesion in a large-diameter artery, such as the aorta or carotid arteries, the thrombus may be small and cause little significant obstruction to blood flow at the site. Fragments of thrombus may, however, become detached and pass into the peripheral circulation to block a smaller vessel and cause ischaemia or infarction in its area of distribution. This phenomenon is known as *thromboembolism* and is more fully described in Chapter 9.

Fig. 8.9 Chapter review

		Main features	Figure
Arteriosclerosis	General term for loss of elasticity and hardening of vessel walls	Modifiable and non-modifiable risk factors	8.1 8.3
Atherosclerosis	Where the underlying process involves atheroma formation	Atheromatous plaques form as a result of endothelial dysfunction, inflammatory cell activity and lipid accumulation	8.2 8.4
Complicated atheroma		Plaque ulceration	8.5
		Stenosis	8.6
		Haemorrhage into plaque	8.7
		Thrombus formation overlying complicated plaque	8.8

9 Thrombosis and embolism

Thrombosis

The vascular system normally contains fluid blood. However, it is often necessary for blood to coagulate to prevent bleeding following injury to a vessel wall. To control this process of **haemostasis**, there are interacting systems which either promote or inhibit the process of blood coagulation. Under certain pathological circumstances these dynamics may be disrupted, leading to the formation of a solid mass of blood products in a vessel lumen. This process is known as **thrombosis** and the mass of blood products is referred to as a **thrombus**. It is important to distinguish thrombosis, a dynamic process occurring in flowing blood, from **coagulation**, which is a process that takes place in static blood to form a blood **clot** and involves coagulation factors only.

A thrombus consists of aggregates of platelets bound together by fibrin strands with variable numbers of erythrocytes and leukocytes trapped in the tangled mass and contributing to the bulk of the thrombus. Thrombosis may occur in any part of the circulation, but most particularly in large veins, large arteries, in the heart chambers and on heart valves. Three major factors, alone or in combination, predispose to thrombosis. These are often referred to as **Virchow's triad**:

- **Damage to the endothelium** is the main cause of arterial and intracardiac thrombosis. This damage may be either through physical endothelial disruption or as a consequence of endothelial cell dysfunction. Hence hypertension, turbulent blood flow and bacterial endotoxins may contribute to endothelial dysfunction and thrombus formation.

- **Disordered blood flow**. Relative stasis is important in initiating thrombus in slow-flowing blood such as in veins. Turbulent blood flow predisposes to thrombus formation in arterial vessels and the heart through disruption of endothelial function and the creation of eddy currents in the blood with focal stasis.

- **Abnormal haemostatic properties of the blood (hypercoagulability)**. Hypercoagulable states may be either inherited or acquired. Of the inherited disorders, abnormalities in the factor V and prothrombin genes are commonest and may present with recurrent venous thrombosis. There are numerous acquired hypercoagulable states, such as those associated with changes in blood viscosity, for example in dehydration, major illness, disseminated carcinoma or in the postoperative state.

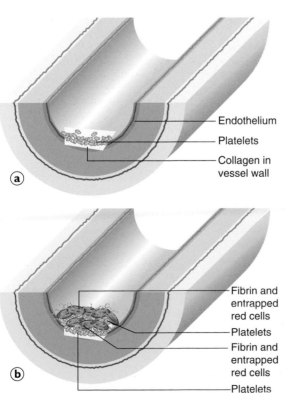

(a)
- Endothelium
- Platelets
- Collagen in vessel wall

(b)
- Fibrin and entrapped red cells
- Platelets
- Fibrin and entrapped red cells
- Platelets

A thrombus has a defined architecture and consistency which reflects the manner and stages of its formation and the nature of blood flow in the vicinity. For example, thrombus formed in an artery is usually dense and composed mainly of aggregated platelets and fibrin, whereas thrombus formed in slowed or static blood more closely resembles clotted blood in that it contains masses of erythrocytes and leukocytes.

Fig. 9.1 Early thrombogenesis

Following endothelial injury (a), platelets adhere to exposed subendothelial collagen (mediated by von Willebrand factor) and become activated, liberating ADP and thromboxane A2 which mediate further platelet aggregation.

Platelets undergo degranulation and their products, together with released tissue factors, activate the coagulation cascade (b). This results in generation of thrombin which converts soluble fibrinogen to insoluble fibrin. Red cells become passively entrapped in the resultant fibrin–platelet mesh, the number depending on the circumstances of thrombus formation. In arteries, there are few red cells and more platelets and fibrin; in veins, where blood flow is slower, there are generally many more red cells.

Fig. 9.2 **Thrombus formation** (*caption opposite*)

Fig. 9.2 **Thrombus formation** **(a)** Early thrombus (HP) **(b)** Enlargement of thrombus (MP) **(c)** Thrombosis in a vein (LP) *(illustrations (a) and (b) opposite)*

Damage to the endothelium exposes intimal collagen, resulting in adherence and then aggregation of platelets at the site of damage. Tissue damage and collagen exposure also activate the extrinsic and intrinsic blood clotting systems, respectively, the latter system also depending on release of platelet factor 3 from aggregated platelets. The result is activation of prothrombin to thrombin, which in turn catalyses the conversion of soluble plasma fibrinogen into insoluble fibrin. Thus, the flimsy platelet aggregates become bound together into a solid, resilient mass, the thrombus.

Micrograph (a) illustrates an arterial wall **W** damaged by atheroma. The endothelium has become ulcerated with the formation of thrombus **T** at the site of injury. This thrombus consists of platelet aggregates within a meshwork of eosinophilic fibrin. Entrapped erythrocytes and leukocytes are present, but are not themselves involved in the specific haemostatic processes.

Small areas of thrombus formed on vessel walls may be dissolved completely by fibrinolytic mechanisms. However, under appropriate conditions, the thrombus continues to enlarge. Micrograph (b)

illustrates this process. The abnormal vessel wall **W** has become coated by a thin layer of fibrin and platelet thrombus T_1, with entrapped red cells **R**. This has formed the basis for the deposition of another layer of fibrin–platelet thrombus T_2, again with entrapped red cells. A third layer T_3 can be seen forming at the left of the picture. Thus, thrombi enlarge by the successive deposition of a number of layers, a feature which is apparent to naked eye in the laminated cut surface seen in an established thrombus (*lines of Zahn*).

In the arterial system, damage to the intimal layer is the most common predisposing factor in thrombus formation, but in the venous system the most important factor is the rate of blood flow; reduced flow rates increase susceptibility to thrombus formation. Vasculitis or inflammation of the vessel wall also causes thrombosis (see Ch. 11).

Micrograph (c) shows a venous thrombus **T** completely occluding the lumen of a vein in a neurovascular bundle from the muscle of the calf. This is known as *deep venous thrombosis (DVT)* and may be encountered in postoperative patients confined to bed.

KEY TO FIGURES
R red cells   **T** thrombus   **W** arterial wall

Fate of vascular thrombi

Once thrombus is formed there are several possible outcomes:

▪ **Propagation**. The thrombus itself is thrombogenic and may attract more platelets and fibrin to the site, resulting in it enlarging and growing along the vessel, ultimately leading to vessel occlusion and/or embolisation if left untreated.

▪ **Embolisation**. In addition to the triad of factors contributing to thrombus generation, Virchow coined the term *embolus* for '*fragments from the end of a softening thrombus which are carried along by the current of the blood and driven into remote vessels*'. This term is now applied not only to fragments of thrombus (*thromboemboli*), but to any material forming in, or entering, the bloodstream and passing with the circulation to lodge in a more distal vessel.

Emboli are most commonly caused by detachment of all or part of a thrombus from its site of formation. Venous thromboembolism is of clinical importance as, for example, following deep venous thrombosis in the leg, the thrombus may propagate as far as the common iliac vein or even the inferior vena cava. Part of such a huge thrombus may readily become detached and pass via the right side of the heart to lodge in the pulmonary arterial tree as a *pulmonary embolus*, which is often fatal (Fig. 9.4).

Systemic arterial thromboemboli most commonly arise from the heart or major arteries. In such cases, the thrombus often covers only part of the luminal wall as a plaque-like structure and is known as *mural thrombus*. Such thrombi may form on the ventricular endocardium following myocardial infarction (Fig. 9.3). Emboli arising in the arterial system impact in peripheral arterial vessels where the most dramatic outcome is necrosis of the tissue supplied (*infarction*); this is described in detail in the next chapter.

Whilst thrombotic emboli are the most common, emboli may also arise from other sources. These include atheromatous debris, tumour cells, bacterial vegetations from infected heart valves, fat and bone marrow after bone fracture (Fig. 9.5), air entering the circulation and, rarely, amniotic fluid in cases of complicated pregnancy.

▪ **Resolution**. This involves the normal physiological phenomenon of fibrinolysis as well as autolytic disintegration of the cellular elements of the thrombus. The end result is complete dissolution with restoration of blood flow. This process may be enhanced by the therapeutic administration of thrombolytic drugs, a principle of the acute management of myocardial infarction.

▪ **Organisation**. Ingrowth of granulation tissue from the vessel wall and subsequent fibrous repair occur when fibrinolysis is ineffective in removing the thrombus. By an extraordinary mechanism, the organised thrombus may undergo recanalisation, a process whereby new vascular channels are formed to re-establish a patent lumen. The processes of organisation and recanalisation are illustrated in Figure 9.7.

Fig. 9.3 **Left ventricular mural thrombus** (LP)

Thrombus within the heart chambers most commonly occurs upon endocardium damaged by myocardial infarction (see Fig. 10.2). This micrograph illustrates infarcted ventricular wall **W** with mural thrombus **T** laid down on the luminal surface; the thrombus surrounds a papillary muscle **P**.

The left ventricle is the most common site of mural thrombosis after myocardial infarction.

KEY TO FIGURES
E embolus   **P** papillary muscle   **T** thrombus   **W** ventricular wall

Fig. 9.4 **Thromboembolism: pulmonary embolus** (LP)

When fragments of thrombus become detached from their site of formation, they travel in the circulation (venous or arterial, according to site of origin) as thromboemboli. On reaching vessels of small enough calibre to prevent further passage, the thromboemboli impact, producing sudden vascular occlusion. Depending on the size of the thromboembolus, the tissue or organ involved and the extent of alternative vascular supply, the result may be either inadequate blood flow for normal sustenance of the tissue

(*ischaemia*) or frank tissue necrosis (*infarction*); these phenomena are described in the next chapter.

This micrograph illustrates lung tissue in which the pulmonary artery branch is occluded by an embolus **E** originating from thrombus in the deep veins of the leg.

This condition, known as *pulmonary embolism*, is an important cause of sudden death, especially in debilitated or immobilised patients predisposed to deep venous thrombosis.

THROMBOLYSIS

To supplement the natural process of fibrinolysis and speed dissolution of thrombus in clinical situations where early restoration of blood flow (***reperfusion***) to an organ may be indicated, a variety of pharmacological agents have been developed which aid breakdown (***lysis***) of the thrombus. Hence this treatment is known as ***thrombolysis*** and the drugs used are termed ***thrombolytics***. These drugs act to increase the conversion of naturally occurring plasminogen to plasmin, which has powerful fibrinolytic properties. Examples of agents in clinical use are streptokinase (an enzyme derived from β-haemolytic *Streptococcus*) and recombinant tissue plasminogen activator (tPA).

Adminstration of these agents has transformed the acute management of myocardial infarction, where they are now in common usage. Similarly, they can have great value in management of acute pulmonary thromboembolism, in acute limb ischaemia and, if administered soon after onset of symptoms, they can be of value in the management of stroke. In each case, the ideal is to achieve reperfusion of the vascular bed as quickly as possible, the aim being to minimise the volume of tissue infarcted.

BASIC PATHOLOGICAL PROCESSES ■ THROMBOSIS AND EMBOLISM

Fig. 9.5 **Bone marrow embolus** (MP)

As noted above, other than thrombus, there are a number of other objects which may embolise. These include atheroma, tumour, fat and bone marrow. Whatever the source, the consequence is obstruction of distal vessels with resultant partial or complete occlusion.

In this micrograph, a fragment of bone marrow has embolised to the pulmonary vasculature and become lodged in a pulmonary artery branch. The lumen of the vessel contains both fat cells of bone marrow **F** and the cellular haematopoietic elements **C**.

Bone marrow/fat embolism is a common complication of trauma, in particular following fracture of a long bone such as the femur. It can also occasionally occur as a complication of orthopaedic surgery. In the majority of cases it passes without symptoms. Where symptoms occur, they most often arise in the days following injury with breathlessness, tachycardia, delirium and a petechial rash; this last observation a useful sign in supporting the diagnosis clinically. In a small proportion of cases (approximately 10%) fat embolisation is fatal.

Fig 9.6 **Therapeutic embolisation** (MP)

Under certain circumstances embolisation may be used as a therapeutic manoeuvre whereby embolic agents, of which there is a variety available, are introduced to the target vasculature through a catheter sited via a peripheral vessel. Indications for this include: to control abnormal bleeding (e.g. complicating fibroids), to occlude vessels supplying a richly vascular tumour prior to chemotherapy or surgery, or to treat a vascular malformation.

In this micrograph taken from a surgical resection specimen several days after embolisation therapy, embolisation spheres **S** are seen almost filling the lumen of a medium-sized artery, the wall of which is clearly visible **A**. As a result of this, thrombus **T** has formed around the spheres. The combination of the spheres and associated thrombus has occluded the vessel. This aids surgery by minimising the risk of intraoperative haemorrhage from a highly vascular tumour.

Fig. 9.7 **Fate of thrombi** **(a)** Organisation (MP)
(b) Recanalisation (MP)

Following occlusion of a vessel by thrombus, there is an initial inflammatory response in the vessel wall. Within a few days, the thrombus becomes *organised* by ingrowth of granulation tissue from the intima of the vessel wall. Micrograph (a) shows a vein occluded by thrombus **T**. At various points, granulation tissue **G** extends from the vessel wall into the thrombus. This eventually results in replacement of the thrombus by fibrovascular granulation tissue. In some cases, larger vessels develop within the fibrovascular granulation tissue of the organising thrombus and may permit passage of blood through the damaged, previously occluded area. This occurs most commonly in arteries and is termed *recanalisation*.

Micrograph (b) illustrates this process in an artery which has been occluded by thrombus and is at a later stage of organisation than in micrograph (a). Note that the granulation tissue in the lumen contains numerous small blood vessels **V**. These vessels may conduct blood across the thrombosed area and some will enlarge with time, acquiring smooth muscle walls.

KEY TO FIGURES
A artery   **C** bone marrow cells   **F** fat   **G** granulation tissue   **S** embolisation sphere   **T** thrombus   **V** blood vessels

Fig. 9.8 Chapter review

	Definition/features	Figure
Thrombus	Aggregate of platelets, fibrin and blood cells formed in vessel lumen by the process of *thrombosis*	9.1 9.2 9.3
Virchow's triad	Factors predisposing to thrombus formation namely damaged endothelium, abnormal blood flow and hypercoagulability	
Fate of thrombi	Propagation – enlargement with growth along vessel, occlusion of vessel and/or embolisation	
	Embolisation – see below	9.4
	Resolution – dissolution of the thrombus by fibrinolysis	
	Organisation – where fibrinolysis is unsuccessful, granulation tissue may form with subsequent fibrous repair and recanalisation	9.7
Embolus	Fragment of thrombus or other material passing with the circulation to lodge in a distal vessel	9.5 9.6

Fig. 10.1 **Renal infarction** **(a)** Early infarct (LP) **(b)** Margin of infarct (MP) **(c)** Old renal infarct (MP) (*illustrations (a) and (b) opposite*)

The kidneys are favoured sites for infarction, often asymptomatic, as a result of the large blood flow to the kidneys and their limited collateral circulation ('*end arteries*'). The majority of renal infarcts result from emboli originating from thrombus in the left ventricle (e.g. mural thrombus after myocardial infarction) or the left atrial appendage (e.g. in atrial fibrillation).

In the very early stages (i.e. within 12 hours of infarction), gross examination shows the infarcted area to be ill-defined and dark. Soon, the lesion becomes paler until it becomes a clearly defined, wedge-shaped, readily identifiable region with the base towards the cortical surface and the apex extending towards the medulla. Such established infarcts may be recognised within 24 hours of onset.

Micrograph (a) shows the histological appearance of a typical early renal infarct. The recently infarcted necrotic area **In** stains less intensely than the normal cortex **N**, but the general architecture of the infarct remains intact with still discernible 'ghosts' of glomeruli and renal tubules. The infarcted area has become demarcated from normal cortex by a narrow hyperaemic zone **H** representing the earliest vascular stages of a typical acute inflammatory response. Between this hyperaemic zone and the necrotic tissue

is a purple-staining band containing the neutrophils of an early cellular acute inflammatory exudate.

Micrograph (b) shows, at higher magnification, the edge of the infarct in micrograph (a). Note that the normal cortical tissue **N**, with its well-defined glomeruli and tubules, gives way to a zone of hyperaemia **H**. Next to this is a purplish band of acute inflammation **I** at the margin of the infarcted area **In** where marked necrotic changes are evident in both glomeruli and tubules (see Fig. 1.8). The acute inflammatory zone exhibits typically dilated and congested capillaries and an influx of small, dark-staining neutrophil polymorphs.

The necrotic tissue is progressively removed by neutrophils and macrophages and replaced by granulation tissue which eventually undergoes fibrous repair to form a small fibrous scar. This is shown in micrograph (c), which illustrates the end result of a renal infarct occurring 2 months previously; the infarct was of a similar size to that shown in (a). All that now remains is a small, narrow, pink-staining, wedge-shaped scar **S** with its broad aspect at the capsular surface. Note that the capsular surface at the site of the scar is depressed as a result of contraction of the collagen fibres within the scar (a process known as *cicatrisation*).

KEY TO FIGURES

H hyperaemic zone   **I** acute inflammation   **In** infarcted region   **N** normal   **S** scar

Ischaemic heart disease

Ischaemic heart disease is a major cause of death in all industrialised countries. Atherosclerosis of coronary arteries accounts for the vast majority of cases, hence the alternative term *coronary artery disease (CAD)*. Four main clinical syndromes are recognised:

■ *Angina (pectoris)* – from the Latin for 'choking pain' of the 'chest'. Angina describes a complex of symptoms arising from paroxysmal, often recurring and brief episodes of reversible myocardial ischaemia. It can be further subdivided into stable, unstable or variant (Prinzmetal's) angina. In the first two, symptoms arise as a consequence of increased load on the heart (e.g. during exercise) in the face of coronary artery stenosis through atheroma. With stable angina, symptoms occur with exercise, there being few or no symptoms at rest. In contrast, unstable angina may be unpredictable, with symptoms at rest, and may progress to myocardial infarction. Hence, unstable angina may be regarded as a medical emergency. In both stable and unstable angina, the underlying pathology is atheromatous plaque, which may be ruptured in unstable angina, hence the increased symptoms. In contrast, variant angina can arise in patients with minimal atheroma and is thought to be a consequence of coronary artery spasm.

■ *Acute myocardial infarction* ('heart attack') – two main pathological forms are recognised:

– *Transmural infarction*. This involves the full thickness of a segment of the ventricular wall and is associated with complete blockage of a main coronary artery by thrombosis, often superimposed on an area of arteriosclerotic narrowing. Fissure or ulceration of an atheromatous plaque is the usual cause of thrombus formation (see Ch. 8).

– *Subendocardial myocardial infarction*. In this case, myocardial necrosis is limited to cells in the inner third of the ventricular wall. The pathogenesis of infarction is limitation of flow to the end arteries supplying the inner part of the ventricular wall, rather than complete occlusion of the main arterial trunks.

■ *Chronic ischaemic heart disease*

■ *Sudden cardiac death* (immediately fatal myocardial infarct or dysrhythmia).

The histological changes following infarction are illustrated in Figure 10.2 and Figure 10.3.

Fig. 10.2 **Myocardial infarction** **(a)** 24-hour infarct (HP) **(b)** 3-day infarct (HP) **(c)** 10-day infarct (HP) **(d)** 14-day infarct (HP) (*illustrations opposite*)

The most common clinical example of infarction is that of the myocardium following occlusion of a coronary artery. Using routine staining methods, the earliest histological features of infarction may be visible some 4 or so hours after infarction and are established at about 12 to 24 hours, as illustrated in micrograph (a). The infarcted cardiac muscle fibres **In** exhibit patchy loss or blurring of cross-striations and tend to become more intensely stained by eosin than normal myocardial fibres **M**. At this stage there may also be a degree of early capillary engorgement, interstitial oedema and a mild neutrophil infiltrate representing the earliest stages of the acute inflammatory response.

By about 2 or 3 days, as shown in micrograph (b), the infarcted fibres are intensely eosinophilic and most have lost their nuclei. There is marked infiltration by neutrophils **N** into the oedematous interstitium. This acute inflammatory process evolves during the succeeding days, during which time the necrotic myocardium undergoes autolysis and fragmentation. By about the 10th day, as illustrated in micrograph (c), most of the necrotic muscle has disappeared as a result of the combined phagocytic activity of neutrophils and macrophages. The infarcted area is now largely occupied by residual macrophages, some lymphocytes and plasma cells in a loose oedematous mesh in which a few capillaries and fibroblasts herald the earliest signs of granulation tissue formation.

By about the 14th day, the infarct is almost wholly replaced by fibrovascular granulation tissue **G**, as illustrated in micrograph (d), and the necrotic myocardium has been almost completely removed by the phagocytic activity of macrophages and neutrophils.

Over succeeding weeks, the fibrovascular granulation tissue becomes progressively more fibrous and less vascular, leading to the formation of a highly collagenous and relatively acellular scar by about the end of the second month following infarction. An example of a myocardial scar is shown in Figure 10.3.

The infarcted myocardium offers the least resistance to pressure around days 5 to 10, at which time the patient is most vulnerable to myocardial rupture. This not uncommon complication is almost invariably fatal, the ruptured ventricle wall spilling blood into the pericardial cavity (*haemopericardium*). If the interventricular septum is involved in the infarct, there may be rupture of the septum with the sudden appearance of a systolic murmur. Similarly, rupture of an infarcted papillary muscle may lead to mitral valve incompetence with the appearance of a characteristic systolic murmur.

Fig. 10.2 **Myocardial infarction** (*caption opposite*)

KEY TO FIGURES
G granulation tissue **In** infarcted fibres **M** normal fibres **N** neutrophils

Fig. 10.3 Old myocardial infarct – full-thickness scar (LP)

This micrograph shows the appearance of a myocardial scar several months after infarction. The site of infarction is marked by densely collagenous, pale pink-staining scar **S**, contrasting with the more eosinophilic, surviving myocardium **M**. Continuing contraction (cicatrisation) of the fibrous scar over succeeding months leads to thinning of the infarcted area. If the scar is inadequate to withstand ventricular pressures, a ventricular aneurysm may develop by ballooning of the wall (most likely after a full-thickness infarct). With or without aneurysm formation, stasis in the region of the non-contractile scar predisposes to formation of a mural thrombus.

If the original infarct involves the endocardium **E**, visceral pericardium **P** or both, as in some full-thickness infarcts, these normally delicate layers become markedly thickened as a result of their involvement in the inflammatory process and subsequent organisation and repair.

Fig. 10.4 Pulmonary infarct (LP)

Pulmonary infarcts often result from emboli arising from fragments of thrombus within the deep veins of the legs. In their early stages, pulmonary infarcts are firm, dark-red, wedge-shaped areas at the lung periphery; their firmness and colour derive from the fact that the alveolar spaces are filled with erythrocytes, partly owing to leakage from damaged capillary walls and partly to blood carried by the unobstructed bronchial arterial circulation. The pleura often become involved in the resulting acute inflammatory response leading to the characteristic sharp pleuritic pain and a pleural friction rub. Larger emboli which obstruct the main pulmonary arteries can result in sudden death through acute right heart failure.

This micrograph illustrates a branch of a pulmonary artery **Pa** containing fragments of fibrin thrombus **T**. Surrounding this vessel there is haemorrhage into air spaces, the walls of which are pale and without nuclei, in keeping with recent infarction.

KEY TO FIGURES

E endocardium   **M** surviving myocardium   **P** pericardium   **Pa** pulmonary artery branch   **S** scar   **T** thrombus

Fig. 10.5 Venous infarction of bowel following volvulus (LP)

Bowel infarction may occur either as a result of arterial occlusion (e.g. mesenteric thrombosis or embolism) or, more commonly, as a result of venous obstruction. Venous obstruction may occur through *torsion* (twisting) of a free loop of bowel around its vascular pedicle (*volvulus*), entrapment in a tight hernial orifice (e.g. *incarcerated indirect inguinal hernia*) or obstruction by fibrous *peritoneal adhesions* (e.g. following previous surgery).

Venous obstruction initially causes the bowel to become intensely congested with blood, giving it a plum-coloured appearance on gross examination. As the dammed-back blood prevents arterial inflow, the bowel becomes progressively ischaemic. Frank necrosis follows unless the venous obstruction is relieved.

In this micrograph of a small bowel volvulus, the necrotic bowel at the top of the picture stains bright red because of massive suffusion with blood; the outline of the necrotic mucosal villi is still apparent. Note the sharp demarcation between normal and necrotic bowel, and the marked engorgement of all vessels.

Fig. 10.6 Chapter review

Disorder	Definition/example	Features	Figure
Infarction	Ischaemic necrosis		
Arterial infarction	Renal infarction	Common and often asymptomatic. Typically wedge-shaped, base towards capsular surface In early stages demarcated from surrounding, non-infarcted tissue by hyperaemic zone Heals leaving fibrous scar	10.1
	Myocardial infarction	Earliest histological changes detected within 4 hours; established by 12 to 24 hours	10.2 10.3
	Pulmonary infarction	Early stages, firm, dark red, wedge-shaped Sharp pleuritic pain plus pleural rub Can result in sudden death	10.4
	Cerebral infarction	Earliest changes within hours of infarction; established at 6 to 12 hours	1.7 23.2
Venous infarction	Torsion of testis	Twisting of spermatic cord leads to compression of thin-walled veins and subsequent infarction	19.1
	Small bowel volvulus	Initially intensely congested with blood Bowel becomes progressively ischaemic. Necrosis unless venous obstruction relieved	10.5

PART 2

BASIC SYSTEMS PATHOLOGY

11 Cardiovascular system

Diseases of the arterial system

The most common pathological abnormality of the arterial tree is thickening and hardening of the walls, known as atherosclerosis (Ch. 8). Among the risk factors for atherosclerosis are hypertension and diabetes mellitus. In both cases, in addition to a contribution to atherogenesis, specific vascular changes of either hypertension or diabetes may be recognised, often superimposed on the changes of atherosclerosis. Some of the important arterial wall changes associated with hypertension are illustrated in this chapter in Figure 11.1 and Figure 11.2, and in relation to the kidney in Figure 15.13.

Fig. 11.1 **Essential hypertension: kidney** **(a)** Medium-sized artery (MP) **(b)** Renal arteriole (HP)

Hypertension, whether idiopathic (primary) or secondary, is frequently associated with changes in peripheral arterial vessels. In larger arteries this can manifest as arterial dissection (Fig. 11.3), which is a life-threatening medical emergency.

More commonly, when the increase in blood pressure is moderate and gradual in onset (*essential* or *benign hypertension*), smaller muscular arteries undergo progressive thickening of their walls. Three features are characteristically seen and are shown in micrograph (a). These are: symmetrical hypertrophy of the muscular media **M**, extensive reduplication of the internal elastic lamina **E** and fibrotic thickening of the intima **In**. All these changes lead to reduction in diameter of the lumen.

Arterioles show a different type of wall thickening, sometimes referred to as *hyaline arteriolosclerosis* and shown in micrograph (b). The normal layers of the wall become ill-defined and replaced by a homogeneous, eosinophilic (pink-stained) material called *hyaline* **H**, thought to consist of basement membrane-like material. This results in reduction in size of arteriolar lumina and may contribute to further hypertension. In the kidney, hypertensive vascular changes may lead to compromised renal blood supply with chronic ischaemic damage of the glomerulus (*hypertensive nephrosclerosis*). This is further discussed in Chapter 15.

KEY TO FIGURES
E internal elastic lamina   **H** hyaline   **In** tunica intima   **M** tunica media   **P** proteinaceous material

Fig. 11.2 Accelerated hypertension: kidney
(a) Medium-sized artery (HP) **(b)** Arteriole (HP)

Accelerated or *malignant hypertension* refers to a situation where the increase in blood pressure is of rapid onset and marked degree (systolic pressure >220 mmHg or diastolic pressure >120 mmHg). Under these circumstances muscular arteries develop severe thickening of the tunica intima **In** by proliferation of intimal cells. This gives the appearance of concentric lamellae ('onion skin' appearance) which encroach upon the arterial lumen as seen in micrograph (a). In contrast to the findings in moderate hypertension, the tunica media **M** and internal elastic lamina **E** remain largely unchanged.

The impact of sudden and severe hypertension on arterioles is even more dramatic, as shown in micrograph (b). The intimal cells undergo rapid proliferation (as in the muscular arteries) which is often complicated by disruption of the vessel wall, with leakage of plasma proteins, including fibrinogen, into and beyond the arteriolar wall. This change, known inaccurately as *fibrinoid necrosis*, is characterised by obliteration of the wall by intensely eosinophilic, amorphous, proteinaceous material **P**; the lumen is often completely occluded. Damage to the vessel wall may lead to thrombosis within the lumen.

Fig. 11.3 Dissection of the aorta (LP)

Aortic dissection most commonly affects the thoracic aorta, with the vast majority of cases associated with hypertension and a smaller number associated with connective tissue disorders (e.g. Marfan's syndrome). A laceration of the tunica intima **In** leads to tracking of blood into the tunica media **M**. The plane of cleavage (dissection) is usually between the middle and outer thirds of the media, as in this example; note the site of intimal laceration is not included in this field. The medial haematoma **H** then frequently bursts through the tunica adventitia **A** with rapidly fatal consequences.

The pathogenesis of dissection is poorly understood but almost all cases exhibit a peculiar type of non-inflammatory degeneration of the smooth muscle and elastic tissue of the tunica media known as **medial myxoid degeneration** or **cystic medial necrosis**. In this condition, areas of the tunica media become replaced by irregular masses of acellular polysaccharide material. Dissection may occur in adults at any age, though it is most common in middle age, with males outnumbering females.

Aneurysms

Abnormal dilatations of the heart or blood vessels are known as **aneurysms**. In clinical practice aneurysms are most often encountered in relation to the aorta, ventricular wall of the heart or vessels of the base of the brain. In respect of aortic aneurysms, the most common aetiology is as a consequence of atherosclerosis, the vessel wall becoming thinned as a consequence of medial destruction. Figure 11.4 lists the types of aneurysm, their aetiology and their most common sites of involvement. The main complications of an aneurysm are rupture, leading to haemorrhage, and thrombus formation, leading to occlusive or embolic phenomena.

Fig. 11.4 Types of aneurysm

Type	Common sites	Aetiology	Common effects of rupture
Atherosclerotic	Abdominal aorta	Weakening of tunica media owing to atheroma	Massive haemorrhage into retroperitoneum and peritoneal cavity
Saccular (Fig. 11.5)	Cerebral arteries	Developmental defects in tunica media and elastic laminae	Subarachnoid haemorrhage
Microaneurysms	Brain, retina	Hypertensive and diabetic small vessel disease	Brain and retinal haemorrhages
Mycotic (infective) aneurysms	Any arterial vessels	Destruction of tunica media by infected thrombus	Haemorrhage from affected vessel
Syphilitic (Fig. 4.11)	Ascending aorta	Damaged tunica media owing to syphilitic arteritis	Massive haemorrhage into mediastinum and thoracic cavity

KEY TO FIGURES

A tunica adventitia   **AC** anterior cerebral artery   **Ad** adventitia   **C** communicating branch   **E** internal elastic lamina   **H** haematoma   **In** tunica intima   **M** tunica media   **S** saccular aneurysm   **W** wall of aneurysm

Fig. 11.5 Saccular aneurysm (Elastic van Gieson; LP)

Saccular (*berry*) aneurysms are a characteristic type of aneurysm found in the cerebral circulation, particularly at junctions in the circle of Willis or at bifurcations of the major cerebral arteries (especially the middle cerebral). Saccular aneurysms most often manifest in middle age by rupturing to cause subarachnoid haemorrhage. These aneurysms are, however, an occasional incidental finding at all ages and are often multiple.

This micrograph illustrates a saccular aneurysm **S** arising from the anterior cerebral artery **AC** just proximal to the point where it gives rise to its anterior communicating branch **C**. The vessel has a normal tunica media **M**, adventitia **Ad** and internal elastic lamina **E** (elastin stains black with this staining method). Note that at the point of origin of the aneurysm, the tunica media is deficient. The wall of the aneurysm **W** is composed of loose fibrous intimal tissue and the lumen contains blood. There is no medial muscle or elastin in the aneurysm wall.

Inflammation of vessels (vasculitis)

Inflammation of the walls of blood vessels may occur in arteries (*arteritis*), capillaries (*capillaritis*) or veins (*phlebitis, venulitis*); the collective term is *vasculitis*. The classification of this group of disorders reflects an increasing understanding of the underlying pathogenic mechanisms.

■ **Direct infection**: Some cases of vasculitis arise from direct infection of the blood vessel wall, for example *syphilitic aortitis* (see Fig. 4.11) and *Aspergillus* infection.

■ **Damage to vessels**: Vascular injury and resulting inflammation may be caused by direct damage to vessels, such as mechanical trauma and radiation injury.

■ **Immunological**: The most common types of vasculitis are caused by a variety of immunological mechanisms.

– The deposition of circulating immune complexes in the walls of blood vessels, as in **Henoch–Schönlein purpura** and **hepatitis B-related microscopic polyarteritis**.

– Direct damage to vessel walls by antibodies which react with endothelial cells (**Kawasaki's syndrome, systemic lupus erythematosus**) or glomerular basement membrane (**Goodpasture's syndrome**).

– Vasculitides associated with **antineutrophil cytoplasmic antibody (ANCA)** such as **Wegener's granulomatosis** and **microscopic polyarteritis** (Fig. 11.8).

■ **Idiopathic**: In a significant proportion of cases the pathogenesis is unknown. In **giant cell arteritis** (Fig. 11.6) and **Takayasu's arteritis** the underlying process may be an abnormality of cell-mediated immunity. Another major type of vasculitis, **classical** or **macroscopic polyarteritis nodosa** (Fig. 11.7), probably belongs to the immunological group, but its aetiology remains unclear.

Fig. 11.6 **Giant cell arteritis** **(a)** LP **(b)** HP **(c)** Elastic stain MP

Giant cell arteritis is the commonest systemic vasculitis in adults. In the majority of cases, the medium-sized arteries of the head are involved (hence the alternative name *temporal arteritis*), though involvement at other sites can occur, including the aorta. The pathogenesis is not known, with an immune-mediated reaction against the vessel wall believed to be responsible.

Histologically, multinucleated giant cells **G** are characteristic and tend to be arranged circumferentially, apparently in relation to degenerate fragments of the internal elastic lamina **E**. This is illustrated in micrographs (b) and (c). There is also an infiltrate of lymphocytes and plasma cells **C** in the vessel wall. Marked fibrous thickening **Fi** of the intimal layer, shown in micrograph (a), may be complicated by thrombosis, which may produce acute blindness if the ophthalmic artery is affected. Occasionally, the involvement can be focal and giant cells may be elusive.

Giant cell arteritis often presents as localised throbbing pain or tenderness over the temporal artery in patients over the age of 50. Alternatively, it presents as more generalised pain involving the muscles of the pelvic and shoulder girdles in the condition known as *polymyalgia rheumatica*. The diagnosis may be confirmed by temporal artery biopsy, although often treatment with immunosuppressive therapy (steroids) is commenced before biopsy because of the risk of ophthalmic artery involvement.

Fig. 11.7 **Polyarteritis nodosa** (MP)

Polyarteritis nodosa (PAN) is a systemic vasculitis affecting mainly medium and small muscular arteries of the kidneys, gut, heart, liver, peripheral nerves and brain. The typical features of an early lesion are shown in this high-power micrograph, where a segment of the vessel wall shows a necrotic area known as *fibrinoid necrosis* **Fn** associated with infiltration of the vessel wall with neutrophils. The lumen of the vessel contains fibrin thrombus **T**, giving rise to one of the common effects of vasculitis, namely ischaemia of the tissue supplied by the affected artery. In addition, the necrotic area of vessel wall may rupture during the healing phase when it is replaced by fibrous tissue, and a small aneurysm may form. These small aneurysms appear as nodules on the affected vessels, hence the term *nodosum*.

Apart from systemic symptoms such as fever, malaise, weakness and weight loss, the clinical presentation is extremely variable, depending on which tissues are involved. For example, kidney involvement may be manifest by pain, haematuria or proteinuria and heart involvement by angina, myocardial infarction or pericarditis. The disease is fatal if untreated, but in the vast majority of cases responds well to immunosuppressive therapy.

Fig. 11.8 Microscopic polyarteritis (MP)

Microscopic polyarteritis, also known as *leukocytoclastic vasculitis* or *hypersensitivity vasculitis*, arises in the context of an immune-mediated reaction to a wide range of precipitants, including drugs, tumour antigens and certain organisms. Typically, it is the smaller vessels that are affected, including arterioles, capillaries and venules, with involvement of the skin (where it causes palpable purpura), mucous membranes, kidneys, lungs and gastrointestinal tract. In contrast to PAN, microscopic polyarteritis causes haematuria, haemoptysis and bloody diarrhoea, rather than frank infarction or major haemorrhage.

This image of the skin shows the typical features of microscopic polyarteritis. Neutrophils infiltrate the vessel walls **V**, which also show fibrinoid necrosis, and nuclear dust **D** (fragmented neutrophil nuclei) is commonly seen, hence the term leukocytoclastic. Neutrophils, nuclear dust and haemorrhage **H** are seen in the surrounding dermis in this micrograph. As in any type of vasculitis, thrombosis of the affected vessels is common although it is not seen in this example.

Antineutrophil cytoplasmic antibody (ANCA) can be detected in the serum of approximately 70% of patients with microscopic polyarteritis. It is also found in most patients with a rare form of vasculitis called *Wegener's granulomatosis* and may somehow directly cause the damage to blood vessel walls.

Malformations and tumours of blood vessels

There are a variety of malformations and tumours which arise from vascular channels. The commonest among these are *haemangiomas*, often regarded as hamartomas or developmental abnormalities (Fig. 11.9). Clinically, benign vascular malformations in the brain are of importance as there is a risk of spontaneous intracerebral haemorrhage. Often, such malformations are composed of both arterial and venous channels and are termed *arteriovenous malformations* (Fig. 11.10).

True neoplasms arising from blood vessels are rare and range from the benign *glomus tumour (glomangioma*; Fig. 11.11) to more aggressive tumours such as *Kaposi's sarcoma* (Fig. 11.12) and *angiosarcoma* (Fig. 11.13).

Fig. 11.9 Haemangioma (MP)

Benign tumours of vascular tissues most commonly occur in the skin and liver but may occur in any tissue. Many are present at birth or soon after and may be considered as hamartomas or developmental disorders. Haemangiomas are usually divided into *capillary* or *cavernous* types, the former composed of small capillary-sized spaces, the latter mainly of large, dilated vascular spaces.

This micrograph shows a typical *cavernous haemangioma* of the liver at low power. In the bottom right-hand corner is normal liver parenchyma L. The upper left half shows the haemangioma consisting of large vascular spaces **S**, some of which contain blood. These are lined by essentially normal endothelial cells, in contrast to angiosarcoma (see Fig. 11.13), and separated by a fibrous stroma **Fs**. These tumours are common in the liver and are often found incidentally at autopsy or laparotomy.

KEY TO FIGURES

C lymphocytes and plasma cells   **D** nuclear dust   **E** internal elastic lamina   **Fi** fibrous thickening   **Fn** fibrinoid necrosis   **Fs** fibrous stroma   **G** giant cell   **H** haemorrhage   **L** liver parenchyma   **S** vascular space   **T** fibrin thrombus   **V** vessel wall

Fig. 11.10 Arteriovenous malformation (LP)

The brain is a clinically important site for vascular malformations, with symptoms related to local mass effect, causing compression of the surrounding brain tissue, and haemorrhage, which may be catastrophic. Commonest among the clinically significant vascular malformations encountered in the brain are arteriovenous malformations (AVMs). These lesions may arise anywhere in the vasculature of the CNS, but are most often associated with superficial branches of the middle cerebral artery.

Macroscopically, AVMs typically appear as a tangle of worm-like vascular channels of varying sizes arising from vessels in the subarachnoid space and extending into superficial brain parenchyma. Occasional examples located exclusively in brain parenchyma may occur.

Histologically, as in this micrograph, AVMs are composed of numerous variably sized vascular channels ranging from thick-walled, recognisable arterial channels **A,** with elastic fibres detectable on special stains, to thinner-walled, irregular venous channels **V.** Between these numerous vascular spaces is reactive brain parenchyma **B.** Often, this surrounding brain parenchyma contains evidence of previous haemorrhage in the form of macrophages containing haemosiderin pigment (not present in this field).

Fig. 11.11 Glomus tumour (glomangioma) (LP)

Glomus bodies are specialised arteriovenous anastomoses in the dermis which have a role in temperature regulation through shunting blood away from the skin surface when exposed to cold temperatures. Benign tumours arising from the specialised smooth muscle of these glomus bodies are known as glomus tumours or glomangiomas. Though benign, they can be exquisitely painful, particularly if the affected region is immersed in cold water.

Macroscopically, they appear as small, raised, red/purple lesions, most commonly on the digits, particularly under the fingernails. In this low-power micrograph it can be appreciated that this well-circumscribed tumour, centred on the dermis, is formed of numerous small vascular spaces **Vs** separated by a fibrous stroma **FS** within which the glomus cells lie. These cells are typically round to cuboidal in shape and arranged around the tumour vessels.

Fig. 11.12 Kaposi's sarcoma (HP)

Kaposi's sarcoma (KS) came to attention in the 1980s as an AIDS-defining illness. Subsequent investigations have identified *Human herpes virus 8 (HHV-8)*, also known as *KS-associated herpes virus*, as the aetiological agent in the vast majority of cases. Four variants are recognised: classical, immunosuppression/transplant-associated, endemic and AIDS-associated. Kaposi's sarcoma lesions are typically found on the skin as slightly raised, red/purple patches, though spread to other sites such as oral cavity, lymph nodes and gastrointestinal tract may occur. As noted above, KS emerged as an important AIDS-defining illness in the 1980s. However, with the introduction of highly active antiretroviral therapy (HAART), AIDS-associated KS is now rare.

A typical lesion, illustrated here, consists of sheets of plump stromal cells **S** interspersed with irregular, slit-like vascular spaces **Vs**. A brisk mixed inflammatory cell infiltrate is typically present. The tumour is seen here infiltrating subcutaneous fat **F**. Extravasation of red blood cells, not seen here, is common. *Bacillary angiomatosis*, caused by infection with *Bartonella quintana*, may appear very similar, except for the presence of numerous neutrophils and nuclear dust. This condition also occurs in AIDS patients, but can be cured by the antibiotic erythromycin.

Fig. 11.13 Angiosarcoma (HP)

Angiosarcomas are rare, occurring most frequently in the skin, soft tissues, breast and liver, with approximately 50% arising in the head and neck. Those in the liver are associated with known carcinogens including arsenic (in some pesticides), thorium dioxide (contrast agent) and vinyl chloride.

The typical appearance is of a raised, purple/red lesion on the face or scalp in the elderly. As the lesion enlarges, it may ulcerate and metastasise to local lymph nodes. On microscopy, angiosarcomas may display a variety of appearances ranging from tumours with numerous vascular spaces lined by plump, atypical endothelial cells to an undifferentiated spindle-celled tumour with few discernible vascular spaces.

In this example the malignant endothelial cells can be seen forming irregular branching vascular spaces **Vs** in some areas and solid sheets of cells **Sc** in other areas. Mitotic figures are common. The difference between these malignant endothelial cells and the benign endothelium lining vascular spaces in the haemangioma of the liver (Fig. 11.9) can be readily appreciated. Malignant tumours arising from the endothelium of the lymphatic system, *lymphangiosarcomas*, are usually similar in appearance except for the absence of blood in the vascular spaces.

KEY TO FIGURES

A arterial channel   **B** brain parenchyma   **F** fat   **FS** fibrous stroma   **S** stromal cells   **Sc** sheets of tumour cells
V venous channel   **Vs** vascular space

Ischaemic heart disease

Of the diseases involving the heart, ischaemic heart disease is the most important in developed countries. In almost all cases the cause of ischaemic heart disease is atherosclerosis of the coronary arteries, with or without accompanying thrombosis. Coronary artery atheroma and thrombosis are illustrated in Figures 8.5 and 8.6, and the stages of myocardial infarction are shown in Figure 10.2.

MYOCARDIAL INFARCTION

A common consequence of coronary artery disease, myocardial infarction is a leading cause of morbidity and mortality in developed countries. Typical symptoms are of central chest pain, often described as tight or pressing, which may radiate to the left arm or jaw. A variety of symptoms, including nausea, vomiting, breathless and sweating, often accompany this chest pain.

Clinical diagnosis of myocardial infarction rests on the demonstration of elevated levels of proteins released into the blood as a result of damaged mycocytes (**cardiac troponin** and/or **myocardial creatine kinase**) combined with at least one of:

■ symptoms of ischaemia

■ typical electrocardiographic changes

■ coronary artery intervention, such as angioplasty.

Treatment is directed towards establishing reperfusion of the ischaemic segment of myocardium as rapidly as possible to minimise the volume of infarcted tissue (see text box 'THROMBOLYSIS' Ch. 9). Complications of myocardial infarction include sudden death, arrhythmia, cardiac failure, ventricular rupture, rupture of papillary muscles with acute valve failure and mural thrombus with potential for thromboembolisation. These complications may arise in the immediate aftermath of the infarction (**acute-phase complications**) or may develop some time later.

Cardiomyopathy

The *cardiomyopathies* are disorders in which there is abnormal myocardial function without an obvious aetiology (a classification is shown in Figure 11.14). The term *secondary cardiomyopathy* is sometimes used to describe cases in which the cause of the myocardial disorder is recognised, for example amyloid deposition, viral myocarditis, alcohol and certain drugs or, rarely, muscular dystrophies. Though strictly speaking, by this definition, myocardial dysfunction as a consequence of chronic ischaemic heart disease should be considered separate from the cardiomyopathies, it is often referred to clinically as *ischaemic cardiomyopathy*.

The abnormalities usually cause progressive cardiac failure, but sudden cardiac death caused by acute dysrhythmia may be the first manifestation.

Fig. 11.14 **Classification and causes of cardiomyopathy**

Classification	Pathology	Aetiology
Dilated (congestive) cardiomyopathy	Defective myocardial contractility leading to atrophy and ventricular dilation and cardiac failure	Post-viral myocarditis (some), unknown (majority)
Hypertrophic (obstructive) cardiomyopathy	Gross hypertrophy of left ventricular wall (particularly interventricular septum) causing outflow obstruction	Autosomal dominant (majority), unknown (some)
Restrictive cardiomyopathy	Abnormal rigidity of myocardium restricts filling and contraction	Deposition of amyloid (some), unknown (majority)

Inflammation of the heart

Inflammation may affect the pericardium, myocardium or endocardium, either separately or concurrently. The causes are numerous, but the most common are ischaemia and infection. Most infections of the pericardium (*pericarditis*) and myocardium (*myocarditis*) are viral, whilst those of the endocardium (*endocarditis*) and valves (*valvulitis*) may be bacterial or fungal (Fig. 11.20).

The main causes of pericarditis are summarised in Figure 11.15. The histological features of most forms of acute pericarditis are virtually identical, whatever the cause, and are illustrated and discussed in Figure 2.4. In tuberculous pericarditis, there is a chronic granulomatous response as described in Chapter 4. In malignant pericarditis, clumps of tumour cells are often mixed with the inflammatory exudate.

The term myocarditis implies inflammatory damage to the myocardium and, by common usage, usually excludes the acute inflammatory reaction to necrotic muscle fibres seen in myocardial infarction (Fig. 10.2). Primary myocarditis can be associated with viral infections, rheumatic fever, and exposure to certain toxins and drugs. In some cases, no causative factor can be identified (*idiopathic myocarditis*).

Endocarditis and valvulitis involve not only inflammation, but also thrombus deposition on the endocardium and/or valves. These are important diseases and have a high mortality rate, their clinical manifestations often resulting from embolic phenomena or from dysfunction of the valves.

Fig. 11.15 Important causes of pericarditis

Myocardial infarction	After transmural myocardial infarction	Common
Cardiac surgery	After surgical opening of pericardial sac	Common
Viral infections	Usually young adults. Coxsackie B virus most common	Common
Malignancy	Local invasion or metastatic tumour deposits	Uncommon
Uraemia	Renal failure	Uncommon
Bacterial infections	Secondary to lung infection, including TB	Uncommon
Rheumatic fever	Part of rheumatic pancarditis	Rare

Fig. 11.16 Viral myocarditis (HP)

Myocarditis presents clinically with symptoms and signs reflecting inflammation or dysfunction of cardiac muscle. Hence, common presenting features include chest pain (stabbing in nature), tachycardia, arrhythmia, fever and cardiac failure. There are many causes, the commonest being as a consequence of viral infection, such as with Coxsackie A and B viruses. Other causes include bacteria, fungi, and immune-mediated reactions, such as in systemic lupus erythematosus or as a drug hypersensitivity reaction.

This micrograph illustrates the appearances of a florid viral myocarditis identified at autopsy. There is a prominent lymphocytic inflammatory cell infiltrate I coursing between myocytes M, many of which are pale, granular and necrotic.

KEY TO FIGURES
I inflammatory cells   M myocytes

Rheumatic fever is a systemic inflammatory disease which, in susceptible individuals, follows several weeks after a *group A β-haemolytic streptococcal* throat infection. The systemic manifestations represent a disordered immunological response resulting in inflammation of connective tissues. All parts of the body may be involved, for example the joints and skin, with painful short-term consequences. Involvement of the heart is of great clinical importance because of potentially fatal acute myocarditis and endocarditis and the long-term consequences of chronic scarring of the heart valves.

Fig. 11.17 Rheumatic carditis (HP)

The characteristic acute myocardial rheumatic lesion is the *Aschoff body* as shown in this image. The fully developed Aschoff body has a central, ill-defined area of degenerate material **D** surrounded by a mixed inflammatory cell infiltrate rich in T lymphocytes. Among these cells can often be seen a so-called *Anitschow myocyte* **A**, recognised by its irregular, ribbon-like nucleus and extensive eosinophilic cytoplasm. Despite the name, these cells are considered to represent large modified macrophages. Aschoff bodies are found in the interstitial connective tissue of the myocardium, particularly near vessels in the subepicardial fibrous tissue and (as in this example) in the subendocardial connective tissue.

Fig. 11.18 Acute rheumatic endocarditis (MP)

The importance of acute rheumatic endocarditis relates to involvement of the heart valves, where endocardial roughening induces formation of fibrin and platelet thrombi. This image illustrates part of a mitral valve leaflet affected by acute rheumatic endocarditis. A small thrombotic vegetation **V** has formed on the upper (atrial) surface of the valve leaflet at the site of the remnants of a large Aschoff body.

Chronic rheumatic valvular disease is the result of organisation and fibrous scarring of affected valves. This continues over many years with eventual thickening and distortion of the valve leaflets as well as the chordae tendineae. Such distortion commonly renders affected valves stenotic or incompetent.

KEY TO FIGURES

A Anitschow myocyte   **D** degenerate material   **L** valve leaflet   **T** thrombus   **V** thrombotic vegetation

Valvulitis (endocarditis of valves)

The heart valves may become subject to a variety of vegetative lesions which have traditionally been described as forms of **endocarditis**. The primary phenomenon underlying all these conditions is the formation of thrombus on the valve leaflets or cusps.

As in the arterial system, roughening of the endocardial surface predisposes to thrombus formation (Ch. 9). This may occur when valve leaflets or cusps have been previously damaged by rheumatic fever or are congenitally abnormal. Thrombus formation may also follow autoimmune valve damage in systemic lupus erythematosus (**Libman–Sacks endocarditis**) and in the acute phase of rheumatic fever (Fig. 11.18). The most frequent type of valve thrombus, however, occurs in so-called **marantic endocarditis** (Fig. 11.19), in which warty, thrombotic vegetations develop on mitral and aortic valves. This phenomenon occurs in seriously ill patients, often those with widely disseminated malignancy, and is usually associated with a hypercoagulable state. Despite use of the term endocarditis in these conditions, inflammation is usually not a feature of the valve at the time of thrombus formation.

True valvular inflammation may arise, however, if these thrombotic vegetations on valves then become infected with bacteria, fungi or other organisms, conditions collectively referred to as **infective endocarditis**. Bacterial endocarditis tends to be divided into two clinicopathological patterns. In the first, traditionally known as **subacute bacterial endocarditis**, the thrombotic vegetations develop on previously damaged valves, which then become colonised by bacteria of low virulence such as *Streptococcus viridans*. Such organisms tend to reach the valves via a transient bacteraemia, for example following dental extraction. The major clinical consequences are those resulting from detachment of small thrombotic emboli, often infected, into the systemic circulation.

In the second type of bacterial endocarditis, known traditionally as **acute bacterial endocarditis** (Fig. 11.20), thrombi form on previously normal valves and become infected by virulent organisms such as *Staphylococcus aureus*. In this case, the patient is usually already severely debilitated and septicaemic, for example from an infected urinary catheter, and the infecting organism is that which is responsible for the septicaemia. In contrast with the subacute pattern, in the acute form the fulminating infection extends into the substance of the valve, causing tissue necrosis. Rapid destruction of the valve leaflet leads to valvular incompetence, with acute cardiac failure as the usual clinical outcome.

Fungal endocarditis, formerly rare, is now appearing more commonly as a complication of immunosuppressive therapy, intravenous drug abuse or AIDS. *Candida albicans* (Fig. 4.15) is the most common organism.

Fig. 11.19 Marantic endocarditis (LP)

This image illustrates a mitral valve lesion of marantic (thrombotic, non-bacterial) endocarditis. Masses of thrombus **T** have developed on the superior surface of the valve leaflet **L**. Such thrombotic masses are only loosely attached to the underlying non-inflamed valve and are therefore readily detached, leading to major embolic consequences such as cerebral, renal and splenic infarction. In practice, this type of endocarditis is rarely diagnosed in life, but is a common autopsy finding.

Fig. 11.20 **Acute bacterial endocarditis** (HP) **(a)** H&E **(b)** Gram stain

This example of **acute bacterial endocarditis** is taken from a patient who presented with acute heart failure following bacterial destruction of his aortic valve. In image (a), the fibrous tissue comprising the valve is seen at the lower left and is infiltrated by sparse inflammatory cells **In**. In the upper right, there is a mass of eosinophilic fibrin **F** containing large colonies of purple-staining bacteria **B**, in this case *Streptococcus bovis*.

Image (b) is from the same specimen and is stained with the Gram stain. This demonstrates large quantities of Gram-positive, purple-staining streptococci embedded in the fibrin. This patient underwent an emergency aortic valve replacement and, with intravenous antibiotic treatment, made an excellent recovery.

Primary tumours of the heart

Whilst metastases to the pericardium and heart are not infrequent in the late stages of systemic malignancies, primary tumours of the heart are rare, the vast majority being benign. Of these, **myxomas** are the most common primary cardiac tumours occurring in adults (Fig. 11.21). In contrast, in children, the commonest primary tumours encountered are **rhabdomyomas**, which are often multiple, present in infancy and have a strong association with **tuberous sclerosis**. Other tumours which may arise in the heart include lipomas, fibromas and angiosarcomas.

Fig. 11.21 **Atrial myxoma** (HP)

Atrial myxomas are the commonest primary tumours of the heart, with the overwhelming majority arising in the atria, particularly the left atrium. The cell of origin of these benign tumours is not known. In large part they are sporadic, though in a small number (approximately 10%) they arise as a manifestation of the autosomal dominant **Carney complex**. Symptoms are rather non-specific, with 'flu-like' symptoms, outflow obstruction and embolic phenomena most common.

Macroscopically, myxomas appear as pedunculated, variably soft to firm masses, often arising in the region of the atrial septum. Histologically, they are formed of stellate tumour cells **S** and abnormal vascular channels **V** set in a myxoid matrix **M**.

KEY TO FIGURES
B bacteria   **F** fibrin   **In** inflammatory cells   **M** myxoid matrix   **S** stellate tumour cells   **V** abnormal vascular channel

Fig. 11.22 Chapter review

Disorder	Main features	Figure
Hypertension	Abnormally raised blood pressure	
Essential hypertension	Walls of small muscular arteries thickened. Hyaline arteriosclerosis in arterioles	11.1
Accelerated hypertension	Severe 'onion skin' thickening of tunica intima of small muscular arteries. Rapid proliferation of intima with accompanying fibrinoid necrosis	11.2
Aortic dissection	Most commonly thoracic aorta. Medial haematoma forms following laceration of intima. Almost all cases show cystic medial necrosis	11.3
Aneurysms	Variety of types summarised in Figure 11.4	11.4
Saccular (berry)	Develop from cerebral arteries. Manifest in middle age as common cause of non-traumatic subarachnoid haemorrhage	11.5
Vasculitis	Classified by presumed aetiology as direct spread of infection, direct trauma to vessel, immune mediated or idiopathic	
Giant cell arteritis	Commonest systemic vasculitis in adults. Most often involves medium-sized vessels of head and neck. Cause unknown. Inflammatory cell infiltrate in vessel wall, including multinucleated giant cells	11.6
Polyarteritis nodosa	Systemic vasculitis of small muscular arteries. Neutrophil-rich inflammatory cell infiltrate with associated fibrinoid necrosis of vessel wall. Small aneurysms may form in relation to weakened vessel wall	11.7
Microscopic polyarteritis	Immune-mediated reaction to variety of agents. Typically, neutrophil infiltrate in walls of small vessels	11.8
Tumours of blood vessels	Common forms benign. Rarer malignant forms	
Haemangioma	Benign tumour of vessels subdivided as capillary or cavernous depending on size of vascular channels	11.9
Arteriovenous malformation	Most often arise in association with superficial vessels of brain and may give rise to neurological symptoms and/or haemorrhage. Irregular vascular channels interspersed among reactive brain tissue	11.10
Glomus tumour	Small, painful, raised lesion most commonly on the digits	11.11
Kaposi's sarcoma	AIDS-defining lesion. Causative agent is HHV-8 in majority. Sheets of stromal cells interspersed with irregular vascular spaces	11.12
Angiosarcoma	Approximately 50% arise in head and neck. Malignant. May metastasise to local lymph nodes. Atypical endothelial cells to undifferentiated spindle cells with irregular vascular spaces	11.13
Ischaemic heart disease	See Chapter 8 (Atheroma) and Chapter 10 (Infarction)	
Cardiomyopathy	Myocardial dysfunction. Various causes, but may be idiopathic	11.14
Inflammation of the heart	May affect pericardium, myocardium, endocardium	
Pericarditis	Inflammation of pericardium. Variety of causes	11.15
Myocarditis	Most often a viral aetiology, but may be bacterial, immune mediated, drug related or idiopathic. Inflammatory cell infiltrate between myocytes with myocyte destruction	11.16
Rheumatic fever	Manifestation of systemic inflammatory disease following streptococcal throat infection. Rheumatic carditis – characteristic Aschoff bodies in myocardium, particularly subendocardial/subpericardial locations. Acute rheumatic endocarditis – inflammation of heart valves with formation of thrombotic vegetations	11.17 11.18
Marantic endocarditis	Non-bacterial endocarditis most commonly associated with systemic illness (e.g. disseminated malignancy). Friable, thrombotic vegetations form on valves	11.19
Acute bacterial endocarditis	Usually complicates systemic sepsis with virulent organism. Can arise on otherwise normal valve. Vegetation forms composed of fibrin containing colonies of causative organism	11.20
Cardiac tumours	Primary cardiac tumour rare, with majority benign	
Atrial myxoma	Benign tumour of unknown histogenesis. Small proportion autosomal dominant as part of Carney's complex. Stellate cells and atypical vascular spaces in a myxoid matrix	11.21

12 Respiratory system

Diseases of the nose, nasopharynx and larynx

Although viral infections (*coryza* – the common cold) and allergic inflammation (*allergic rhinitis* – hay fever) commonly affect the nose, nasal sinuses and nasopharynx, there are only a few conditions of general histopathological interest in the upper respiratory tract. *Nasal polyps* (Fig. 12.1) are a common sequel of prolonged or recurrent inflammation, particularly allergic inflammation. Malignant tumours of the nasal passages and sinuses are rare but *nasopharyngeal carcinoma* (Fig. 12.2) is of special interest because of its association with Epstein–Barr virus (EBV) infection.

The stratified squamous epithelium of the larynx may undergo hyperplastic or dysplastic change to form benign *squamous papillomas* or *invasive squamous cell carcinoma* (Fig. 12.3). Cigarette smoking and alcohol consumption predispose to the development of carcinoma of the larynx.

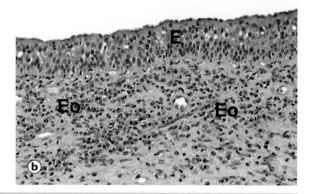

Fig. 12.1 Nasal polyp (a) LP (b) HP

Nasal polyps are a consequence of chronic inflammation of the nasal mucosa, commonly infective or allergic in nature. Simple polyps of this type are generally bilateral and the finding of unilateral involvement suggests alternative diagnoses. There is marked oedema and engorgement of mucosal connective tissue and infiltration by chronic inflammatory cells. Eosinophils are prominent in allergic rhinitis.

In the low-power view of a nasal polyp in micrograph (a), note the grossly oedematous stroma **S** and the stretched but otherwise relatively normal covering of respiratory-type epithelium **E**. As seen in micrograph (b), the connective tissue contains an inflammatory cell infiltrate in which eosinophils **Eo** and plasma cells predominate. Eosinophils are also present in the surface respiratory epithelium.

Fig. 12.2 Nasopharyngeal carcinoma (MP)

In the nasal cavities and nasopharynx, most malignant tumours take the form of *keratinising* or *non-keratinising squamous cell carcinoma*s or *undifferentiated carcinomas*. This undifferentiated group is associated with a dense, reactive lymphoid infiltrate in the stroma (the origin of the older term *lymphoepithelioma*).

In this micrograph, an undifferentiated nasopharyngeal carcinoma is shown. Note the island **I** of invasive carcinoma with surrounding lymphoid cells and overlying dysplastic epithelium **D**. The EBV genome can usually be identified in the epithelial cells of these tumours, as well as in many non-keratinising squamous cell carcinomas of the nasopharynx.

KEY TO FIGURES

B bone **D** dysplastic epithelium **E** epithelium **Eo** eosinophils **K** keratin pearl **I** island of carcinoma **S** stroma **Sq** squamous epithelium

Fig. 12.3 Carcinoma of the larynx (a) LP (b) MP

Squamous cell carcinomas form the vast majority of malignant tumours of the larynx, most commonly originating in the vocal cords (intrinsic), but also occasionally arising in epiglottis, aryepiglottic folds and piriform fossae (extrinsic carcinoma of larynx). Squamous carcinomas of the larynx are usually well differentiated and exhibit keratin pearl formation. Laryngeal carcinomas can usually be seen to arise from dysplastic surface epithelium.

Micrograph (a) shows a low-power view of a well-differentiated squamous carcinoma arising from the vocal cord. The section also shows part of the normal laryngeal wall including bone **B**.

At higher power in micrograph (b), it is possible to see occasional keratin pearls **K**. Normal stratified squamous epithelium **Sq** is seen at one edge, but dysplastic epithelium **D** overlies the main part of the tumour.

Inflammatory diseases of the airways and lungs

The trachea and bronchi may become acutely inflamed as a result of infections by viruses or pyogenic bacteria, causing *acute tracheobronchitis* (Fig. 12.4). Bacterial infections of airways are frequently complicated by extension of inflammation into the surrounding lung parenchyma to cause a pattern of lung infection known as *bronchopneumonia* (Fig. 12.5), a common cause of illness and death in the debilitated and elderly. Another pattern of bacterial lung infection is *lobar pneumonia* which involves a whole segment or lobe. In this setting, usually a more virulent bacterium, such as the pneumococcus (*S. pneumoniae*) is involved, and fit young people may be almost as susceptible as the elderly and debilitated. Lobar pneumonia illustrates many important principles of acute inflammation and the phenomenon of resolution and is discussed in Chapter 2 (see Figs 2.3 and 2.8). In contrast, *tuberculosis* and *sarcoidosis* are classical examples of specific chronic inflammations and are discussed fully in Chapters 3 and 4.

Recurrent or persistent suppurative bacterial infections of bronchi may lead to irreversible dilatation of airways with marked thickening and chronic inflammation of the walls, a condition known as *bronchiectasis* (see Fig. 3.4). Abscess formation in the lungs is a serious complication of certain pneumonias, particularly staphylococcal and *Klebsiella* pneumonias. Lung abscesses may also result from septic emboli causing infarction of the lung, from bronchiectasis, bronchial obstruction (e.g. by tumour or foreign body) or as a complication of pulmonary tuberculosis.

The term *chronic obstructive pulmonary disease (COPD)* refers to conditions characterised by chronic or recurrent obstruction of air flow and includes chronic bronchitis and emphysema. Recurrent episodes of acute bronchitis or persistent, non-infective irritation of bronchial mucosa (e.g. as a result of cigarette smoking) may produce *chronic bronchitis* (Fig. 12.7), which is frequently associated with persistent dilatation of air spaces and destruction of their walls, a condition known as *emphysema* (Fig. 12.6). *Asthma* (Fig. 12.8) is a disorder of the airways characterised by reversible bronchoconstriction, often provoked by allergens in susceptible individuals, but also triggered by physical agents or infection. There is also increased secretion of bronchial mucus, leading to plugging of the bronchial lumina.

The massive capillary bed of the lungs makes them vulnerable to a variety of haemodynamic and other vascular disorders. Left ventricular failure results in engorgement of pulmonary capillaries and fluid transudation into the alveolar spaces causing *pulmonary congestion* and *oedema* (Fig. 12.9). Two other common vascular disorders of great clinical importance are *pulmonary embolism* and its sequel *pulmonary infarction*, illustrated in Figures 9.4 and 10.4, respectively.

BASIC SYSTEMS PATHOLOGY ■ RESPIRATORY SYSTEM

Fig. 12.4 Acute purulent bronchitis (MP)

Bacterial infections of the upper respiratory tract (often following a transient viral infection) tend to spread down the respiratory tract where they may produce an acute, purulent *tracheobronchitis* and *bronchiolitis*. The mucosa of the airways becomes acutely inflamed and congested, and the smaller lobular bronchi and bronchioles become filled with purulent exudate **P** composed of protein-rich fluid and numerous neutrophils. Strips of necrotic epithelium are often shed into the pus. The inflammatory process inhibits ciliary activity but promotes secretion of mucus which, with the dead and dying neutrophils, pools in the airways and is coughed up as yellow-green sputum. In the early stages, the lung parenchyma is usually unaffected, but the alveolar spaces adjacent to the affected bronchioles often become filled with oedema fluid. In susceptible patients, this may then progress to *bronchopneumonia* (Fig. 12.5).

Fig. 12.5 Bronchopneumonia (MP)

Extension of bacterial infection from bronchioles into the surrounding lung parenchyma leads to a patchy pattern of purulent pneumonic consolidation known as bronchopneumonia. This is in contrast to the involvement from the outset of a whole lobe or lobule, as occurs in lobar pneumonia (see Fig. 2.3).

Each peribronchial focus of pneumonic consolidation has within it a small bronchus or bronchiole exhibiting the features of acute purulent bronchitis **P** (see Fig. 12.4). As each focus of bronchopneumonia expands, it tends to merge with adjacent foci until the consolidation becomes confluent.

Bronchopneumonia is a threat to the very young, the elderly or those debilitated by pre-existing illness, such as congestive cardiac failure or carcinomatosis, and is a very common terminal event. No single organism is responsible, but *Streptococcus pneumoniae* and *Haemophilus influenzae* are the most common.

KEY TO FIGURES
B bullae **G** mucinous glands **In** chronic inflammatory cells **M** mucosal smooth muscle **P** purulent exudate

Fig. 12.6 **Pulmonary emphysema** (a) Normal lung (LP) (b) Emphysematous lung (LP)

Emphysema is a condition characterised by permanent enlargement of the respiratory spaces distal to the terminal bronchioles, accompanied by destruction of their walls. Comparison with normal lung (shown in micrograph (a) at the same magnification) demonstrates the marked increase in alveolar volume and consequent reduction in area of alveolar wall available for gaseous exchange in emphysema (b). This problem is compounded by the loss of elastic 'guy rope' support which alveolar walls normally provide to the airways. As a result, the airways tend to collapse during expiration. Emphysema is often associated with recurrent or chronic infection of the airways (*chronic bronchitis*) and some degree of reversible airways obstruction caused by bronchospasm. In micrograph (b), two small subpleural bullae **B** are present. These are common in emphysema and may rupture into the pleural space causing a *pneumothorax* (the presence of air in the pleural cavity).

Fig. 12.7 **Chronic bronchitis** (a) Normal bronchial wall (MP) (b) Bronchial wall in chronic bronchitis (MP)

Chronic bronchitis is defined as excess sputum production on most days for at least 3 months in at least 2 consecutive years.

Although well defined as a clinical term, pathological changes in chronic bronchitis are variable and relatively non-specific. Chronic irritation of the bronchial mucosa, by tobacco smoke, atmospheric pollution or by repeated episodes of infection, induces chronic inflammatory and hyperplastic changes resulting in marked thickening of the bronchial wall. This feature is the main abnormality in cases of chronic bronchitis and is well illustrated in micrograph (b) compared to the normal bronchial wall shown in micrograph (a) at the same magnification. Three factors contribute to the increased thickness of the bronchial wall: infiltration of the submucosa by chronic inflammatory cells **In**, marked hypertrophy of mucosal smooth muscle **M** and marked hyperplasia of the mucinous glands **G** with the production of copious mucus.

In addition, the surface epithelium undergoes hyperplasia and often squamous metaplasia (not shown here). The consequent loss of ciliary activity then compounds the problem of excessive mucus production by destroying the 'mucociliary escalator', providing an ideal environment for superimposed bacterial infection.

BASIC SYSTEMS PATHOLOGY ■ RESPIRATORY SYSTEM

Fig. 12.8 Chronic asthma (MP)

Asthma is a common respiratory disorder characterised by instability of the smooth muscle of bronchial walls leading to *paroxysmal bronchoconstriction*. This results in diminution of airway diameter, causing marked resistance to air flow, particularly on expiration. Clinically, there is shortness of breath, wheezing and cough. There are several aetiological and trigger factors for bronchospasm, including IgE-mediated hypersensitivity reactions to allergens, bacterial or viral infections, exertion, changes in air temperature and non-allergic sensitivity to specific environmental agents (often through occupational exposure). In severe asthma, reduction in bronchial diameter has three components: bronchospasm, mucosal oedema and luminal occlusion due to excessive mucus production.

Single acute asthma attacks resolve with therapy, leaving no apparent structural disorder. In chronic asthma, as in this example, the bronchial walls become thickened via the process of *airway remodelling*. There is hypertrophy of smooth muscle **M**, hyperplasia of submucosal mucinous glands **G**, protracted oedema of submucosa and marked infiltration by eosinophils. The bronchial lumen becomes obstructed by mucus **Mu** containing numerous eosinophils.

Fig. 12.9 Pulmonary oedema (LP)

Any condition in which the left ventricle or atrium fails to empty adequately increases pressure in the affected chamber, which is transmitted back to the pulmonary venous system and pulmonary capillaries. The pulmonary capillaries become dilated and congested with erythrocytes and the increased hydrostatic pressure results in *transudation* of plasma fluid into the alveolar spaces, causing pulmonary oedema.

As progressive cardiac failure is a terminal event in many diseases, pulmonary congestion and oedema are common post-mortem findings. This condition also provides an ideal environment for the growth of pathogens of relatively low virulence, so superimposed bronchopneumonia is a common sequel (see Fig. 12.5). Chronic pulmonary congestion, for example owing to mitral stenosis, may result in numerous small intra-alveolar haemorrhages, followed by red cell lysis. Phagocytosis of released iron pigments, mainly haemosiderin, leads to the gross appearance known as *brown induration*.

Interstitial diseases of the lung

A wide range of pathogenic stimuli may cause interstitial lung inflammation, i.e. inflammation primarily involving the alveolar walls. This contrasts with the pneumonic or intra-alveolar inflammation seen in pneumonia.

Acute interstitial inflammation is often called *pneumonitis*. The clinical picture may be of catastrophic acute respiratory distress as seen in *adult respiratory distress syndrome (ARDS)* which has a wide range of causes, including viral and atypical pneumonias, shock, drugs and hypersensitivity reactions. Respiratory distress syndrome of premature infants (IRDS) is a similar phenomenon and both the adult and infant forms are characterised by the formation of hyaline membranes on the alveolar walls (Fig. 12.10).

At the chronic end of the spectrum, interstitial lung disease usually presents with the insidious onset of breathlessness secondary to *pulmonary fibrosis* (Fig. 12.11). The development of pulmonary fibrosis again may be due to a wide range of agents and may be preceded by an acute phase. The common causative factors are inorganic dusts such as silica, coal dust and asbestos, organic dusts such as mouldy hay in 'farmer's lung', and disorders of unknown cause such as *sarcoidosis* and *idiopathic pulmonary fibrosis* (see Fig. 3.6).

The disorders caused by inhalation of inorganic dusts are known as *pneumoconioses* and follow inhalation of mineral dusts (e.g. silica and asbestos), usually over a long period of industrial exposure, leading to fibrotic reactions in the lung. Inhalation of organic dusts (e.g. fungal spores and plant dusts) usually causes pulmonary fibrosis by the development of chronic allergic responses termed *extrinsic allergic alveolitis*.

The end result of these diseases is the development of interstitial fibrosis in the lungs. Pulmonary fibrosis of this type results in thickening of the barrier between blood and air, causing reduced gas transfer. As the disease progresses this may cause pulmonary hypertension and respiratory failure may develop. In most of these diseases, there are few clues to the causative agent when the fibrosis is well developed. Exceptions to this rule include *silicosis* (Fig. 12.12), which has a distinctive pattern of fibrosis, *asbestosis* (Fig. 12.13), where the presence of plentiful asbestos bodies is diagnostic, and *sarcoidosis*, where characteristic granulomas may be seen (Fig. 3.9).

Fig. 12.10 Hyaline membrane disease (HP)

At the very acute end of the spectrum of interstitial lung diseases, the histological appearances of the lung are characterised by the formation of '*hyaline membranes*' H, which represent accretions of protein and necrotic cell debris upon the alveolar surface of the alveolar walls **A**. The other name sometimes used for this condition is *diffuse alveolar damage (DAD)*. Characteristically, the alveolar walls are thickened, owing to a mixed inflammatory infiltrate, oedema, congestion of capillaries and haemorrhage. In combination with the hyaline membranes, this greatly inhibits gaseous exchange and results in respiratory failure. Occasionally, there are characteristic histological features of a particular aetiological agent, such as caseating granulomas in miliary TB (see Fig. 4.6) or nuclear inclusion bodies in Cytomegalovirus infection (see Fig. 4.13).

In most cases, the histological appearance is non-specific and a careful history is important in defining the cause. In premature infants (IRDS), the cause is a deficiency of pulmonary surfactant. In adults there is a wide variety of causes. This condition is often fatal, but may resolve completely with treatment or progress to pulmonary fibrosis.

Fig. 12.11 Pulmonary fibrosis (LP)

This condition may represent the end stage of acute diffuse alveolar damage or of subacute disease as in extrinsic allergic alveolitis. Often, however, the condition presents with insidious breathlessness and lung biopsy shows established pulmonary fibrosis. The alveolar walls **A** are markedly thickened due to the deposition of collagen. There is a variable chronic inflammatory infiltrate **In** consisting mainly of lymphocytes. In addition, the alveolar epithelium consists mainly of type 2 pneumocytes. When no aetiological factors can be established from the biopsy and careful recording of the clinical history, the condition is called *cryptogenic fibrosing alveolitis* or *idiopathic pulmonary fibrosis*. The histological pattern associated with this diagnosis is described as *usual interstitial pneumonitis*, as in this case. In other cases, there maybe distinctive histological features, such as granulomas in sarcoidosis and asbestos bodies in asbestosis. Some cases are associated with exposure to particular drugs, for example bleomycin-induced pulmonary fibrosis. In the late stages, the normal lung parenchyma may be densely fibrotic with macroscopically visible spaces. In this situation, it is known as *honeycomb lung*.

KEY TO FIGURES
A alveolar walls   **G** mucinous glands   **H** hyaline membranes   **In** inflammatory infiltrate   **M** smooth muscle   **Mu** mucus

Fig. 12.12 Silicosis (MP)

Silicosis is a form of pneumoconiosis which tends to occur in miners and others with industrial exposure to silica dusts. Initially, the inhaled silica particles are phagocytosed by macrophages which accumulate in clumps, very occasionally forming granuloma-like masses. The presence of silica-laden macrophages excites a vigorous focal fibrotic reaction, resulting in the formation of nodules of collagenous tissue. The centre of each focus becomes progressively acellular and hyaline **H** and is surrounded by a variable zone of more cellular fibrous tissue **F**, exhibiting a relatively sparse chronic inflammatory cell infiltrate in which black, carbon-laden macrophages abound. Usual histological methods do not reveal the presence of silica which can, however, be demonstrated as refractile particles by polarised light microscopy. As the process continues, the fibrotic nodules may coalesce, resulting in widespread pulmonary fibrosis.

Silicosis is the most common of the pneumoconioses. Other examples are asbestosis (Fig. 12.13) and berylliosis, in which the inhaled particles excite a giant cell granulomatous reaction similar to that seen in sarcoidosis (see Fig. 3.9).

All of the clinically significant inorganic dust diseases of the lung lead to progressive fibrosis with respiratory failure and diminished gaseous exchange. Disruption of the pulmonary microvasculature may lead to pulmonary hypertension.

Fig. 12.13 Asbestosis (a) HP (b) HP

Asbestos, a complex silicate, occurs in the form of long needle-like or serpentine fibres. The needle-like forms are more pathogenic and, when inhaled into the lung parenchyma, they become coated with proteinaceous material to form segmented *asbestos bodies*. The presence of asbestos fibres excites a macrophage and giant cell response which ultimately leads to fibrosis in a similar manner to that of silicosis (Fig. 12.12). The major fibrotic lesions initially occur in the subpleural zone of the lower lobes.

Micrograph (a) shows an alveolar space containing a giant cell **G** in which there are typical asbestos bodies **A**. The brownish colour of the asbestos bodies derives from the incorporation of haemosiderin in the proteinaceous coat. Micrograph (b) shows the beaded appearance of this encrusted iron at higher magnification, with a very fine central core representing the actual fibre.

Apart from its tendency to produce lung fibrosis, exposure to asbestos predisposes to neoplastic change. *Mesotheliomas* of the pleura (Fig. 12.21) and less often the peritoneum may occur many years after exposure to asbestos. This latent period often exceeds 20 years and so disease usually occurs in older patients, long after the period of industrial exposure. Asbestos exposure also greatly increases the risk of lung carcinomas, especially in cigarette smokers.

KEY TO FIGURES
A asbestos body   **F** fibrous tissue   **G** giant cell   **H** hyaline centre

Genuinely benign lung tumours are rare. Most 'bronchial adenomas' are in fact *carcinoid tumours*, arising from lung neuroendocrine cells. These may be locally invasive and occasionally metastasise. Their histological appearance is similar to that of carcinoid tumours in the gastrointestinal tract (see Fig. 13.13).

The great majority of primary malignant tumours of the lung are carcinomas which arise in the bronchi and are thus often called *bronchogenic carcinomas*. Carcinogens in cigarette smoke are the major aetiological agents. Other less important factors include exposure to radiation, asbestos (especially when combined with smoking), as well as other minerals such as nickel and chromium. Air pollution and genetic predisposition are other possible factors. Occasionally, tumours may arise in a pre-existing lung scar.

Bronchogenic carcinomas are of various histological types but in clinical and therapeutic terms, the most important distinction is between two broad groups: *small cell carcinoma* (Fig. 12.15) versus *non-small cell carcinomas*. The World Health Organization (WHO) classification of lung tumours further divides non-small cell lung carcinomas into several histological groups, including squamous cell carcinoma (Fig. 12.16), adenocarcinoma (Figs 12.17 and 12.18) and large cell carcinoma (Figs 12.19 and 12.20). There are further subtypes within some of these groups, but only common or important forms which are listed in Figure 12.14 are illustrated here. It should also be noted that mixtures of these tumour types occur quite commonly, most often in the form of adenosquamous carcinoma. Metastatic tumours, usually blood-borne from distant organs, are also very common in the lungs (see Fig. 7.19).

The pleura is the site of an uncommon but fatal tumour known as *malignant mesothelioma* (Fig. 12.21). Mesothelioma occurs almost exclusively in those exposed to asbestos.

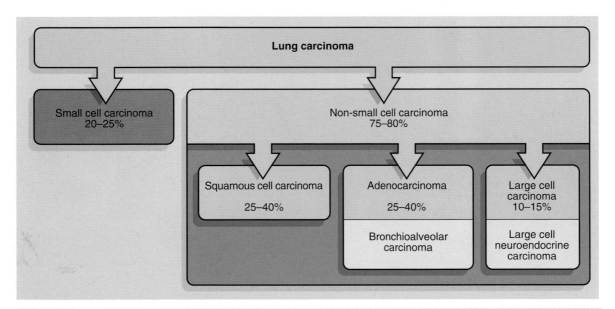

Fig. 12.14 **Relative frequencies and main histological subtypes of lung carcinoma**

For clinical purposes, the most important therapeutic distinction is between small cell and non-small cell carcinoma. The term non-small cell carcinoma encompasses large groups of tumours with different histological appearances but for which current therapy is similar. In general, small cell carcinoma is widely disseminated at the time of presentation and so it is treated primarily by systemic chemotherapy. In contrast, non-small cell tumours are more likely to be localised, so these are usually treated using combinations of surgery and radiotherapy in the first instance.

There is geographical variation, both in the incidence of lung cancer and also in the relative frequency of different histological types. This is reflected in the range of figures provided here for some tumour types. Lung adenocarcinoma is now more frequent than squamous carcinoma within the United States, but squamous carcinoma remains the most common diagnosis in Europe at present. It has been suggested that these trends may reflect changes in patterns of cigarette smoking, but further epidemiological study is required. Adenocarcinoma is less strongly associated with cigarette smoking and many of the lung cancers which occur in non-smokers are of this type.

DIAGNOSIS OF LUNG CARCINOMA

The diagnosis of lung carcinoma is usually first suspected due to symptoms such as weight loss, breathlessness and *haemoptysis*, often in patients who are cigarette smokers. Initial investigation typically involves obtaining a chest radiograph, followed by more detailed imaging using other modalities such as CT scanning. If a lung mass is identified, formal diagnosis is usually made on the basis of small amounts of material obtained by minimally invasive techniques, such as bronchoscopic biopsy or radiologically guided needle biopsy for peripherally situated lung masses. This is because management of lung carcinoma is highly dependent upon initial classification as small cell or non-small cell type. During bronchoscopy, samples for cytological examination are often obtained as well as small biopsies, because bronchial washings and brush cytology samples can allow retrieval of cells from sites which are not visible or accessible for biopsy. This means that cytological and histological techniques have complementary roles in the pathological diagnosis of lung cancer. Cytological preparations are illustrated here alongside the biopsy findings for comparison.

Fig. 12.15 **Small cell carcinoma** **(a)** Biopsy (HP) **(b)** Cytology (Papanicolaou stain) (HP)

Small cell carcinoma (or *oat cell carcinoma* as it is sometimes termed) is an important and highly malignant tumour which most commonly arises centrally within the lung. As seen at high magnification in micrograph (a), the name derives from the supposed resemblance of the small, tightly packed, darkly stained, ovoid tumour cells to oat grains. In areas, the cells appear crushed and there is brisk mitotic and apoptotic activity. In clinical practice, immunohistochemical staining is commonly used to confirm this diagnosis, revealing evidence of *neuroendocrine differentiation*.

These tumours rapidly and extensively invade the bronchial wall and surrounding parenchyma and may compress and invade nearby pulmonary veins. Early lymphatic and blood-borne spread is a feature of these tumours. Small cell tumours have the worst prognosis of all bronchogenic carcinomas because, although they are the most responsive to chemotherapy, they almost always relapse early.

Apart from their local and metastatic effects, these tumours may also secrete peptide hormones, such as anti-diuretic hormone and adrenocorticotrophic hormone (*ectopic hormone secretion*), giving rise to various *tumour-related endocrine syndromes*.

Micrograph (b) shows typical bronchial cytology from a case of small cell carcinoma. The tumour cells **T** have scant cytoplasm and hyperchromatic nuclei and typically show moulding of adjacent nuclei **M**. Nucleoli are inconspicuous. Some normal bronchial epithelial cells **E** are also present for comparison.

KEY TO FIGURES

B bronchus   **E** bronchial epithelial cells   **K** keratinisation   **In** tumour infiltration   **M** moulding of nuclei
T tumour cells

Fig. 12.16 Squamous cell carcinoma of bronchus
(a) Biopsy (LP) **(b)** Biopsy (MP)
(c) Cytology (Papanicolaou stain)
(HP)

Squamous cell carcinoma usually arises in the main bronchi or their larger branches, close to the lung hilum and often in an area of epithelium which has previously undergone *squamous metaplasia*, for example as a result of cigarette smoking. Bronchial mucosa adjacent to tumours frequently shows evidence of *squamous dysplasia*. Micrograph (a) shows a centrally arising carcinoma which protrudes into the lumen of a large bronchus **B** (*endobronchial*), as well as infiltrating **In** into the surrounding parenchyma. Eventually, such tumours tend to obstruct the involved airway as well as spreading via local lymphatics to regional lymph nodes. These tumours have the typical features of squamous cell carcinoma, but vary widely in degree of differentiation.

At one end of the spectrum is the well-differentiated keratinising type as illustrated in Figure 7.6, where the likeness to normal stratified squamous epithelium is evident and there is formation of keratin in areas. Micrograph (b) shows a moderately differentiated squamous cell carcinoma. There is no keratinisation in this example, but the tumour is still recognisably squamous, forming islands of large, eosinophilic cells with central whorling and with intercellular bridges (*desmosomes*) between the cells. At the other end of the spectrum are poorly differentiated tumours in which squamous characteristics, such as desmosomes, are difficult to identify and are seen only at high magnification (see Fig. 7.6). Some tumours arc so poorly differentiated that squamous features cannot be seen by light microscopy and these tumours are classified as *large cell undifferentiated carcinomas* (see Fig. 12.19).

Well-differentiated squamous cell carcinomas are readily identifiable using cytological methods. Image (c) shows numerous large, highly atypical squamous cells with evidence of cytoplasmic keratinisation. Keratin **K** appears orange in colour when stained by the Papanicolaou method. Comparison of these images with those of Figure 12.15 highlights the difference in cell size.

Fig. 12.17 **Adenocarcinoma of the lung** **(a)** Biopsy with H&E stain (MP) **(b)** Biopsy with staining for TTF-1 (MP) **(c)** Cytology (Papanicolaou stain) (HP)

Adenocarcinomas tend to arise more peripherally in the lung and have a particular predilection for old areas of scar tissue, such as healed tuberculosis. Adenocarcinoma of the lung is not as closely linked with cigarette smoking as other primary lung tumours.

The main histological feature of this type of tumour is the formation of a glandular pattern **G** by the tumour cells, the glands often being filled with mucus. The tumour excites a surrounding fibroblastic and inflammatory response.

Many different organs can give rise to adenocarcinoma and some of these may metastasise to lung, giving rise to similar histological appearances. Micrograph (b) illustrates the use of specific immunohistochemical staining for *thyroid transcription factor-1 (TTF-1)*.

This transcription factor (despite its name!) is important in the embryological development of lung tissue and is strongly expressed in the nuclei of most primary lung adenocarcinomas (as well as thyroid tissue). This can be useful in diagnostic practice.

In the cytological preparation shown in micrograph (c), note the groups of large adenocarcinoma cells **A** with prominent nucleoli. These contrast with occasional normal ciliated bronchial epithelial cells **E**. A few of the tumour cells include cytoplasmic vacuoles **V** containing mucin.

Very poorly differentiated variants of adenocarcinoma are included in the category of large cell undifferentiated carcinoma (see Fig. 12.19). Only electron microscopy can demonstrate the glandular origin of such tumours.

Fig. 12.18 **Bronchioloalveolar carcinoma** (MP)

This is an uncommon subtype of adenocarcinoma which may appear as a solitary, well-defined mass in the lung periphery on X-ray or, more commonly, as a diffuse infiltrate. The characteristic feature of this tumour is that malignant cells grow along the alveolar walls, as shown here. The alveolar epithelium on the right of the image is replaced by crowded, atypical cells with enlarged, hyperchromatic nuclei. The more normal alveolar walls on the left are somewhat fibrotic and inflamed.

Fig. 12.19 Large cell undifferentiated carcinoma (a) Biopsy (HP) (b) Cytology (HP)

Micrograph (a) shows a large cell undifferentiated carcinoma of the lung. As mentioned earlier, large cell undifferentiated carcinomas include extremely poorly differentiated squamous cell carcinomas and adenocarcinomas with no discernible features of squamous or glandular differentiation by light microscopy, although such features can be seen on electron microscopy. These tumours consist of large, anaplastic epithelial cells growing in islands and sheets. By definition, no evidence of keratinisation, intercellular bridges or intracytoplasmic mucin is seen.

Micrograph (b) shows large, undifferentiated malignant cells **C**. In contrast to those seen in the previous examples of squamous carcinoma and adenocarcinoma, these cells lack any evidence of specific differentiation. Normal ciliated bronchial epithelial cells **E** are present and there are scattered neutrophil polymorphs **NP**.

Fig. 12.20 Large cell neuroendocrine carcinoma (MP)

This is a highly malignant form of non-small cell lung carcinoma which shows evidence of *neuroendocrine differentiation*. The tumour cells are arranged in nests and islands and have abundant, rather granular cytoplasm. Central zones of necrosis **N** are also commonly seen and the tumour cell nuclei show peripheral *palisading* **P**. Immunohistochemical staining may be useful in confirming this diagnosis. Demonstrating neuroendocrine differentiation is important in planning therapy, since these patients may benefit from specific types of chemotherapy.

KEY TO FIGURES

A adenocarcinoma cells **C** undifferentiated malignant cells **E** bronchial epithelial cells **G** glandular formations
N necrosis **NP** neutrophil polymorphs **P** nuclear palisading **V** cytoplasmic vacuole

EFFUSIONS

An accumulation of fluid within the pleural cavity is termed *pleural effusion*. Similar collections of fluid can also occur within the other serous cavities, described as *ascites* within the peritoneal cavity or as *pericardial effusion* when within the pericardium.

Such collections of fluid are divided into two broad groups on the basis of their protein content. *Transudates* have a low protein content and their formation reflects altered hydrostatic or colloid osmotic pressures (*Starling forces*). Common causes include congestive cardiac failure and hypoalbuminaemia. In contrast, *exudates* have a high protein content and, in broad terms, are a result of damage to the integrity of the microvasculature, allowing leakage of plasma proteins across capillary walls. The causes of exudates are diverse but include infection, infarction, inflammation and malignancy.

Cytological examination of fluid from effusions is frequently used in clinical practice, often as a means of guiding further investigation. Malignant cells can be identified in such samples and the type of tumour can often be determined by a combination of morphological examination and use of immunostaining. Distinguishing carcinoma cells from reactive mesothelial cells and from malignant mesothelioma can be extremely challenging.

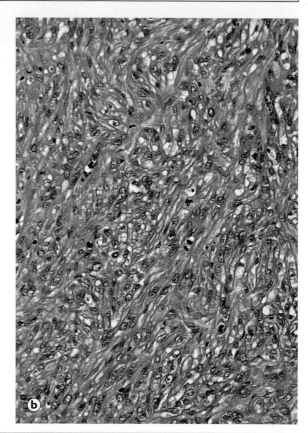

Fig. 12.21 Malignant mesothelioma of pleura (a) Epithelioid (HP) **(b)** Sarcomatoid (HP)

The pleura is frequently involved in secondary spread of tumours such as bronchial and breast carcinoma. Involvement of the pleura by tumour usually gives rise to a *pleural effusion* (see above).

Primary malignant tumours of the pleura, known as *mesotheliomas* because of their origin from mesothelial cells, are rare, but are of great interest since they are related to exposure to asbestos, often in the distant past. Even more rarely, mesotheliomas arise from the peritoneum and these are also often associated with a history of asbestos exposure.

Pleural mesothelioma forms a dense sheet of tumour over the pleural surface, often encasing the lung in a hard, white shell. Mesothelioma may extend into the lung parenchyma but more frequently, tumour invades through the tissues of the chest wall, often at sites of previous biopsy or chest drain insertion. Metastatic spread is uncommon.

Micrograph (a) shows pleura which is involved by a malignant mesothelioma with an *epithelioid* growth pattern. The tumour can be seen to involve the pleural surface **PS**, where it adopts a papillary architecture **P**, as well as infiltrating in a tubular, gland-like pattern **T**. This may be difficult to distinguish from metastatic adenocarcinoma. Most mesotheliomas have both epithelioid components and sarcomatoid spindle cell components. Mesotheliomas of this type are said to be *mixed* or *biphasic*. Occasionally, one pattern predominates. Image (b) shows a different area of the same tumour as illustrated in (a). In this field, the tumour is composed of plump spindle-shaped cells with no epithelioid elements. Both the epithelioid and spindle-cell components of this tumour exhibit the pleomorphism characteristic of malignancy.

KEY TO FIGURES
P papillary architecture   **PS** pleural surface   **T** tubular architecture

Fig. 12.22 Chapter review

Disorder	Main features	Figure
Nose, nasopharynx & larynx		
Nasal polyps	Oedematous, polypoid respiratory mucosa with vascular congestion, numerous eosinophils and plasma cells	12.1
Nasopharyngeal carcinoma	Various types, including keratinising squamous, non-keratinising squamous and undifferentiated carcinoma. EBV association	12.2
Laryngeal carcinoma	Mostly squamous and well differentiated, strongly associated with smoking and alcohol consumption	12.3
Inflammatory lung disease		
Acute purulent bronchitis	Purulent exudate within lumina of bronchi and bronchioles, some surrounding oedema in parenchyma	12.4
Bronchopneumonia	Extension of purulent material into alveolar spaces around bronchi, may become confluent (compare with lobar pneumonia, Fig. 2.3)	12.5
Emphysema	Abnormal permanent dilatation of airspaces with reduced alveolar area for gas exchange, peripheral bullae may form	12.6
Chronic bronchitis	Clinical definition. Histological changes include thickened bronchial wall due to inflammation, smooth muscle and bronchial gland hyperplasia	12.7
Asthma	Paroxysmal bronchoconstriction. No acute changes but, when chronic, smooth muscle hyperplasia, excess mucus and eosinophils	12.8
Pulmonary oedema	Alveolar spaces filled with fluid transudate due to altered Starling forces. Foci of alveolar haemorrhage with haemosiderin in macrophages	12.9
Interstitial lung disease		
Hyaline membrane disease	Result of diffuse alveolar damage (DAD). Fibrin within alveolar exudate forms hyaline membranes. May be fatal, resolve or progress to fibrosis	12.10
Pulmonary fibrosis	Deposition of collagen within alveolar walls, reducing gas exchange. Many causes, e.g. end stage of DAD and extrinsic allergic alveolitis	12.11
Silicosis	Inorganic dust deposition resulting in collagenous scars with hyaline centre and surrounding fibrosis. Silica visible on polarisation	12.12
Asbestosis	Complex silicate causing fibrosis in lower lobes, often subpleural. Asbestos bodies formed due to protein and iron encrustation	12.13
Tumours of lung and pleura		
Small cell carcinoma	Highly malignant but chemosensitive. Small cells with little cytoplasm showing nuclear moulding	12.15
Squamous cell carcinoma	Central tumours arising from squamous metaplasia and dysplasia. Endobronchial growth may cause obstruction	12.16
Adenocarcinoma	More often peripheral, some associated with scars. Glandular formations, often with mucin formation	12.17
Bronchioloalveolar carcinoma	Rare type of adenocarcinoma with spread along alveolar walls. May form mass or diffusely involve lung	12.18
Large cell undifferentiated carcinoma	No evidence of clear line of differentiation. Includes very poorly differentiated forms of squamous and adenocarcinoma	12.19
Large cell neuroendocrine carcinoma	Islands of large cells with zones of necrosis and granular cytoplasm. Confirm with immunostaining because of treatment implications	12.20
Malignant mesothelioma	Important association with asbestos. Epithelioid and spindle cell components. Spreads along pleural surfaces	12.21

13 Gastrointestinal system

Introduction

The alimentary system includes the mouth and its associated salivary glands, the oesophagus, stomach, small and large bowels, appendix and anus. The function of the alimentary tract is the ingestion, digestion and absorption of nutrients, along with the storage and expulsion of waste products. A wide range of congenital and acquired diseases may affect all parts of the tract.

Diseases of the oral tissues and salivary glands

The mouth and associated structures may be involved in a wide variety of disease states that may be loosely divided into three categories. First, many systemic diseases, particularly dermatological conditions, exhibit oral manifestations (e.g. lichen planus (see Fig. 21.7), syphilis (see Fig. 4.11)). Second, all oral tissues may be subject to acute or chronic inflammatory states, the most common being dental caries and its sequelae, periapical abscess formation and periodontal disease (i.e. inflammation of the gums). Of more general histopathological interest is inflammation of the salivary glands leading to chronic sialadenitis (Fig. 13.2). Third, many benign and malignant tumours may arise in the oral tissues, the most common being squamous cell carcinomas of the lips, oral mucosa and tongue (Fig. 13.1). A wide range of salivary tumours, both benign (Figs 13.3 and 13.4) and malignant (Figs 13.5 and 13.6), can arise in both major and minor salivary glands. A fascinating but fairly esoteric range of benign and malignant tumours arises in the jaws.

Fig. 13.1 Carcinoma of the tongue (LP)

Malignant tumours of the mucosa of the lips, tongue, cheeks and gums are almost invariably squamous cell carcinomas; they tend to be well differentiated and metastasise to regional lymph nodes (see also Fig. 7.6).

This micrograph illustrates a squamous carcinoma involving the tongue. The tumour has arisen from adjacent normal stratified squamous epithelium **Ep** and has deeply infiltrated the tongue. It exhibits keratin pearl formation **K**. These tumours are usually preceded by dysplasia of the epithelium (see Fig 7.1) that may be identifiable clinically as thickened or reddish patches of mucosa.

Fig. 13.2 Chronic sialadenitis (LP)

Prolonged obstruction of a large salivary gland duct by a calculus (*sialolith*) results in chronic inflammation and acinar atrophy in the gland, termed *chronic sialadenitis*.

This micrograph is from the submandibular gland, the gland most frequently involved. Two salivary duct branches **D** are dilated, with periductal fibrosis **F** and infiltration by lymphocytes and formation of lymphoid follicles **L**. The surrounding secretory acini **A** are markedly atrophic and the interstitial spaces have become expanded by fibrous tissue **F**.

INFLAMMATION OF THE SALIVARY GLANDS
Sialadenitis may also be caused by viral infections (most commonly mumps), bacterial infections (*Staph. aureus* and *Strep. viridans*), autoimmune disease (**Sjögren's syndrome**) and **sarcoidosis**, as well as other rarer causes. A dry mouth, due to dehydration, various drugs or Sjögren's syndrome, also predisposes to bacterial sialadenitis, as do calculi as mentioned above.

(a)

(b)

Fig. 13.3 **Pleomorphic adenoma of the salivary glands** **(a)** Typical pleomorphic form (MP) **(b)** Monomorphic variant (HP)

The most common salivary gland tumour is the **pleomorphic adenoma**, formerly known as **mixed salivary tumour**. The latter term was acquired from the histological appearance of columns and islands of benign epithelial cells, separated by loose myxoid connective tissue stroma in which areas resembling cartilage may be found.

Pleomorphic adenomas occur most commonly in the parotid gland. They are usually encapsulated but irregular in shape; in the parotid gland, this leads to difficulty in achieving total excision (bearing in mind the course of the facial nerve) and local recurrence can happen. Almost all pleomorphic adenomas are benign but, very rarely, malignant change may supervene after many years.

Micrograph (a) demonstrates the typical features of benign pleomorphic adenomas, namely a strongly staining neoplastic epithelial element with glands **G** and a pale blue-stained, loose connective tissue stroma **S**, somewhat resembling cartilage. Note that the tumour is circumscribed by a thin fibrous capsule **C**.

Much less commonly, salivary adenomas are entirely composed of the glandular epithelial component and contain none of the myxomatous stromal component which often dominates the picture in the typical pleomorphic salivary adenoma; this variant is described as a **monomorphic salivary adenoma** and an example is shown in micrograph (b).

KEY TO FIGURES
A acini   **C** capsule   **D** duct   **Ep** epithelium   **F** fibrosis/fibrous issue   **G** gland   **K** keratin pearl   **L** lymphoid follicle   **S** stroma

Fig. 13.4 Warthin's tumour (MP)

This unusual benign tumour occurs almost exclusively in and around the parotid gland; it commonly arises in middle-aged and older men and mostly in smokers.

The tumour, which is often cystic, is composed of large glandular acini **A** embedded in dense lymphoid tissue **L** in which typical germinal centres **GC** are often seen. The glandular element consists of a surface layer of tall columnar epithelium, rather resembling that of large salivary ducts, overlying a layer of cuboidal cells.

The histogenesis of this tumour is not understood but the glandular element may represent hamartomatous salivary duct tissue within lymph nodes in and around the parotid gland. Warthin's tumours are also known as *adenolymphomas* or *papillary cystadenoma lymphomatosum*, but the former may give an erroneous impression of malignancy and Warthin's tumour is the preferred term.

Fig 13.5 Mucoepidermoid carcinoma (MP)

Mucoepidermoid carcinoma is the most common malignant tumour of the salivary glands, but is still relatively rare, comprising about 15% of all salivary gland tumours. As the name indicates, the tumour consists of a mixture of squamous (epidermoid) **E** and glandular (muco) elements **M**. Intermediate cells with both squamous and glandular features can also be identified at higher magnification. These tumours most often occur in the parotid gland but may also arise in the minor salivary glands. They may be low, intermediate or high grade, the grade indicating the likely clinical course. Low-grade tumours pursue an indolent course with local invasion, whereas high-grade tumours are locally invasive and may metastasise to distant sites.

KEY TO FIGURES

A acinus **E** epidermoid (squamous) elements **F** fibrous stroma **GC** germinal centre **L** lymphoid tissue
M mucous (glandular) elements **S** spaces in tumour cell masses

Fig. 13.6 Adenoid cystic carcinoma (MP)

Another important malignant tumour of salivary tissue is the *adenoid cystic (adenocystic) carcinoma*. This tumour is seen most often in the submandibular and sublingual glands and also in the minor salivary glands. Histologically, it has a characteristic cribriform (sieve-like) appearance owing to the presence of small spaces **S** in a mass of tightly packed tumour cells. The tumour cells are arranged in clumps and cords, separated by a fibrous stroma **F** which may exhibit a marked degree of hyalinisation.

These tumours are locally invasive and prone to recurrence following surgical excision. Spread to regional lymph nodes is frequent and wide local spread is common, although the rate of growth is often slow. Perineural invasion, which is often extremely painful, is a common feature of this tumour.

Other malignant tumours of the salivary glands include acinic cell tumour, epithelial myoepithelial carcinoma and many others. As in almost every other tissue or organ in the body, always consider whether a mass lesion could be a metastasis from a primary malignant tumour at another site. Also, lymphoma can arise in or spread to almost any organ. The most common lymphoma arising in the salivary glands is of the MALT lymphoma type and usually occurs on a background of chronic inflammation.

Oesophageal diseases

Infections of the oesophagus are rare in healthy individuals, but in debilitated or immunosuppressed patients, infection with Herpes simplex virus (see Fig. 4.12) or *Candida albicans* (see Fig. 4.15) can occur. The lower oesophagus frequently becomes inflamed as a result of gastric acid reflux, producing either *oesophagitis* or sometimes *chronic peptic ulceration*, analogous to that seen in the stomach and duodenum (Figs 3.3 and 13.8). This condition is known as *gastro-oesophageal reflux disease (GORD* or *GERD*, depending on how you spell oesophagus). In response to reflux of acid, the squamous mucosa of the lower oesophagus may undergo metaplastic transformation into a form of glandular epithelium similar to that seen in the stomach or small intestine. This metaplastic condition is termed *Barrett's oesophagus* (Fig. 13.7).

CARCINOMA OF THE OESOPHAGUS

The most common oesophageal neoplasm used to be *squamous cell carcinoma*, which is similar to squamous cell carcinomas at other sites (see Figs 7.6 and 17.7). However, the incidence of *adenocarcinomas* arising in Barrett's oesophagus at the lower end of the oesophagus is increasing and comprises almost 50% of oesophageal carcinomas in developed countries. Both adenocarcinoma and squamous cell carcinoma of the oesophagus have a very poor prognosis. The lower oesophagus may also be involved by local spread of adenocarcinoma of the upper stomach.

Patients with long-standing GORD/GERD are at risk of developing adenocarcinoma of the oesophagus. The sequence of events appears to be oesophagitis → Barrett's oesophagus without dysplasia → low-grade dysplasia → high-grade dysplasia → invasive carcinoma. High-grade dysplasia is a premalignant condition and oesophagectomy often reveals coexisting superficially invasive carcinoma. Because of the grim prognosis of oesophageal carcinomas, Barrett's oesophagus is usually regularly monitored by endoscopy and biopsy. High-grade dysplasia and superficially invasive carcinomas can be locally resected or ablated by photodynamic therapy (PDT), laser therapy or other means before reaching an advanced stage.

Fig. 13.7 Barrett's oesophagus
(a) No dysplasia (LP) **(b)** Low-grade dysplasia (HP) **(c)** High-grade dysplasia (HP)

Micrograph (a) shows a longitudinal section of the lower oesophagus in which there is an abrupt transition from stratified squamous epithelium **S** to metaplastic glandular epithelium **G**. An infiltrate of lymphocytes and plasma cells with occasional lymphoid aggregates **L** is indicative of chronic inflammation which is commonly seen in this condition. The detail of the glandular epithelium cannot be seen at this magnification but it generally consists of a mucus-secreting glandular mucosa, similar to that seen in the cardia of the stomach. The goblet cells that characterise intestinal metaplasia are often found in a patchy distribution so that some biopsies may miss them. By definition, glandular epithelium found within the oesophagus (as opposed to within a hiatus hernia) is diagnostic of Barrett's oesophagus.

At high magnification in micrograph (b), glands with intestinal metaplasia **In** are seen as well as low-grade dysplasia. Low-grade dysplasia **LG**, with enlargement, crowding and disorganisation of the nuclei of the epithelial cells, can be difficult to differentiate from the reactive changes in inflamed mucosa. When a clear determination cannot be made, the biopsy is classified as *indefinite for dysplasia* to signal the need for follow-up and repeat biopsy. In micrograph (c), high-grade dysplasia **HG** is shown at high power. The pleomorphism and hyperchromasia of the epithelial cell nuclei is easily appreciated and there are prominent mitotic figures **M**. Again, intestinal metaplasia **In** is easily identified.

KEY TO FIGURES

G glandular mucosa **HG** high-grade dysplasia **In** intestinal metaplasia **L** lymphoid aggregate
LG low-grade dysplasia **M** mitotic figure **S** stratified squamous epithelium

Diseases of the stomach

Gastritis

Inflammation of the stomach is termed *gastritis* and may be divided into acute and chronic forms.

■ **Acute gastritis** may be associated with the use of aspirin or other non-steroidal anti-inflammatory drugs (NSAIDs). It also occurs with excessive alcohol consumption and in severely debilitated patients. It may present with nausea and vomiting but is also an important cause of haematemesis. Although not uncommon, acute gastritis rarely requires biopsy.

■ **Chronic gastritis** can be divided into distinct subtypes, each of which has particular histological features (Fig. 13.8):

– **Chronic infection**: *Helicobacter pylori* is the usual infective agent.

– **Chronic chemical gastritis** (also known as **reactive** or **reflux gastritis**) is associated with reflux of bile or alkaline duodenal secretions into the stomach, especially following surgical procedures, and with chronic alcohol consumption or with use of gastrotoxic drugs such as NSAIDs.

– **Chronic autoimmune gastritis** is associated with autoantibodies to various components of gastric parietal cells and with pernicious anaemia.

– Less common causes include *Crohn's disease, graft-versus-host disease* and *gastric outlet obstruction*.

Peptic ulceration

The histological details of chronic peptic ulceration in the stomach are described in Chapter 3 (see Fig. 3.3). Acid-induced necrosis of the gastric wall, the acute inflammatory response, organisation, granulation tissue formation, and fibrous scarring occur concurrently. *H. pylori* infection is almost always present in chronic duodenal ulceration and most cases of chronic gastric ulceration and must be eradicated for permanent healing. The outcome of this dynamic process depends on which is the dominant element, i.e. the damaging stimulus or the attempts of the body to heal the damage.

There are three main complications of chronic peptic ulceration:

■ **Perforation**: If tissue destruction outstrips attempts to confine or repair it, the process may extend rapidly through the wall, leading to perforation (Fig. 13.9).

■ **Haemorrhage**: Tissue necrosis may extend deeply enough to involve the wall of a large artery. This is most common in long-standing chronic gastric ulcers on the posterior wall, in the region of the left gastro-epiploic artery. This vessel tends to become incorporated in the fibrous scar on the serosal aspect of a chronic gastric ulcer and may then be eroded during a subsequent acute exacerbation of ulceration (Fig. 13.9). This may produce torrential haemorrhage, presenting as *haematemesis* and/or *melaena*, which may be fatal.

■ **Obstruction**: Persistent attempts at repair lead to progressive fibrous scarring which undergoes shrinkage and ultimately causes distortion and thickening of the wall of the viscus, commonly at the lower end of the oesophagus or in the pyloric region of the stomach. The narrowing may cause *stricture* formation with partial or even complete obstruction of the lumen. When the ulcerative process is still active, obstruction may be compounded by inflammatory oedema of the mucosa surrounding the ulcer.

Neoplasia

By far the most common malignant tumours of the stomach are *adenocarcinomas* (90–95%). These may assume a variety of gross morphological forms, including *malignant ulcers* with heaped-up edges, *fungating polypoid tumours* or *diffuse infiltration* of the wall *(linitis plastica)*, giving rise to the so-called 'leather bottle stomach'. Gastric adenocarcinomas are classified histologically as *intestinal type* (Fig. 13.11) or *diffuse type* (Fig. 13.12). *Gastric lymphoma* (see Fig. 16.8) and *carcinoid tumours* (Fig. 13.13) make up a small percentage of stomach malignancies. Both adenocarcinoma and gastric lymphoma are associated with *H. pylori* infection. Of the benign tumours, gastric adenomas comprise only a small proportion of gastric polyps, most of which are inflammatory or regenerative. Mesenchymal tumours occur in the stomach and other parts of the gastrointestinal tract including lipomas, leiomyomas and *gastrointestinal stromal tumours (GIST)* (Fig. 13.14), which are found mainly in the gastrointestinal tract; rare examples occur at other sites such as the mesentery, the retroperitoneum and the pelvis.

Fig. 13.8 **Chronic gastritis** **(a)** *H. pylori* infection (MP) **(b)** *H. pylori* infection (Cresyl violet) (HP) **(c)** Autoimmune gastritis (MP) **(d)** Chemical gastritis (MP)

Helicobacter pylori infection is the most common cause of chronic gastritis, typically affecting the mucosa of the gastric antrum, but extending to the body of the stomach in some cases (pangastritis). The histological features, as shown in micrograph (a), include a mixed inflammatory infiltrate in the lamina propria, with neutrophils, plasma cells, lymphocytes and eosinophils. Typically, neutrophils **N** are seen infiltrating the epithelium of the gastric glands: this is often described as ***active, chronic gastritis***, indicating a combination of acute and chronic inflammation. ***Intestinal metaplasia*** is quite common in association with this type of gastritis and it may lead to dysplasia (see Fig. 13.10). In intestinal metaplasia, the gastric epithelial cells are replaced with goblet cells and columnar absorptive cells typical of the small intestine. *H. pylori* organisms can sometimes be seen in routine H&E preparations but a range of special stains will highlight the organisms. The Cresyl violet stain shown in micrograph (b) at high magnification demonstrates the *H. pylori* organisms **H** in the mucous layer at the

surface of the epithelium. Bacterial invasion of the mucosa is not a feature.

In contrast, autoimmune-type chronic gastritis primarily affects the body of the stomach. As seen in micrograph (c) from the gastric body, the histological features include atrophy of the gastric glands with loss of parietal cells. The glands **G** are small and the mucosa is thinned. The lamina propria is infiltrated mainly with lymphocytes and plasma cells, and intestinal metaplasia **M** is a prominent feature. Chronic autoimmune gastritis in its late stages is often termed ***chronic atrophic gastritis***.

Chemical or reactive gastritis, as shown in micrograph (d), is characterised by inflammation of the superficial mucosa with a scanty infiltrate of inflammatory cells **In** (lymphocytes and plasma cells). The gastric glands show hyperplasia of the foveolae of the glands **Hy,** the part of the gland where cell division occurs, and characteristically the lamina propria is oedematous with marked vasodilatation **V.** Spurs of smooth muscle **S** branch from the muscularis mucosae into the lamina propria.

KEY TO FIGURES

A artery   **Ex** inflammatory exudate   **F** fibrous scar tissue   **G** glands   **H** *H. pylori* organisms
Hy foveolar hyperplasia   **In** inflammatory cells   **M** intestinal metaplasia   **MP** muscularis propria   **Mu** mucosa
N neutrophils   **S** smooth muscle spurs   **SM** submucosa   **V** vasodilatation

COMPLICATIONS OF CHRONIC GASTRITIS

Chronic gastritis is very common and, in untreated patients, was often associated with the development of peptic ulceration and its complications (see below). However the recognition and treatment of *H. pylori* infection, as well as the widespread use of **proton pump inhibitors (PPIs)** to reduce gastric acid secretion, has greatly changed the incidence of serious complications. Gastric adenocarcinoma, which is usually preceded by intestinal metaplasia and dysplasia (Figs 13.10–13.12) is known to have a strong association with *H. pylori* gastritis but may also occur with any other form of chronic gastric inflammation. *H. pylori* is also associated with gastric lymphoma (MALT lymphoma) (see Fig. 16.8).

Fig. 13.9 **Complications of peptic ulceration** **(a)** Perforated gastric ulcer (LP) **(b)** Bleeding gastric ulcer (LP)

Perforation of peptic ulcers has become less common with the advent of effective medical treatment for gastritis and peptic ulcer. It results in discharge of gastric contents into the peritoneal cavity with resulting *acute peritonitis*. In the perforated gastric ulcer shown in micrograph (a), tissue necrosis has extended through the full thickness of the wall, with complete destruction of the mucosa **Mu**, submucosa **SM** and muscle layers **MP**. Peritonitis is manifest by an acute inflammatory exudate **Ex** on the serosal surface of the stomach. The margins of the perforated ulcer are lined by necrotic tissue, beneath which is a zone of acute inflammation, similar to that found in the floor of a more chronic ulcer (see Fig. 3.3). There is no evidence of fibrous granulation tissue or fibrous scar since the destructive process has been too acute. Perforations such as this occur most commonly in peptic ulcers in the first part of the duodenum, but also occur in the stomach, as in this example.

Haemorrhage from erosion of a large artery in the base of an ulcer may occur in untreated chronic gastric ulcers as shown in micrograph (b). Note the eroded artery **A** trapped in the fibrous scar tissue **F** forming the floor of the ulcer. Part of the arterial wall is undergoing necrosis as a result of acid attack and massive haemorrhage will follow.

Fig. 13.10 Gastric dysplasia (LP)

Dysplasia is defined as an epithelial change with many similarities (morphological and molecular) to invasive carcinoma, but which does not breach the basement membrane of the epithelium. In the stomach dysplasia goes by many names, including *carcinoma in situ*, *non-invasive neoplasia*, *intraepithelial neoplasia*, *borderline lesions* and *category 4 lesions*, depending on which classification is in use. Dysplasia may arise in association with long-standing chronic gastritis of any type. Generally, the sequence of events seems to be gastric atrophy, intestinal metaplasia, low- then high-grade dysplasia and finally invasive carcinoma, usually of intestinal type. However, the individual steps in this progression remain to be elucidated.

This micrograph shows *high-grade dysplasia* D of the gastric mucosa, arising on a background of *intestinal metaplasia* I. There is marked irregularity of the glands with nuclear enlargement, hyperchromasia and crowding of the epithelial cells. There is little evidence of mucus production by epithelial cells and cellular polarity (basal alignment of nuclei) is completely lost. Note the similarity to dysplasia in Barrett's oesophagus (Fig. 13.7).

The importance of detecting gastric dysplasia is that treatment can prevent progression to gastric carcinoma.

Fig. 13.11 Gastric carcinoma: intestinal type (a) LP (b) MP

Gastric adenocarcinomas of the *intestinal type* are well or moderately differentiated and usually form a polypoid tumour mass or an ulcer with heaped-up edges. As mentioned above, this type of gastric carcinoma is usually preceded by gastric dysplasia and its precursors (Fig. 13.10). The low-power view in micrograph (a) shows irregular malignant glands G infiltrating the gastric wall beneath a dysplastic mucosa with focal intestinal metaplasia I. Deeper in the gastric wall in micrograph (b), malignant glands G can be seen infiltrating the muscularis propria M.

KEY TO FIGURES

D high-grade dysplasia   **E** neuroendocrine cell   **G** malignant glands   **I** intestinal metaplasia   **M** muscularis propria   **N** nucleus   **Ne** nest of tumour   **T** tumour cells   **Tr** trabeculae   **V** mucin vacuole

Fig. 13.12 **Gastric carcinoma: diffuse type** (a) MP (b) HP

Diffuse-type gastric carcinomas are poorly differentiated adenocarcinomas with little or no discernible gland formation. This pattern tends to take the form of a diffuse infiltration of the stomach wall starting as a flat localised area of infiltration, but in advanced cases giving rise to *linitis plastica* or *leather bottle stomach*. In micrograph (a), the tumour cells **T** can be seen forming a diffuse sheet infiltrating between bundles of smooth muscle in the muscularis propria **M**. At high power in micrograph

(b), the tumour includes many *signet ring cells*, so named because the cytoplasm is occupied by a mucin-filled vacuole **V** pushing the nucleus **N** to the periphery of the cell. If the tumour consists of more than 50% of signet ring cells overall, it is called a signet ring carcinoma. These tumours are generally more poorly differentiated than the intestinal type (Fig. 13.11). Some gastric carcinomas produce large amounts of extracellular mucin giving rise to *mucinous adenocarcinomas* (see Fig. 7.8).

GASTRIC CARCINOMA

There are large differences in the incidence of gastric cancer in different parts of the world. As well as different rates of *H. pylori* infection, the other major aetiologic factor appears to be diet and, in particular, high consumption of smoked and salted foods. Diffuse type carcinomas seem to have different risk factors and, unlike the intestinal type, are not thought to be associated with preceding inflammation, atrophy, metaplasia or dysplasia. Carcinoma of the stomach may be staged histologically as *early* or *late*, with early carcinomas infiltrating into the submucosa but not into the muscularis propria. Early gastric carcinomas have an excellent prognosis, in contrast to late gastric carcinomas.

Fig. 13.13 **Gastrointestinal carcinoid tumour** (a) H&E (MP) (b) Chromogranin (MP)

These tumours are found in the appendix, small intestine, rectum, stomach and colon in that order of frequency, and in many other sites such as pancreas and lung. The behaviour of carcinoid tumours ranges from benign to malignant, depending on site of tumour, size, depth of invasion into the wall of the gut and mitotic activity. They may secrete a variety of hormone products, such as *serotonin (5-HT)*, which may cause *carcinoid syndrome*.

In carcinoid tumours, the tumour cells form nests **Ne** and trabeculae **Tr** as in micrograph (a), glandular structures or diffuse sheets of cells. The cells are

characteristically small and uniform with round nuclei, stippled chromatin and pinkish granular cytoplasm. Immunoperoxidase staining will often reveal the hormone products within the cells, as in micrograph (b) of duodenal mucosa, where tumour cells **T** have been stained for *chromogranin A*, a protein associated with the secretory granules. Note also the positive staining of normal neuroendocrine cells **E** scattered in the adjacent normal duodenal epithelium. These are classified as a type of neuroendocrine tumour, a group which also includes small cell carcinoma (see Fig. 12.15).

Fig 13.14 **Gastrointestinal stromal tumour** (a) H&E (MP) (b) Immunohistochemistry for CD117 (MP)

Gastrointestinal stromal tumours (GISTs) are a specific type of mesenchymal tumour found mainly in the gastrointestinal tract. Previously, many of these tumours were misdiagnosed as leiomyomas, neurofibromas, Schwannomas and leiomyosarcomas. However, although instances of the above tumours do occur in the gastrointestinal tract, the majority of these tumours turn out to be GISTs. GISTs are thought to be derived from the interstitial cells of Cajal or a precursor cell. One of the key features of these tumours is that they are positive for *CD117* (c-kit) (>95%) and may also be positive for CD34, nestin and smooth muscle actin (SMA) by immunostaining.

They are composed of spindled, epithelioid or pleomorphic cells that may resemble smooth muscle or nerve sheath tumours. The cells may be arranged in fascicles, nests or sheets, with variable amounts of collagen in the stroma. Micrograph (a) shows a typical GIST with spindle cells **S** arranged in randomly orientated fascicles **F**. The histological features, however, can be very variable, and immunostaining for CD117 and CD34 is important to confirm the diagnosis. Positive immunostaining for CD117 in the same tumour is shown in micrograph (b).

MOLECULAR BIOLOGY AND SPECIFIC TREATMENTS FOR GISTs

GISTs have a wide spectrum of clinical behaviour. About a quarter of gastric GISTs and half of small intestinal GISTs are frankly malignant. The most useful pathological features that predict malignant behaviour are site, size of tumour and high mitotic rate. Most are treated by complete excision, but where this is not possible, treatment with a specific monoclonal antibody, imatinib is indicated. c-kit is a membrane receptor protein for stem cell factor. When stem cell factor binds to c-kit, it is activated and acts as a tyrosine kinase, an enzyme that activates other intracellular proteins by phosphorylation of the amino acid tyrosine. Mutations in c-kit lead to constitutive activation of this signalling pathway, resulting in cell proliferation and in time formation of tumours. Imatinib is a tyrosine kinase inhibitor, and so blocks the activity of the mutated c-kit protein. Most GISTs are responsive to imatinib initially, although with time many become resistant and so the tumour recurs. A small proportion of tumours have no c-kit mutation but have activating mutations in a very similar cell surface receptor/tyrosine kinase enzyme, called platelet-derived growth factor receptor-α (PDGFRα); this acts, and is treated, in the same way.

KEY TO FIGURES

C crypts **F** fascicle **In** inflammatory cells **L** intraepithelial lymphocytes **P** plasma cells **S** spindle cells
V villi

Inflammation of the small intestine due to self-limiting infections is very common but rarely biopsied. *Giardiasis* (see Fig. 4.19) is a common infective cause of inflammation in some countries and is often diagnosed on biopsy. Other inflammatory conditions affecting the small intestine include *coeliac disease* (Fig. 13.15) and *Crohn's disease* (Fig. 13.17). *Appendicitis* (Fig. 13.16) is extremely common and is a classical example of acute inflammation.

Primary tumours of the small intestine and appendix are very rare, with the exception of *carcinoid tumours* (Fig. 13.13) and *lymphomas*, which may be MALT lymphomas (see Fig. 16.8) or occasionally of Burkitt lymphoma type (see Fig. 16.9). Carcinoid tumours occur in the appendix, as do rare adenomas, similar in appearance to colonic adenomas. However, the anatomy of the appendix means that mucin-producing adenomas may produce enough mucin to distend the appendix and form a *mucocoele* or *mucinous cystadenoma*. Very rarely, these tumours may become malignant.

Fig. 13.15 Coeliac disease (gluten enteropathy)
(a) Normal jejunal mucosa (MP) **(b)** Atrophic jejunal mucosa (MP) **(c)** Atrophic jejunal mucosa (HP)

Hypersensitivity to gluten (a constituent of wheat, rye and barley) gives rise to *coeliac disease (gluten-sensitive enteropathy, coeliac sprue)*, a condition in which the patient's own immune system damages the small bowel mucosa. Clinically, this results in a malabsorption syndrome with very variable symptoms, including weight loss, anaemia and *steatorrhoea* (diarrhoea containing unabsorbed lipid) in severe cases.

The diagnosis is usually confirmed by endoscopic biopsy of the proximal small intestine. Micrograph (a) shows normal mucosa with villi **V** and short crypts **C**. In coeliac disease, as shown in micrograph (b), there is infiltration of the mucosa by inflammatory lymphocytes and plasma cells **In**, loss of villi (villous atrophy), and hyperplasia (elongation) of crypts **C**. The result is a flat small bowel mucosa. At high power, micrograph (c) shows the preponderance of plasma cells **P** in the lamina propria with the typical increase in *intraepithelial lymphocytes* **L**. These lymphocytes are mainly T cells and represent a cell-mediated immune reaction to gluten. Specific antibodies to various antigens are also a characteristic indication of a humoral component to the aberrant immune response.

DIAGNOSIS OF COELIAC DISEASE
The histological changes in coeliac disease are also found in a wide range of other disorders, including other infections such as *Giardia lamblia* (see Fig. 4.19) and allergies to other foods. The combination of serological tests (IgA antibodies specific for transglutaminase and endomysium) with biopsy features is significantly more specific for diagnosis. Change to a gluten-free diet results in eventual restoration of the normal villous mucosal pattern, which is also very helpful in confirming the diagnosis. Accurate diagnosis is important for correct treatment. Patients with coeliac disease are at risk of developing lymphoma and adenocarcinoma of the small bowel.

Fig. 13.16 **Acute appendicitis** (*caption opposite*)

KEY TO FIGURES

Ex fibrinopurulent exudate   **F** fibrinous exudate   **G** mucosal gland   **M** muscular layer   **Mu** smooth muscle fibres
N neutrophils   **Ne** necrosis   **P** pus   **S** serosa   **SM** submucosa   **U** ulceration

Fig. 13.16 Acute appendicitis (a) Early acute appendicitis (MP) (b) Later acute appendicitis (MP) (c) Established acute appendicitis (HP) (d) Gangrenous appendicitis (MP) *(illustrations opposite)*

Acute inflammation of the appendix is one of the most common surgical emergencies and is a typical example of acute inflammation (see Ch. 2). The earliest change, shown in micrograph (a), is ulceration of the mucosa **U** with an overlying acute fibrinopurulent inflammatory exudate **Ex** and pus **P** within the lumen. At this stage, the patient may experience vague central abdominal pain.

As the condition progresses, the inflammation spreads through all layers of the wall of the appendix and the mucosal ulceration becomes more extensive. This is illustrated in micrograph (b). Few of the original mucosal glands **G** now remain intact and large numbers of neutrophils have infiltrated through the submucosa **SM** and muscle layer **M** to the serosa **S**, where at one point a fibrinous exudate **F** is beginning to form on the peritoneal surface. This *peritonitis*, involving the parietal peritoneum in the right iliac fossa, is responsible for the classical clinical features of acute appendicitis, with localisation of the pain to the right iliac fossa. The peritoneal exudate often spreads to cover most of the serosal surface of the appendix and the mesoappendix, even though the

point at which the inflammation spreads through the appendix wall may remain localised. At high power, micrograph (c) shows the acute inflammatory infiltrate in the muscular layer of the wall of the appendix; the inflammatory infiltrate consists mainly of neutrophils **N**. The smooth muscle fibres **Mu** are separated by inflammatory oedema. Severe continuing inflammation of the appendix wall often leads to extensive necrosis of the muscle layer (*gangrenous appendicitis*) which predisposes to perforation of the appendix with more widespread peritonitis. This feature can be seen in micrograph (d) where the muscle layer **M** is identifiable up to a point where it has undergone necrosis **Ne**. Perforation of the appendix is imminent and will almost certainly take place at this site. The pus **P** that fills the lumen will then be discharged into the peritoneal cavity, leading to a more severe and extensive peritonitis which is infective. In the absence of appropriate treatment, the complications of perforation may ensue, including appendiceal abscess, subdiaphragmatic abscess, septicaemia, shock and death.

CHRONIC INFLAMMATORY BOWEL DISEASE

This term describes a group of conditions including *Crohn's disease* and *ulcerative colitis*. These are chronic inflammatory conditions of unknown aetiology with a typically relapsing course. Both conditions may lead to surgical removal of large parts of the bowel. Other conditions may mimic these two diseases, such as diverticulosis-related colitis, radiation colitis and ischaemic colitis. Infections, including TB, must also be ruled out before a diagnosis of chronic inflammatory bowel disease is made. Ulcerative colitis and Crohn's disease can occasionally be very difficult to differentiate from each other clinically and pathologically and often the distinction can only be made at the time of colectomy. Unlike ulcerative colitis, Crohn's disease may affect any part of the gastrointestinal tract, so the diagnostic difficulty only arises when disease is limited to the colon and rectum. In this situation, the term *indeterminate colitis* may be used until there is enough information for a definitive diagnosis; thus the term indeterminate colitis does not indicate a specific disease, only that there is idiopathic chronic inflammatory bowel disease that cannot yet be fully classified. The distinction is important as different treatment options are appropriate for the different conditions. Both ulcerative colitis and Crohn's disease may have extraintestinal manifestations, such as arthritis, sacroileitis and sclerosing cholangitis. Both may be associated with the development of adenocarcinoma of the bowel, but this risk is particularly high in long-standing ulcerative colitis.

Fig. 13.17 **Crohn's disease** **(a)** Fissured ulcer (MP) **(b)** Crohn's granuloma (HP)

Crohn's disease is a chronic inflammatory disease of unknown aetiology which mainly involves the small intestine, especially the terminal ileum, but which also often affects the large bowel and anus and occasionally the upper gastrointestinal tract. When it is restricted to the colon, it may be confused clinically with *ulcerative colitis* (see Fig. 13.19) and, in the anus, with anal fissures and fistulae. Crohn's disease is characteristically patchy in distribution, affecting short segments with lengths of normal bowel in between (*skip lesions*).

As shown in micrograph (a), the affected segments of intestine show gross thickening of the wall, mainly because of marked oedema and inflammation of the submucosa **SM**. This oedema produces the typical 'cobblestone' macroscopic appearance of the mucosa, in which domed areas of swollen mucosa and submucosa are criss-crossed by linear depressions caused by narrow *fissured ulcers*. A typical fissured ulcer **U** can be seen here. Fissured ulcers may extend into and even through the muscularis propria, giving

rise to *fistulae* (abnormal connections) between different parts of the bowel or between the bowel and bladder, vagina or even the skin surface. Micrograph (a) also demonstrates two other characteristic features of Crohn's disease. First, the chronic inflammatory changes are *transmural* (i.e. affecting all layers of the bowel wall). Second, non-caseating granulomas **G**, often containing giant cells, may be found in all layers. A granuloma in the submucosa is illustrated at higher magnification in micrograph (b). The granulomas in Crohn's disease resemble those seen in sarcoidosis (see Fig. 3.9). Granulomas such as these may also be found in lymph nodes draining the affected segment of bowel. The result of long-standing transmural inflammation is widespread fibrosis, which may cause the characteristic strictures seen in Crohn's disease, leading to bowel obstruction. Patients who have repeated operations to remove segments of small bowel may eventually develop short bowel syndrome, characterised by malabsorption and rapid intestinal transit time.

KEY TO FIGURES

C collagen band **G** granuloma **In** inflammatory infiltrate **L** lymphocytes **SM** submucosa **U** ulcer

Diseases of the large intestine

The colon and rectum are subject to various viral, bacterial and parasitic infections that are usually short-lived and readily diagnosed by microbiological methods; important exceptions are **amoebic colitis** (see Fig. 4.22), and various infections in immunosuppressed individuals, which are often diagnosed in biopsy specimens. Of great importance is chronic inflammatory bowel disease i.e. **ulcerative colitis** (Fig. 13.19) and **Crohn's disease**. Other causes of chronic diarrhoea include **microscopic colitis** (Fig. 13.18), radiation-induced colitis, ischaemic colitis and diverticulitis-associated colitis, among others.

Raised intraluminal pressure in the colon, probably as a result of a low-residue diet, may lead to saccular herniation of mucosa through the muscle layers of the bowel wall; the diverticula so formed may become inflamed, giving rise to **diverticulitis** (Fig. 13.20) which may have serious sequelae.

The large intestine may undergo infarction, either as a result of mesenteric artery occlusion by thrombus or embolus, or, more commonly, by venous infarction following hernial strangulation or **volvulus** (see Fig. 10.5).

Colonic polyps are very common. By far the most common is the **hyperplastic polyp** (Fig. 13.21). Less common, non-neoplastic polyps include **inflammatory pseudopolyps** as seen in ulcerative colitis (Fig. 13.19) and polypoid hamartomas such as **Peutz–Jeghers polyps**. Neoplastic benign polyps include **tubular adenomas**, **villous adenomas**, **tubulovillous adenomas** (Fig. 13.22) and **serrated adenomas** (Fig. 13.21), all of which have a definite risk of malignant transformation.

Malignant tumours of the colon and rectum are very common and almost all are **adenocarcinomas** (Fig. 13.23); most appear histologically moderately differentiated with a clearly defined glandular pattern. The anal canal, being lined by squamous epithelium, is occasionally the site of **squamous cell carcinoma**, identical to squamous cell carcinomas at other sites (see Fig. 7.6), although local invasion of the anal canal by adenocarcinoma of the lower rectum also occurs.

Fig. 13.18 Microscopic colitis (a) Collagenous colitis (HP) **(b)** Lymphocytic colitis (HP)

Microscopic colitis is the collective term for **collagenous** and **lymphocytic colitis**, conditions that typically cause watery, non-bloody diarrhoea with a normal-appearing bowel at colonoscopy. The two conditions have similarities but their exact relationship and aetiologies are unknown. There is a connection with autoimmune disease, and in particular coeliac disease, and also with certain drugs, including H_2-receptor antagonists and non-steroidal anti-inflammatory drugs (NSAIDs). **Collagenous colitis**, found mainly in middle-aged and elderly women, is shown in micrograph (a). It is characterised by a band of collagen **C** deposited immediately below the epithelial basement membrane. There is also inflammation **In** of the lamina propria with

occasional inflammatory cells and erythrocytes trapped within the collagen band. The surface epithelium contains increased numbers of intraepithelial lymphocytes **L**. The changes may be patchy throughout the colon and are generally least prominent in the distal colon and rectum.

Lymphocytic colitis, shown in micrograph (b), occurs in both men and women and generally affects the whole colon. Typically, there is a marked increase in intraepithelial lymphocytes **L** in both the surface epithelium and glands, with degenerative changes in the surface epithelium. There is also an inflammatory infiltrate **In** in the lamina propria. The changes are, in fact, similar to those of collagenous colitis, but without the collagen band.

Fig. 13.19 **Ulcerative colitis** (*caption opposite*)

KEY TO FIGURES
A crypt abscess **B** branched crypt **CM** circular muscle layer **D** diverticulum **G** colonic crypt or gland
L lymphoid tissue **LP** lamina propria **M** muscularis propria **P** Paneth cells

Fig. 13.19 Ulcerative colitis (a) Active disease with pseudopolyp formation (LP) **(b)** Acute disease (HP)
(c) Quiescent-phase disease (HP) *(illustrations opposite)*

Ulcerative colitis is a chronic relapsing inflammatory disease of unknown cause affecting the large bowel. The disease always involves the rectum but often extends proximally to involve the whole colon. It is sometimes accompanied by systemic features such as anaemia, arthritis and uveitis.

In active disease, there is acute inflammation of the mucosa with neutrophils accumulating in the lamina propria and in the lumina of the colonic glands (crypts) to form *crypt abscesses*; ulceration of the mucosa occurs, but the ulcers are superficial rather than fissured as in Crohn's disease (see Fig. 13.17).

In severe cases, ulceration may develop extensively throughout the length of the colon as shown in micrograph (a). Note that the ulcerative process has destroyed much of the mucosa and submucosa in this field, leaving isolated islands of non-ulcerated mucosa which is swollen by acute and chronic inflammatory changes; some of the colonic glands **G** remain. Non-ulcerated areas such as this project above the surrounding ulcerated areas to produce so-called *inflammatory pseudopolyps*. Despite the severity and extent of the inflammation and ulceration, the changes are mainly confined to the mucosa and submucosa. The muscularis propria **M** is not involved. The inflammatory changes are rarely transmural, a useful distinguishing feature from Crohn's disease.

Micrograph (b) illustrates features indicative of acute-on-chronic inflammatory activity, namely the presence of crypt abscesses **A** in the glands, depletion of mucus-containing goblet cells and the presence of neutrophils, as well as chronic inflammatory cells, in the lamina propria.

During quiescent periods between acute exacerbations, the mucosa damaged by earlier severe inflammation or ulceration shows mixed features of chronic inflammation and attempts at restitution. Micrograph (c) shows a mucosal biopsy taken during a quiescent phase. The lamina propria **LP** is infiltrated by lymphocytes, plasma cells and eosinophils. The colonic glands usually show reduction in the numbers of mucin-secreting goblet cells (although that is not a major feature in this example) and there is mild reactive change in the epithelial cells. The crypts are shortened and often branched **B**. Paneth cell metaplasia **P** may be seen.

Repeated episodes of inflammation, ulceration and epithelial regeneration may lead to dysplastic change in the constantly irritated epithelium. This factor may contribute to the high incidence of colonic adenocarcinoma arising in patients with a long history of ulcerative colitis.

Fig. 13.20 Diverticular disease (LP)

Diverticular disease is a common condition in the elderly which is often asymptomatic; it may involve any part of the colon, although the sigmoid colon is the most frequently and most severely affected part.

The normal muscular wall of the colon consists of an inner circular layer and a discontinuous outer longitudinal layer represented by the *taeniae coli*. Diverticula are formed by herniation of pouches of colonic mucosa **D**, including mucosal lymphoid tissue **L**, through unsupported areas of the circular muscle between the taeniae coli. The diverticula bulge towards the serosal surface and often contain faecal material. This probably results from abnormally high intraluminal pressure associated with low-residue diets and subsequent constipation. A characteristic histological feature is marked hypertrophy of the circular muscle layer **CM**.

Acute inflammation, *diverticulitis*, may develop following obstruction of the narrow neck of a diverticulum. Complications include acute haemorrhage, perforation, peritonitis, paracolic abscess formation and fistula formation with other viscera such as bladder and vagina. Diverticulosis-associated colitis may mimic ulcerative colitis but tends to be localised to the area adjacent to the openings of the diverticula.

Fig. 13.21 **Hyperplastic polyp and serrated adenoma** **(a)** Hyperplastic polyp (LP) **(b)** Hyperplastic polyp (HP) **(c)** Serrated adenoma (HP)

Hyperplastic (metaplastic) polyps are very common in the large bowel. They are usually small, often multiple and occasionally bleed. They may coexist with neoplastic polyps and malignant tumours but most do not themselves have malignant potential. An exception is the rare hereditary *hyperplastic polyposis syndrome*; these patients may develop invasive adenocarcinoma. At low magnification, micrograph (a) shows a typical hyperplastic polyp, composed of crypts with a characteristic 'sawtooth' outline **S**; this is also seen at medium power in (b). Apart from mild crowding, i.e. hyperplasia, the epithelial cells lining the crypts are very similar in appearance to normal colonic epithelium and exhibit no evidence of dysplasia. A related lesion, the *serrated adenoma* shown in micrograph (c), has a very similar sawtooth architecture but this is combined with cytological dysplasia ranging from low-grade (as in this micrograph) to high-grade. These polyps are associated with a significant risk of developing adenocarcinoma, which may also have a serrated architecture.

Fig. 13.22 **Colonic adenomatous polyps** **(a)** Tubular adenomas: polyposis coli (LP) **(b)** Villous adenoma (LP) **(c)** Tubulovillous adenoma (LP) **(d)** Villous adenoma (HP) *(illustrations opposite)*

Classical adenomatous polyps (as distinct from the serrated type) of the colonic mucosa are of three main histological patterns: *tubular adenoma*, *villous adenoma* and *tubulovillous adenoma*.

Tubular adenomas are by far the most common type and usually have a pedicle or stalk, the adenoma proper being connected to the mucosa by a narrow stalk of normal tissue. The adenoma consists of dysplastic colonic epithelium arranged in branched tubular glands. When seen with the naked eye, these tumours have a smooth or slightly bosselated surface. Tubular adenomas may be either solitary or multiple. In one heritable condition known as *familial adenomatous polyposis (FAP)*, numerous tubular adenomas develop throughout the colon with a high rate of progression to adenocarcinoma.

Micrograph (a) shows two tubular adenomas **T** in a segment of colon from a patient with FAP. Note the darkly stained adenomatous masses connected to the underlying mucosa by stalks, which merely represent extensions of the normal mucosa and submucosa.

Villous adenomas, which are much rarer, are usually sessile; that is to say they arise from a broad base. They are composed of narrow, frond-like outgrowths of epithelial cells supported by a delicate connective tissue stroma giving a papillary

appearance both histologically and with the naked eye. A typical sessile villous adenoma is illustrated in micrograph (b).

Tubulovillous adenomas exhibit intermediate features and contain at least 25–50% villous architecture. In the example shown in micrograph (c), note that the stalk is covered by normal colonic-type mucosa that contrasts markedly with the intensely staining dysplastic epithelium of the adenoma.

Cytologically, all three types of adenoma show varying degrees of dysplasia ranging from low to high grade (sometimes also called carcinoma in situ). Micrograph (d) shows a high-power view of low-grade dysplasia in a colonic villous adenoma. The cells are enlarged and crowded, with large pleomorphic nuclei, increased nuclear to cytoplasmic ratio, palisading of nuclei and increased mitotic figures.

By definition, adenomas exhibit no evidence of invasive carcinoma. However, although classified as benign, all adenomas have the potential to develop invasive adenocarcinoma. This occurs more frequently in villous adenomas than in the other types and is more likely with increasing size and high-grade dysplasia.

Fig. 13.22 **Colonic adenomatous polyps** (*caption opposite*)

KEY TO FIGURES
S sawtooth outline   **T** tubular adenoma

BASIC SYSTEMS PATHOLOGY ■ GASTROINTESTINAL SYSTEM

Fig. 13.23 **Adenocarcinoma of the colon** (*caption opposite*)

KEY TO FIGURES

F pericolic fat   **M** muscularis propria   **N** normal epithelium   **SM** submucosa   **T** tumour epithelium

Adenocarcinoma of the colon is a common malignant tumour, arising most frequently in the sigmoid colon and the rectum. There are three common macroscopic patterns of growth: tumours may consist of a central ulcer with raised margins, some tumours may infiltrate the entire circumference of the bowel forming an annular stricture or they may develop as a protuberant, cauliflower-like (exophytic) mass, most commonly seen in the caecum and proximal colon.

Micrograph (a) shows an ulcerated adenocarcinoma of the rectum; the tumour has infiltrated deeply through the submucosa SM, muscularis propria M and out into the pericolic fat F. Micrograph (b) shows the raised, everted edge of this tumour at higher magnification. There is an abrupt transition between normal rectal mucosa N and the malignant tumour epithelium **T**. In this area, the tumour has infiltrated into the submucosa SM, but not the muscularis propria M. Micrograph (c) shows a vein in the adventitial fat of the colon; it is filled with colonic adenocarcinoma which is growing along it as a solid cord.

The prognosis of colonic and rectal carcinomas depends on a number of factors, the most important being tumour stage as assessed by the depth of invasion of the bowel wall, the presence of lymph node and distant metastases and evidence of tumour invasion into veins and lymphatics.

Staging is vital for optimal management of all tumours. *Dukes' classification* has been in general use for staging colorectal carcinomas since 1932. This system, initially applied to rectal tumours only, divides tumours into three stages designated A to C. In *Dukes' stage A*, the tumour is confined to the bowel wall, if the tumour extends into the pericolic fat, it is classified as *Dukes' stage B* and the presence of metastases in lymph nodes automatically classifies it as *Dukes' stage C*. However, the more detailed TNM staging is often used in conjunction with or instead of the Dukes' classification. In addition, features such as grade, circumferential margin involvement, extramural vascular invasion and the number of positive lymph nodes are used to help determine whether additional chemotherapy is required following surgery.

MOLECULAR PATHWAYS TO COLORECTAL CARCINOMA

The recognition and investigation of various hereditary colorectal cancer syndromes such as *familial adenomatous polyposis (FAP)*, *non-polyposis hereditary colon cancer (NPHCC)* and *hyperplastic polyposis syndrome* has led to huge advances in the understanding of the development of adenocarcinoma in the large bowel. It has long been understood that adenomas may develop into adenocarcinomas through the stepwise accumulation of genetic mutations. In the case of typical adenomas, the first step seems to be the loss of both copies of the APC gene. Individuals with FAP already have one copy of this gene inactivated as a germline mutation (the 'first hit' according to Knudson's hypothesis – see Ch. 7); individuals with sporadic carcinomas must lose both copies to develop disease. Activation of the oncogene KRAS is also an early event, as is inactivation of p53. A second, more recently discovered, pathway is the *serrated pathway*. In this pathway, serrated adenomas with increasing degrees of dysplasia develop into invasive adenocarcinoma. Other characteristic features include increased DNA methylation and high levels of microsatellite instability (MSI-H) due to mutations in mismatch repair genes. This is a fast-advancing field and further pathways and subtypes of carcinoma are under investigation. Apart from the intrinsic fascination of these mechanisms, they may prove useful in determining optimal methods of treatment for different types of adenocarcinoma.

Fig. 13.24 Chapter review

Disorder	Clinical presentation	Main features	Figure
Mouth			
Squamous cell carcinoma	Non-healing ulcer	Nests of epithelial cells with eosinophilic cytoplasm, intercellular bridges, squamous pearls, keratinisation	13.1
Salivary glands			
Sialadenitis	Pain and swelling, especially after food if there is a calculus Mainly submandibular	Chronic inflammatory cell infiltrate, fibrosis, atrophy of gland tissue	13.2
Pleomorphic adenoma	Painless swelling, mainly parotid	Mixed epithelial and connective tissue components	13.3(a)
Monomorphic adenoma	Painless swelling, often male smokers, mainly parotid	Epithelial cells forming nests, trabeculae and glands	13.3(b)
Warthin's tumour	Painless swelling, may be cystic, almost exclusively parotid	Glandular element consisting of tall columnar cells with lymphoid tissue, including reactive germinal centres	13.4
Mucoepidermoid carcinoma	Painless swelling, usually parotid or minor glands	Mixed squamous and glandular (mucus-producing) components	13.5
Adenoid cystic carcinoma	Initial painless swelling, later nerve pain	Epithelial cells arranged in cribriform pattern with hyalinised, fibrotic stroma, perineural invasion common	13.6
Oesophagus			
Barrett's oesophagus	Heartburn	Metaplastic glandular (intestinal) epithelium at lower end of oesophagus	13.7(a)
Dysplasia	Heartburn	Atypical epithelial cells with pleomorphic nuclei, architectural distortion, increased mitotic activity	13.7(b),(c)
Carcinoma	Obstruction, dysphagia	May be squamous cell carcinoma or adenocarcinoma	Like 7.6 Like 13.11
Stomach			
Chronic gastritis – *H. pylori* associated	Dyspepsia, haemorrhage	Chronic inflammation of lamina propria with neutrophils infiltrating glands, *H. pylori* in surface mucus	13.8(a),(b), 3.3
Chronic gastritis – autoimmune type	Megaloblastic (macrocytic) anaemia	Atrophic body of stomach with reduction or absence of parietal cells, intestinal metaplasia	13.8(c)
Chronic gastritis – reflux or chemical type	Dyspepsia, haemorrhage	Foveolar hyperplasia of glands with saw tooth outline, minimal inflammation, smooth muscle bundles in lamina propria	13.8(d)
Peptic ulceration	Dyspepsia, haemorrhage, perforation	Discontinuity of epithelial surface with necrotic slough, granulation tissue and fibrosis lining the defect	13.9
Gastric dysplasia	Dyspepsia	Atypical epithelial cells with pleomorphic nuclei, architectural distortion, increased mitotic activity	13.10
Gastric carcinoma – intestinal type	Dyspepsia, weight loss abdominal pain, anaemia	Atypical invasive glands with atypical epithelial cells, mucus production	13.11
Gastric carcinoma – diffuse type	Dyspepsia, weight loss abdominal pain, anaemia	Malignant signet ring cells forming sheets with no gland formation (linitis plastica appearance)	13.12
Small intestine			
Coeliac disease	Anaemia, weight loss, steatorrhoea	Blunting/flattening of small bowel villi, increased lymphocytes and plasma cells in the lamina propria, increased intraepithelial lymphocytes, crypt hyperplasia	13.15
Giardiasis	Diarrhoea, steatorrhoea	Mucosa normal or inflamed with villous atrophy, sickle-shaped parasitic *Giardia lamblia* organisms on epithelial surface	4.19

CHAPTER 13

Fig. 13.24 Chapter review—cont'd

Disorder	Clinical presentation	Main features	Figure
Appendix			
Acute appendicitis	Right iliac fossa pain, fever, vomiting	Ulceration of mucosa, transmural acute inflammatory infiltrate	13.16
Enterobius vermicularis (pinworm)	Incidental finding	Pinworm sections seen within lumen of appendix	4.24
Large intestine			
Microscopic colitis (lymphocytic and collagenous colitis)	Watery, non-bloody diarrhoea with normal colonoscopy	Subtle inflammation of lamina propria, increased lymphocytes and apoptotic bodies in epithelium, subepithelial collagen band n collagenous subtype	13.18
Ulcerative colitis	Bloody diarrhoea, pain, fever, toxic megacolon	Inflammation and ulceration of mucosa, crypt abscesses, distortion of crypt architecture	13.19
Diverticular disease	Altered bowel habit, pain in left iliac fossa, rectal bleeding, often asymptomatic	Herniation of mucosa through muscularis propria with surrounding inflammation and fibrosis	13.20
Hyperplastic polyp	Incidental finding, bleeding	Polypoid glandular lesion with saw tooth architecture but no dysplasia	13.21(a).(h)
Serrated adenoma	Incidental finding, bleeding	Polypoid glandular lesion with saw tooth architecture and variable dysplasia	13.21(c)
Tubular adenoma	Incidental finding, bleeding	Polyp, usually with stalk, glandular architecture with variable dysplasia	13.22(a)
Villous adenoma	Incidental finding, bleeding	Polyp, usually sessile, villous architecture with variable dysplasia	13.22(b)
Tubulovillous adenoma	Incidental finding, bleeding	Polyp, glandular and villous architecture with variable dysplasia	13.22(c)
Adenocarcinoma	Haemorrhage, obstruction, anaemia	Invasive glands with atypical epithelial cells, mucus production, 'dirty' necrosis in lumina	13.23
Various sites throughout GI tract			
Gastrointestinal stromal tumour (GIST)	GI haemorrhage, mass lesion, incidental finding, usually stomach or small intestine	Mainly spindle cells in collagenous stroma, less commonly epithelioid or pleomorphic	13.14
Carcinoid tumour	Incidental finding, commonly appendix, or small bowel obstruction, rarely carcinoid syndrome	Small uniform cells with round nuclei, stippled chromatin and pinkish, granular cytoplasm	13.13
Crohn's disease	Diarrhoea, weight loss, obstruction, fistula formation, usually small bowel/colon but can affect mouth to anus	Transmural inflammation, granulomas, fibrosis, fissuring ulceration, skip lesions	13.17

14 Liver and pancreaticobiliary system

Disorders of the liver

The liver is affected by a wide range of disorders, the most important of which are listed below. The liver performs many different metabolic functions and so liver disease produces diverse clinical symptoms and signs. The pathophysiology of the more common symptoms and signs is described in Figure 14.1.

■ **Acute hepatic necrosis** has been described in Chapter 1. This usually results from exposure to certain drugs or poisons, or occurs as part of a fulminant viral infection.

■ **Acute hepatitis** has many causes. It may resolve or become persistent (*chronic hepatitis*).

■ **Chronic hepatitis** is diagnosed when biochemical manifestations of liver cell damage have persisted for more than 6 months. It may eventually progress to cirrhosis.

■ **Cirrhosis** is the end stage of various types of liver disease in which there is liver cell loss and architectural distortion over a long period. It is characterised by destruction of normal liver architecture which is replaced by regenerative nodules of hepatocytes, separated by bands of fibrous tissue. There may be evidence of continuing active damage to liver cells. Eventually, liver function is impaired or fails totally (*chronic liver failure*). The distortion of vascular architecture leads to *portal hypertension*. Various different types of cirrhosis are illustrated and discussed in Figure 14.7.

■ **Malignant disease** frequently involves the liver, most commonly as metastatic spread, especially from primary lesions in the gut, breast and lung (see Fig. 7.19). Less frequently, the liver becomes diffusely infiltrated in haematolymphoid malignancies such as Hodgkin and non-Hodgkin lymphomas.

■ **Primary malignancy** of the liver, *hepatocellular carcinoma* (Fig. 14.9), is uncommon and most often arises on a background of pre-existing cirrhosis.

■ **Right-sided cardiac failure** involves the liver when raised venous pressure is transmitted to the central hepatic venules, resulting in congestion of the sinusoids with blood. Hepatocytes in the centrilobular area (zone 3 of the liver acinus) may then undergo atrophy or even frank necrosis.

■ **Inborn errors of metabolism**, often reflecting single gene defects, can result in the abnormal accumulation of various metabolites within hepatocytes. These are known as *storage diseases* and include *glycogen storage diseases*, *mucopolysaccharidoses*, *lipidoses*, *haemochromatosis* (see Fig. 14.8) and *Wilson's disease*. Liver biopsy may be useful in the diagnosis of such disorders.

Fig. 14.1 Clinical features of hepatobiliary diseases and their pathophysiology

Sign/symptom	Clinical feature	Mechanism
Jaundice	Yellow colouration of tissues owing to bile pigments	Failure of metabolism or excretion of bile
Bleeding	Easy bruising and prolonged clotting time of blood	Failure of hepatic synthesis of clotting factors
Oedema	Swelling of dependent parts owing to extracellular accumulation of water	Failure of hepatic synthesis of albumin resulting in reduced plasma oncotic pressure
Ascites	Fluid in peritoneal cavity	Low serum albumin and portal hypertension
Gynaecomastia	Enlarged male breasts	Failure to detoxify endogenous oestrogens
Encephalopathy	Altered consciousness, lack of coordination, may lead to coma	Failure to detoxify ammonia and excitatory amino acids which result from protein breakdown
Haematemesis and/or melaena	Vomiting blood and/or passing blood	Bleeding from oesophageal varices or per rectum, owing to portal hypertension

KEY TO FIGURES
C Councilman body   **H** hydropic degeneration   **In** inflammatory cells

Acute inflammation of the liver

Hepatocytes, with their high degree of metabolic activity, are readily disturbed by toxins and demonstrate the histological cellular responses known as cloudy swelling, fatty change and necrosis, as described in Chapter 1. Acute inflammation of the liver parenchyma is usually marked by focal accumulation of inflammatory cells, usually in relation to necrotic hepatocytes. The exception to this is in the formation of *hepatic abscesses* which usually develop, either as a result of bacterial infections from the biliary tract or from a septic focus in the abdomen, drained by the portal venous system to the liver.

Acute hepatitis is a general term for inflammation of the liver parenchyma which can then be further classified according to aetiology. The four most important groups of conditions causing acute hepatitis are:

■ **Viral hepatitis**: This is illustrated in Figure 14.2 and its various subtypes are outlined in Figure 14.3.

■ **Toxins**: Alcohol is the most common hepatic toxin (Fig. 14.4).

■ **Drugs**: Hepatitis may be caused by the anaesthetic gas halothane, particularly after repeated exposure. Isoniazid, a drug commonly used in the treatment of tuberculosis, results in acute hepatitis in a small proportion of cases. Many other drugs occasionally cause acute hepatitis.

■ **Systemic infections**: Infections caused by *Leptospira* and *Toxoplasma* usually involve the liver as part of disseminated disease. Other systemic infections may cause multiple minute infective lesions, as in bacterial septicaemia and miliary tuberculosis.

Fig. 14.2 Acute viral hepatitis (HP)

The viral agents causing acute hepatitis all produce a similar histological picture in the acute phase.

There is widespread swelling and ballooning of hepatocytes owing to hydropic degeneration **H** and this progresses to focal or *spotty necrosis* throughout the lobule. The areas of necrosis are identified by aggregates of inflammatory cells **In** surrounding eosinophilic (pink-stained) bodies called *Councilman bodies* **C**, representing the cytoplasm of necrotic liver cells. The Kupffer cells are very active and, within portal tracts, there are increased numbers of chronic inflammatory cells (not illustrated here).

In time, regeneration of the dead hepatocytes occurs. In hepatitis A and E, complete resolution is the rule but, in hepatitis B, C and D, activity may persist or the disease may progress to chronic hepatitis (Fig. 14.5).

Rare cases of viral hepatitis occur in which there is massive liver necrosis instead of the focal type seen here. This is particularly seen with hepatitis E in pregnancy. Such fulminant cases are usually fatal.

Fig. 14.3 Viral causes of hepatitis

Virus type	Mode of transmission	Acute hepatitis	Chronic hepatitis	Chronic carrier	Notes
Hep A	Faecal–oral	Yes	No	No	Mild, self-limiting (rarely fulminant)
Hep B	Blood, saliva, semen	Yes	Yes	Yes	Transmission – needle sharing, sexual, transfusion
Hep C	Blood, saliva, semen	Yes	Yes	Yes	Transmission – needle sharing, sexual, transfusion
Hep D	Blood, saliva, semen	Yes	Yes	Yes	Only in association with hepatitis B
Hep E	Faecal–oral	Yes	No	No	Usually mild, self-limiting (rarely fulminant)

Fig. 14.4 **Alcoholic hepatitis** **(a)** MP **(b)** HP

Alcohol is a potent hepatotoxin when taken in large quantities and liver changes occur even after isolated bouts of heavy drinking. Early evidence of metabolic injury to the hepatocytes is the appearance of *steatosis* or *fatty change* **F**, manifest by the accumulation of lipid in the form of large cytoplasmic vacuoles within some hepatocytes, usually displacing the nucleus to one side (see also Fig. 1.6). With more severe metabolic disruption, the hepatocytes undergo hydropic degeneration (see Fig. 1.5) and become swollen and vacuolated, an appearance described as *ballooning degeneration* **B**. In some cases, the metabolic disruption may be irreversible and some hepatocytes undergo necrosis. The location of necrotic hepatocytes **N** is marked by foci of neutrophils and lymphocytes. Some hepatocytes accumulate an eosinophilic material, derived from cytokeratin intermediate filaments, termed *Mallory's hyaline* **H**. This is illustrated at high magnification in micrograph (b). This material forms irregular cytoplasmic globules, usually near the nucleus, and stains a glassy pink colour which is slightly darker than the normal cytoplasm. The hepatocytes around the centrilobular veins appear to be most vulnerable to alcohol toxicity and in some individuals delicate fibrosis may be seen around the central veins and perivenular hepatocytes.

With prolonged alcohol abuse, there is progressive fibrosis because of hepatocyte necrosis and regeneration of liver cells and this can develop into alcoholic cirrhosis (Fig. 14.7). Fatty change, alcoholic hepatitis and hepatic cirrhosis may all occur in the same individual. Some individuals develop recurrent alcoholic hepatitis and are likely to proceed to cirrhosis, whilst others may develop cirrhosis insidiously with no preceding episodes of acute hepatitis. Reversible fatty change may occur in a healthy individual after a single drinking binge. The presence of fatty change in a known alcoholic is an indicator of continuing alcohol intake.

NON-ALCOHOLIC FATTY LIVER DISEASE

This is a relatively common disorder which closely resembles alcoholic liver disease but which occurs in the absence of excessive alcohol intake. It is often diagnosed incidentally due to the discovery of deranged liver function tests upon routine blood testing. Patients may have no symptoms or clinical signs of liver disease at the time of diagnosis. It is thought that this process may account for a large proportion of patients who present with cirrhosis or end-stage liver disease without any preceding history of overt liver pathology (a pattern of disease often referred to as *cryptogenic cirrhosis*).

Of interest, epidemiological studies suggest that non-alcoholic fatty liver disease is very prevalent in Western populations and it is strongly associated with other common metabolic disorders such as obesity, dyslipidaemia, impaired glucose tolerance and non-insulin dependent diabetes mellitus. As with alcoholic liver disease, there is a spectrum of pathological changes from simple steatosis through *non-alcoholic steatohepatitis* (known as **NASH**) to eventual hepatic fibrosis and cirrhosis. Clearly, given the morphological similarity to alcohol-related liver disease, this diagnosis can only be made after correlation of the clinical and pathological findings.

Chronic hepatitis

When inflammation of the liver continues without improvement for 6 months or more, the condition is described as *chronic hepatitis*. Conventionally, this term excludes chronic inflammation of the liver caused by alcohol, bacterial agents and biliary obstruction. The main causes of chronic hepatitis are summarised below.

■ **Viral infection**
  – *Hepatitis B*: chronic hepatitis occurs in ~5–10% of cases (but ~80% if hepatitis D superinfection)
  – *Hepatitis C*: chronic hepatitis occurs in ~85% of cases
  – Other hepatitis viruses

■ **Autoimmune disease**
  – *Autoimmune hepatitis*
    • Usually occurs in middle-aged women
    • Positive serum autoantibodies (anti-nuclear antibodies, anti-smooth muscle antibodies)
    • Often associated with other autoimmune diseases, e.g. rheumatoid arthritis, thyroid disease
  – *Primary biliary cirrhosis*
    • Usually occurs in middle-aged women
    • Positive anti-mitochondrial antibodies in most patients
    • Autoimmune destruction of intrahepatic bile ducts
    • Despite name, cirrhosis occurs only with end-stage disease
  – *Primary sclerosing cholangitis*
    • Usually young or middle-aged, more common in men
    • Strongly associated with inflammatory bowel disease
    • Fibrous obliteration of intrahepatic and extrahepatic bile ducts

■ **Toxic/metabolic**
  – *Wilson's disease*: disorder of copper metabolism with CNS effects (*hepatolenticular degeneration*)
  – *α_1-antitrypsin deficiency*: protease inhibitor deficiency causing chronic lung and liver damage
  – *Drug-induced hepatitis*: many causes and various histological patterns.

Histologically, chronic hepatitis is characterised by:

■ the presence of inflammatory cells (mainly lymphocytes) in portal tracts or scattered within the liver lobules, or both

■ necrosis of hepatocytes, either concentrated upon the *limiting plate* of hepatocytes around the portal tracts (*interface hepatitis*, previously called *piecemeal necrosis*) or scattered within the liver lobules (*lobular hepatitis*, previously called *spotty necrosis*), or both

■ the presence of fibrosis, either in the portal tracts, or extending from the portal areas into the adjacent parenchyma as short septa, or forming 'bridges' across the lobular structure, causing architectural distortion

■ assessment of these features can be used to determine how active the disease is (*grade* of chronic hepatitis) and how far the disease has progressed (*stage* of disease). The general principles of grading and staging are outlined below.

STAGING AND GRADING OF CHRONIC HEPATITIS

Various scoring systems have been devised for grading and staging hepatitis. These aim to give information about appropriate treatment and likely disease prognosis. In this context, *grade* is used to reflect the severity of any ongoing inflammation or necrosis. The extent of such damage can be assessed within portal areas and within the liver lobule. When there is significant inflammation, drug treatment may be initiated to reduce continuing liver damage and to prevent the development of progressive disease with fibrosis.

Stage is a means of assessing the degree of damage to the connective tissue framework of the liver. Fibrosis tends to begin within the portal areas and fine septa then extend out into the parenchyma. Eventually, if disease continues to progress, bands of collagen form between adjacent portal tracts, dividing the liver parenchyma into distorted nodules and culminating in *cirrhosis.*

KEY TO FIGURES
B ballooning degeneration   **F** fatty change   **H** Mallory's hyaline   **N** necrosis

Fig. 14.5 **Chronic hepatitis** (a) LP (b) MP (c) HP (d) HP

Micrograph (a) shows inflammation confined to a portal tract. The periportal hepatocytes (called the *limiting plate* L) show no necrosis. Bile duct B, artery A and vein V are easily seen. This corresponds to low-grade disease. In contrast, micrograph (b) shows higher-grade disease. Inflammation and necrosis extend out from the portal tract to involve periportal hepatocytes P which show necrosis N. This pattern is described as *interface hepatitis*. In addition to changes around the portal tract, there is necrosis of individual hepatocytes in the liver lobule LN, a feature described as *lobular hepatitis*. This is shown in micrographs (b) and (c). Regeneration of liver cells may be seen, reflected in binucleate cells Bn or liver cell plates two cells wide. In more severe cases, liver cell necrosis and inflammation may become confluent

to form bands of *bridging necrosis* extending between adjacent portal tracts.

If disease progresses, there is fibrosis in the liver, with continued liver cell regeneration that ultimately leads to cirrhosis.

In chronic hepatitis caused by hepatitis B virus, the cytoplasm of hepatocytes may assume a pale pink, '*ground-glass*' appearance G, seen in micrograph (d), caused by accumulation of viral proteins. In hepatitis C infection, lymphoid follicles and focal fatty change may be clues to diagnosis.

Previous classifications have used the terms chronic persistent and chronic aggressive hepatitis. These are no longer used. Current classifications define chronic hepatitis in terms of aetiology and histological grade.

CHRONIC VIRAL HEPATITIS

On a global scale, chronic viral hepatitis is an important public health problem. Both hepatitis B and hepatitis C may give rise to symptomatic chronic hepatitis or to an asymptomatic carrier state. Normally, when hepatitis B is acquired in adulthood, the risk of chronic viral carriage is around 1–10%. In the developing world, transmission of hepatitis is commonly from mother to child (**vertical transmission**). This is important because when infection occurs at the time of childbirth, chronic carriage will occur in 90–95% of cases. These patients may develop chronic liver fibrosis with eventual cirrhosis. Cirrhosis is a major risk factor for the development of **hepatocellular carcinoma** and, in some areas where hepatitis B infection is highly prevalent, hepatocellular carcinoma (a rare tumour in most Western countries) is the most common form of malignancy.

KEY TO FIGURES

A artery   **B** bile duct   **Bn** binucleate cell   **C** chronic inflammation   **D** bile ductules   **F** fibrosis
G ground glass hepatocytes   **Gr** granuloma   **L** limiting plate   **LN** lobular necrosis   **N** necrosis
P periportal hepatocytes   **V** vein

Fig. 14.6 **Primary biliary cirrhosis** **(a)** Early lesion (MP) **(b)** Granuloma (HP) **(c)** Later lesion (MP)

Primary biliary cirrhosis is a chronic inflammatory disease of the liver in which destructive inflammatory changes are centred primarily on bile ducts. The earliest changes are seen in the epithelium of the larger bile ducts **B** as shown in micrograph (a). There is vacuolation of the epithelial cells and infiltration of the wall and surrounding tissues by lymphocytes. A characteristic feature at this stage is the formation of *granulomas* **Gr** in relation to damaged bile ducts, illustrated in micrograph (b). Portal tracts then become expanded by chronic inflammatory cells **C**.

As seen in micrograph (c), the inflammatory cells extend from the portal tracts into the liver parenchyma, resulting in *interface hepatitis* (previously called *piecemeal necrosis*), occurring along the limiting plate in a manner similar to chronic hepatitis (Fig. 14.5). As liver cells are destroyed, the portal tracts also become expanded by fibrosis **F**. Large bile ducts are no longer visible, having been destroyed. At the periphery of the portal tracts, there is proliferation of small bile ductules **D** which do not appear to be canalised. This feature is best seen in micrograph (a).

If primary biliary cirrhosis proceeds unchecked, true cirrhosis develops (Fig. 14.7). Note that this disease is referred to as primary biliary cirrhosis even in its earlier stages when there is no evidence of cirrhotic change.

Fig. 14.7 **Cirrhosis** (*caption opposite*)

KEY TO FIGURES
F fibrous tissue   **In** inflammation   **N** nodules   **P** portal areas

Fig. 14.7 **Cirrhosis** **(a)** Alcoholic cirrhosis (MP) **(b)** Cryptogenic cirrhosis (MP) **(c)** Cryptogenic cirrhosis (van Gieson stain) (MP) **(d)** Cirrhosis due to progressive chronic hepatitis (MP) (*illustrations opposite*)

Cirrhosis is the end result of continued damage to liver cells from a great many causes. It is characterised by wholesale disruption of the liver architecture, with the formation of nodules of regenerating liver cells separated by fibrous bands. There are two main effects of this altered liver architecture and cellular damage, namely disordered hepatocyte function (Fig. 14.1) and disturbance of blood flow through the liver from portal vein to hepatic vein.

The effect of vascular obstruction within the liver is an increase in portal venous pressure termed ***portal hypertension***. Anastomoses open up between the portal circulation and the systemic venous system, resulting in large, dilated veins called *varices*. The most important site of varices is in the lower oesophagus, but they can occur elsewhere. These dilated thin-walled veins are liable to rupture and this is a common fatal event in patients with cirrhosis.

The classification of cirrhosis is based on the disease which caused the underlying liver damage. The most important causes are chronic alcohol abuse, chronic hepatitis and biliary cirrhosis (primary and secondary to obstruction). In a small percentage of cases no underlying disease can be found. This is known as ***cryptogenic cirrhosis*** (see text box on non-alcoholic fatty liver disease).

The diagnosis of cirrhosis is confirmed by percutaneous liver biopsy. Histological examination is directed towards identifying the nature of any underlying disease process, as well as establishing evidence of cirrhosis.

In micrograph (a), the features of cirrhosis are broad fibrous bands **F** connecting portal areas **P** and intervening nodules **N** of liver cells showing marked fatty change. This is an example of alcoholic cirrhosis.

Micrograph (b) shows a typical cirrhotic pattern, with bands of fibrous tissue **F** disrupting the lobular architecture. Here, there is no inflammation, fatty change or specific features. If there are also no clinical pointers to the aetiology, this is classified as cryptogenic cirrhosis. Micrograph (c) is from the same case, this time stained using the van Gieson method, which emphasises the fibrosis (stained red).

Cirrhosis following progressive chronic hepatitis is illustrated in micrograph (d). The portal tracts **P** contain large numbers of chronic inflammatory cells, and in some areas these inflammatory cells spill over the limiting plate into nodules of hepatocytes. There are also focal areas of inflammation **In** in the liver parenchyma. The portal tracts show evidence of fibrosis and fibrous bands **F** containing chronic inflammatory cells have formed bridges between adjacent portal areas. These features are characteristically seen in the more active forms of chronic hepatitis (see Fig. 14.5).

Once fibrous tissue has been deposited, cirrhosis has traditionally been viewed as a virtually irreversible process, but there is emerging evidence that, in some cases, treatment which achieves control of the underlying liver disease may result in some restitution of the liver architecture. Repeated liver biopsy can be used to monitor progress.

Older classifications of cirrhosis grouped the diseases according to the size of the regenerative nodules seen at post-mortem or laparotomy. In ***macronodular cirrhosis***, large nodules up to several centimetres in diameter are present. ***Micronodular cirrhosis*** is characterised by small and uniform regenerative nodules, up to 1 cm in diameter. Whilst it is useful to describe macroscopic features, this classification does not help in assessing disease type or progression. In active cirrhosis as seen in micrograph (d), there is evidence of continuing damage to liver cells, whereas in inactive cirrhosis there is no evidence of continuing liver damage.

Fig. 14.8 **Haemochromatosis (Perls' stain)** (MP)

Haemochromatosis is a condition characterised by excessive deposition of iron in the tissues. It is due to an inherited defect of iron transport, such that excessive iron is absorbed from a normal diet. Pathologically, excessive iron is deposited in many tissues, especially myocardium, liver, adrenal glands, pancreas and synovial joints. Hepatic involvement causes cirrhosis. As seen in this micrograph, liver cells accumulate enormous amounts of iron which are stained blue by Perls' stain. Excessive iron may also be stored in the liver in conditions where frequent blood transfusion is required. This is termed *secondary haemosiderosis*.

CLINICAL FEATURES OF IRON OVERLOAD

Genetic haemochromatosis is an autosomal recessive disorder which occurs due to a single amino acid substitution within the protein encoded by the HFE gene. Clinical presentation tends to be earlier in men than in women because normal menstrual blood loss in premenopausal females reduces the extent of iron deposition within the tissues and so exerts a degree of physiological control. The diagnosis may be first suspected from deranged liver function tests, but other clinical signs include skin pigmentation and the development of diabetes mellitus due to chronic pancreatic damage. These features gave rise to the old clinical description of haemochromatosis as **bronzed diabetes**, a term which serves as a useful *aide memoire*.

Fig. 14.9 **Hepatocellular carcinoma** (a) MP (b) HP (c) HP

In developed countries, primary carcinoma of the liver is a relatively uncommon condition compared to metastatic tumours from other sites. On a worldwide basis, the incidence of **hepatocellular carcinoma** (often confusingly called **hepatoma**) is closely related to the prevalence of hepatitis B virus infection and, in some parts of Africa, it accounts for up to 40% of all cancers. In Europe and the USA, it accounts for only around 2%. Cirrhosis from any cause also predisposes to the development of hepatocellular carcinoma. These tumours are associated with rapid clinical progression and average survival from diagnosis is only around 6 months.

The tumour may form a single massive nodule, multiple small nodules, or exhibit a diffuse infiltrating pattern. Micrograph (a) shows normal hepatocytes **H** on the left and malignant hepatocytes **T** on the right.

Sometimes, poorly differentiated tumours form irregular duct-like structures **D** as shown in micrograph (b) and may resemble metastatic adenocarcinoma. In this situation, immunohistochemical staining may be helpful (see below).

In contrast, very well-differentiated hepatocellular carcinomas may produce well-formed ducts **D** and even secrete bile **B** as shown in image (c).

Alpha-fetoprotein (AFP) is secreted by a large proportion of hepatocellular carcinomas and is a useful tumour marker.

METASTATIC TUMOUR IN THE LIVER

The liver is very commonly affected by metastatic malignant tumours, particularly metastatic carcinomas. For this reason, **staging** of most newly diagnosed malignant tumours involves biochemical testing of liver function, as well as careful radiological assessment to identify any evidence of tumour deposits. When such tests do reveal mass lesions, percutaneous liver biopsy may sometimes be undertaken to confirm the diagnosis histologically. More often, liver biopsy is used when a patient is found to have multiple tumour deposits in the liver but without any known primary site of tumour. In this setting, the pathologist plays a vital role in confirming the diagnosis of malignancy and in investigating the likely site of origin of the tumour.

The pathological examination of a liver biopsy which is obtained from a mass lesion begins with assessment of a routine H&E-stained section to confirm whether the biopsy has successfully targeted the tumour mass. If tumour is present, it is then necessary to decide whether it could be a primary liver tumour, either a hepatocellular carcinoma or possibly a benign liver lesion such as a haemangioma (see Fig. 11.9). If it is a metastatic malignant tumour, then it is necessary to determine the type of tumour, e.g. carcinoma, melanoma, lymphoma, etc. Immunohistochemical staining is useful but is always guided by the histological appearance on H&E staining.

Metastatic adenocarcinoma is very common and immunostaining can help to distinguish likely sites of origin such as colon, lung, breast etc. This allows the pathologist to direct further investigation of the patient. Sometimes, confirming a diagnosis in this way is sufficient to guide further management, allowing immediate treatment of the tumour with appropriate chemotherapy and avoiding the need for further biopsy.

Cholestasis is the term applied to accumulation of bile within the liver. This is illustrated in Figure 14.10. Gallbladder disease is a common surgical problem in developed countries and is often associated with stone formation and chronic obstruction of the cystic duct leading to *chronic cholecystitis* (Fig. 14.11). *Cholesterolosis* describes the deposition of cholesterol and other lipids within the lamina propria of the gallbladder. This is commonly seen in cholecystectomy specimens and is illustrated in Figure 14.12. Tumours of the biliary system are relatively rare and usually take the form of highly malignant adenocarcinomas (Fig. 14.13).

Fig. 14.10 Cholestasis (HP)

Cholestasis, or accumulation of bile within the liver, is a consequence of obstruction to bile flow. This may occur in the extrahepatic biliary tree (most commonly as a result of gallstones), in the intrahepatic biliary tree because of destruction of bile ducts (as in primary biliary cirrhosis) or at the level of the hepatocytes, owing to failure to secrete bile. The last is a common feature of liver cell damage from any cause or may be a reaction to certain drugs.

In all types of cholestasis, there is accumulation of bile **B** within the hepatic parenchyma. In ductal obstruction, there are also plugs of bile within the canaliculi **C**. Hepatocytes containing bile show *feathery degeneration* **FD**, where the cytoplasm becomes foamy.

Acute biliary obstruction predisposes to the development of bacterial infection in the stagnant bile, a very serious condition called *ascending cholangitis*. Long-standing obstruction of the biliary tract may result in *secondary biliary cirrhosis*.

Fig. 14.11 Chronic cholecystitis (LP)

Many gallbladders containing stones are removed surgically because of abdominal pain. *Gallstones* are formed from the constituents of bile and may be composed of cholesterol, bile pigments or a mixture of these. In broad terms, they occur because of an imbalance in the ratio of these normal bile constituents. This is well illustrated by the frequent occurrence of pigment stones in patients with chronic *haemolytic anaemias*. Excess breakdown of erythrocytes results in increased excretion of the haem breakdown products bilirubin and biliverdin in bile. These then precipitate to form dark, crystalline gallstones which may cause biliary obstruction.

On histological examination, there is low-grade chronic inflammation with marked muscle hypertrophy **M** and an infiltrate of lymphocytes and plasma cells in the submucosal layer. Irregular gland-like mucosal pockets extend deep into and beyond the thickened muscle layer and are known as *Rokitansky–Aschoff sinuses* **R**. Outside the muscle layer, there is fibrosis **F** and mild chronic inflammation beneath the serosa. If bile becomes inspissated and concentrated within the gallbladder, it may cause an acute chemical cholecystitis with many neutrophils and often extensive haemorrhage within the gallbladder wall.

KEY TO FIGURES

B bile   **C** canalicular bile plugs   **D** duct-like structures   **F** fibrosis   **FD** feathery degeneration   **H** normal hepatocytes   **M** muscle hypertrophy   **R** Rokitansky–Aschoff sinuses   **T** malignant tumour cells

Fig. 14.12 Cholesterolosis (MP)

This micrograph shows accumulation of foamy, lipid-laden histiocytes **H** within the lamina propria of the gallbladder. Macroscopic examination of the mucosa reveals many tiny flecks of yellow upon a background which may be red and congested or green-stained with bile pigments. This appearance (like so many other pathological processes!) is likened to food and is termed *strawberry gallbladder*.

Cholesterolosis often coexists with cholesterol gallstones and probably reflects the presence of increased cholesterol levels in the bile. It is commonly seen in cholecystectomy specimens.

Fig. 14.13 Carcinoma of gallbladder (LP)

Carcinoma of the gallbladder usually occurs in the elderly. The micrograph shows a moderately differentiated adenocarcinoma which invades through the full thickness of the gallbladder wall, from the lumen **L** to the serosal surface **S**. The wall is replaced by adenocarcinoma with a glandular pattern **G**. There are zones of necrotic debris **N** within the islands of infiltrating tumour cells. Invasion has occurred through the submucosa into the muscularis propria **M** of the gallbladder and beyond into the outer serosa **S**. In addition, there is tumour within a large vein **V** in the subserosa. An adjacent muscular artery **A** is visible.

Gallbladder carcinoma is often seen to arise from surface epithelium which has undergone intestinal metaplasia and subsequent dysplasia. Similar carcinomas can also occur in the intrahepatic and extrahepatic bile ducts (intrahepatic and extrahepatic *cholangiocarcinomas*). These tumours tend to cause early obstructive jaundice, but tumours in the gallbladder rarely cause obstruction to the bile flow and therefore usually present late in the disease or are identified incidentally at the time of cholecystectomy. Gallbladder carcinoma frequently infiltrates directly into the liver, often rendering the tumour inoperable.

Pancreatic disorders

Inflammation of the pancreas (*pancreatitis*) may present in acute or chronic form. *Acute pancreatitis* has a high mortality, partly because of the release of pancreatic enzymes into surrounding tissues causing severe local tissue destruction. This is discussed in Figure 14.14. *Chronic pancreatitis* is frequently associated with intractable pain and, in some cases, it causes chronic pancreatic insufficiency.

Pancreatic adenocarcinomas (Fig. 14.15) are highly malignant lesions. When these occur in the head of pancreas, the typical presentation is with painless jaundice due to obstruction of the distal part of the extrahepatic biliary system. Metastases are almost always present by the time of diagnosis and the prognosis is poor.

KEY TO FIGURES
A artery **F** necrotic fat **G** malignant glands **H** lipid-laden histiocytes **L** lumen **M** muscularis propria
N necrotic debris **P** pancreas **S** serosa **T** tumour **V** vein with tumour

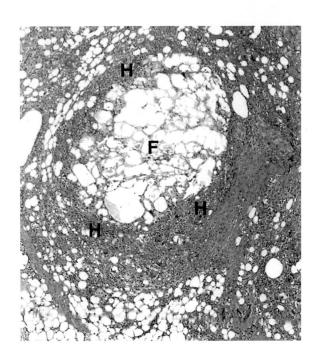

Fig. 14.14 **Fat necrosis in acute pancreatitis** (MP)

Acute pancreatitis is a condition in which there is destruction of the pancreas because of liberation of pancreatic enzymes. Severe cases result in a massive chemical peritonitis causing severe abdominal pain and shock. Patients with acute pancreatitis are at high risk of developing multi-organ failure, including adult respiratory distress syndrome (ARDS), severe coagulopathy and acute renal failure. The two most important predisposing conditions are alcohol abuse and biliary tract disease (usually gallstones).

Histologically, there is extensive haemorrhagic necrosis of the pancreas and surrounding tissues. Release of pancreatic enzymes gives rise to *fat necrosis*, a characteristic feature. With the naked eye, numerous chalky-white spots are seen in peripancreatic and omental fat. Histologically, these represent foci of necrotic adipose tissue **N**, surrounded by a rim of foamy histiocytes **H** which contain phagocytosed lipid within their cytoplasm.

Fig. 14.15 **Adenocarcinoma of the pancreas (a)** LP **(b)** HP

Pancreatic adenocarcinomas usually arise in the head of the gland and present with obstructive jaundice. Micrograph (a) shows tumour **T** with normal pancreas **P** on the upper right. Note the characteristic tortuous, irregular glands **G** within a dense, fibrous stroma. Macroscopically, the tumours are hard and white because of this stromal reaction.

At higher magnification in micrograph (b), the tumour is seen to have a ductal pattern, with marked variation in the size and shape of neoplastic glands **G**.

PANCREATIC TUMOURS

Pancreatic adenocarcinomas usually arise from the pancreatic ductal epithelium and are of great importance because of their insidious manner of growth, often remaining undetected until a very advanced stage. Most arise in the head of the gland where they tend to obstruct the common bile duct, thus presenting with painless obstructive jaundice.

This pattern of presentation is basis of the old clinical adage known as Courvoisier's Law: 'A *painless jaundice in the presence of a palpable gallbladder is rarely due to gallstones*'. The preceding discussion helps explain the pathological basis of this rule. Chronic gallstone disease typically causes scarring and fibrosis of the gallbladder wall and, as a result, obstruction of the biliary tree due to gallstones will not result in dilatation of the shrunken, scarred gallbladder. In contrast, occlusion of the biliary tree due to a tumour in the head of pancreas will cause back pressure and so the (presumably) normal, thin-walled gallbladder will become distended with bile such that it can be palpated.

Tumours arising in the body and tail of the pancreas are very difficult to detect, and frequently these are only identified following autopsy examination in patients with disseminated malignancy of unknown origin.

Other tumours may arise from the islets of Langerhans'. These lesions belong to the *neuroendocrine* group of tumours (see Fig. 13.13) and are usually named according to their secretory products, for example *insulinoma* and *glucagonoma*.

Fig. 14.16 Chapter review

Disorder	Main features	Figure
Inflammatory liver diseases		
Acute hepatitis	Cloudy swelling, fatty change, liver cell necrosis – various causes Many resolve or persist as chronic hepatitis	14.2
Viral hepatitis	Hepatotropic viruses (A, B, C, D, E, etc.) or others (CMV, EBV, HSV, etc.) Hep A and E faecal–oral transmission, no chronicity or carrier state Hep B (D) and C bloodborne, chronic hepatitis and carrier states	14.3
Alcoholic liver disease	Steatosis – fat droplets in hepatocytes Steatohepatitis – ballooning degeneration, neutrophils, Mallory's hyaline Fibrosis/cirrhosis – initially perivenular and pericellular collagen	14.4
Non-alcoholic fatty liver disease	Same morphological spectrum as alcoholic liver disease Association with obesity, dyslipidaemia, NIDDM	Like 14.4
Chronic hepatitis	Persisting more than 6 months, various causes Portal/interface/lobular inflammation (grade) Extent of fibrosis (stage)	14.5
Primary biliary cirrhosis	Early autoimmune damage to bile ducts with granuloma formation Later interface hepatitis, ductular proliferation and progressive fibrosis	14.6
Cirrhosis	Diffuse process, end stage of chronic liver damage Formation of regenerative nodules divided by fibrous bands	14.7
Haemochromatosis	Defect of HFE gene, iron overload with deposition in liver, heart, endocrine organs, joints and skin – progressive cirrhosis	14.8
Liver tumours		
Haemangioma	Benign proliferation of blood vessels in the liver Common incidental finding on imaging	11.9
Hepatic metastases	Usually carcinoma, especially GI tract (portal drainage), breast, lung Tendency to be multiple	7.19
Hepatocellular carcinoma	Primary malignant tumour arising from hepatocytes – may secrete bile Serum α-fetoprotein useful serum marker. Often single nodule	14.9
Biliary disease		
Cholestasis	Extrahepatic or intrahepatic obstruction to bile flow Plugs of bile in liver canaliculi Feathery degeneration of hepatocytes	14.10
Chronic cholecystitis	Usually due to gallstones – cholesterol, pigment or mixed types Chronic scarring, muscle hypertrophy, Rokitansky–Aschoff sinuses	14.11
Cholesterolosis	Deposition of lipid-laden histiocytes in lamina propria Gross appearance of 'strawberry gallbladder'	14.12
Gallbladder carcinoma	Uncommon, usually elderly patients Origin from surface intestinal metaplasia and dysplasia Presents late, often liver infiltration	14.13
Cholangiocarcinoma	Adenocarcinoma arising in intrahepatic or extrahepatic bile ducts Typically causes intense fibrous stromal reaction	
Pancreatic disease		
Acute pancreatitis	Gallstones and alcohol main risk factors Pancreatic enzymes cause tissue damage and necrosis High risk of multi-organ failure	14.14
Chronic pancreatitis	May follow repeated episodes of acute pancreatitis Commonly alcohol related Scarring and loss of gland tissue Back pain, risk of diabetes	
Pancreatic adenocarcinoma	Usually head of pancreas, insidious growth Presents late with obstructive jaundice Poor prognosis	14.15
Pancreatic endocrine tumours	Origin from islet cells Resemble carcinoid tumours seen at other sites Uncommon Named for secretory product, e.g. insulinoma, glucagonoma.	Like 13.13

15 Urinary system

Introduction

The *urinary tract* comprises the kidneys, pelvicalyceal systems, ureters, bladder and urethra. The kidney is responsible for the excretion of waste products from body metabolic processes, the waste products being excreted in the form of an aqueous solution called *urine*. The urine passes from the kidneys into the pelvicalyceal systems and thence via the ureters to the bladder, which acts as a reservoir. Urine is held in the bladder by a series of muscular sphincters until sufficient volume has accumulated. Relaxation of the sphincters and contraction of smooth muscle in the bladder wall allows the urine to be voided to the exterior through the urethra (*micturition*) at a convenient time.

The kidney

Disorders of the kidney arise from a wide range of pathological causes, many of which are common in other organ systems (e.g. infections, tumours, drug reactions, vascular disorders). However, the kidney is unusual in that it is much more prone to immunological disorders than most other organs. Vascular diseases such as hypertension and vasculitis and the common metabolic disease, diabetes mellitus, may also have profound effects on renal function. Disorders of the kidney can be conveniently divided into categories according to which structural component of the kidney is primarily affected.

- **Glomerulus**
  - *Glomerulonephritis* of various types, most of which are due to deposition of immunoglobulins and/or complement components (collectively called *immune complexes*) within the glomerulus (Figs 15.3–15.8).
  - *Vasculitis*: strictly speaking this is a vascular disorder, but some forms affect the glomerular capillaries giving the clinical and pathological appearances of a glomerulonephritis (Fig. 15.8).
  - *Diabetes mellitus*: deposition of abnormal glycosylated proteins causes irreversible structural and functional abnormalities in the glomerulus (Fig. 15.3).
  - *Amyloidosis*: deposition of amyloid proteins in the glomerulus alters the structure and therefore the function of the glomerulus (Fig. 5.31).

- **Tubules and interstitium**
  - *Acute tubular necrosis (ATN)* is usually due to profound hypotension causing ischaemic damage to tubular epithelial cells.
  - *Infections* include acute pyelonephritis, renal abscesses and TB.
  - *Drug toxicity* usually causes tubulointerstitial nephritis due to a hypersensitivity reaction, but other patterns may occur, including direct toxicity to tubular epithelial cells giving an appearance similar to ATN.
  - *Mechanical obstruction* of the ureters or bladder may lead to *hydronephrosis* and recurrent infection.

- **Blood vessels**
  - *Hypertension* causes marked changes to both large and small renal vessels.
  - *Vasculitis* may affect larger vessels as well as glomerular capillaries.

Irreversible damage to one component of the kidney inevitably damages the other parts, eventually leading to **chronic renal failure**, a condition invariably fatal until the advent of renal dialysis and transplantation. Severe reversible damage to any of the above components of the kidney may lead to *acute renal failure*.

- **Chronic renal failure**: Progressive retention of nitrogenous metabolites manifests as a slow rise in serum creatinine levels owing to insufficient glomerular filtration. Concomitant failure of tubular function produces widespread abnormalities in biochemical homeostasis, including salt and water retention, metabolic acidosis and other electrolyte imbalances, particularly hyperkalaemia.

- **Acute renal failure**: Abrupt cessation of activity of the nephrons usually manifests initially as a marked fall in urine production (*oliguria*) which may even be total (*anuria*). This is accompanied by an abrupt rise in urea and potassium. Disturbances of fluid and electrolyte balance soon follow, particularly a rise in the serum potassium level and metabolic acidosis.

Fig. 15.1 End-stage kidney (MP)

Many kidney diseases, whatever the underlying cause, may progress to chronic renal failure. Macroscopically, the kidneys are usually found to be small and firm with symmetrical thinning of the cortex and poor demarcation of cortex from medulla. This condition is known as *end-stage kidney*. In both gross and histological appearance, there is often little clue to the original renal pathology.

In the cortex, the non-functioning or *obsolescent* glomeruli are replaced by avascular, acellular hyaline material **H** (*hyalinisation*). The cortical tubules **T** also become shrunken and atrophic and the relatively expanded interstitial spaces **In** undergo fibrosis; some atrophic tubules may become cystically dilated with *casts* of inspissated proteinaceous material **P**, which is highly eosinophilic (pink-staining) and resembles thyroid follicles, hence often called *thyroidisation*.

Diseases of the glomerulus

Glomerular disorders arise from a variety of causes, the two major causes being *immunological* (including disorders confined to the kidney and systemic diseases) and *metabolic* (the most important being diabetes mellitus). It is confusing to many students that there is not a direct one-to-one relationship between a particular mechanism of damage and a particular histological appearance and/or clinical syndrome. In fact, most causes of glomerular damage will give rise to one of five clinical syndromes summarised in Figure 15.2 below, along with the glomerular diseases with which they are most commonly associated. Acute and chronic renal failure are described above and may supervene in any of these conditions. For example, an individual with a very severe nephritic syndrome may progress quickly to acute renal failure, or an individual with undiagnosed diabetes, who has had undetected proteinuria for some time, may first be diagnosed in chronic renal failure.

Fig 15.2 Clinical syndromes associated with glomerular disease

Syndrome	Clinical features	Histological changes	Associated disease
Acute nephritis	Haematuria Hypertension Uraemia (↑BUN) Oedema (often periorbital) Oliguria or anuria	Hypercellular glomerulus with obstructed capillary loops	Diffuse proliferative glomerulonephritis (GN)
Nephrotic syndrome	Proteinuria (3.5g/24h) Hypoalbuminaemia Oedema Hyperlipidaemia	Changes to the structure of the glomerular filtration mechanism – most often the glomerular basement membrane (GBM)	Diabetes mellitus Amyloidosis Minimal change nephropathy Focal segmental glomerulosclerosis Membranous nephropathy Systemic lupus erythematosus (SLE)
Mixed nephritic–nephrotic syndrome	Features of both nephritic and nephrotic syndromes	Both cellular proliferation and GBM alterations	Mesangiocapillary GN (membranoproliferative GN) SLE
Asymptomatic haematuria	Periodic dark-coloured urine or microscopic haematuria	Proliferation of glomerular cells or structural abnormalities of GBM	IgA nephropathy Thin basement membrane disease SLE
Asymptomatic proteinuria	Proteinuria	Early stages of the changes in the GBM seen in the nephrotic syndrome	Early phases of all of the conditions which cause the nephrotic syndrome

ROLE OF RENAL BIOPSY

The introduction of safe and reliable techniques of percutaneous needle biopsy of the kidney has greatly increased knowledge about the natural history of renal diseases, particularly by elucidating the underlying lesion early in the course of glomerular diseases when treatment might be applied effectively. It is of limited value in chronic renal failure when the kidney is shrunken and histological changes are non-specific, i.e. **end-stage kidney** (Fig. 15.1). Renal biopsy is also frequently used in the assessment of renal transplants to detect the presence of transplant rejection, drug toxicity and a number of other conditions which may cause reduced function of the graft. Maximum information is obtained from a needle biopsy of renal tissue using a combination of the following methods:

- **light microscopy**, including special stains to define glomerular structures

- **electron microscopy** to show the presence and precise location of immune complexes, which appear as irregular deposits of electron-dense material (**dense deposits**)

- **immunofluorescence microscopy** to localise and identify the class of immunoglobulins and complement components.

The immunofluorescence and electron microscopic patterns of immune complex deposition can be vital to differentiate between different types of glomerulonephritis, which have similar patterns of glomerular damage by light microscopy. Examples include:

- **IgA nephropathy**: granular deposits of IgA in the mesangium

- **Membranous nephropathy**: granular deposits of IgG and complement on the epithelial side of the glomerular basement membrane (GBM)

- **Goodpasture's syndrome**: linear deposits of IgG along the GBM

- **Systemic lupus erythematosus**: deposits of most classes of immunoglobulin and many complement components at any site in the glomerulus

- **Mesangiocapillary glomerulonephritis type I**: granular deposits of complement component 3 (C3) on the endothelial side of the GBM.

Interpretation of a renal biopsy also requires information about the clinical history, physical examination and other investigations to arrive at a correct diagnosis. For example, a membranous pattern of GN might be idiopathic, related to use of certain drugs (e.g. gold, penicillamine) or may be part of the spectrum of systemic lupus erythematosus (SLE) (Class V lupus nephritis).

Glomerulonephritis

Most types of glomerulonephritis (GN) are caused by immune complex deposition in the glomerulus. This applies to *primary glomerulonephritis*, where the condition is confined to the kidney (e.g. *membranous nephropathy*, *mesangiocapillary GN*), and to diseases with a systemic component (for example *Goodpasture's syndrome*, *SLE*, *Henoch–Schönlein purpura*). The site of immune complex deposition is dependent on the size of the complexes, which is in turn dependent on the type of antigen and on the class of immunoglobulin produced, i.e. the host response. The antigen may be either a normal component of the body (a self antigen as in Goodpasture's) or an external antigen such as a bacterial product (as in *post-streptococcal GN*). Immune complexes may be deposited from the circulating blood or may be formed in situ. In the latter situation, the complexes may involve intrinsic glomerular antigens (basement membrane components in Goodpasture's) or antigens which have been deposited there from the circulation (e.g. DNA in the case of SLE). An important exception to this rule is minimal change nephropathy, where the podocytes are thought to be damaged by a cell-mediated immune response rather than by immune complex deposition. Whatever the mechanism of damage to the glomerulus, the various immunological insults alter the structure and therefore the function of the glomerulus and, ultimately, of the nephron as a whole.

In response to damaging stimuli, the glomerulus appears to react in one or more of the following ways:

- Swelling and/or proliferation of the normally flat endothelial cells lining the glomerular capillaries

- Proliferation of the epithelial cells investing the outer surface of the glomerular capillary tuft (the podocytes) and the cells lining Bowman's capsule (*crescent formation*)

- Thickening of glomerular basement membrane

- Proliferation of the cells of the mesangium and excessive production of acellular mesangial material.

KEY TO FIGURES
H hyalinised glomerulus **In** interstitial space **P** protein cast **T** tubule

These reactions give rise to various histological patterns of glomerulonephritis, which can be identified by light microscopy. This is then put together with the immunofluorescence and electron microscopy findings, clinical history and other investigations to come to a definitive diagnosis. As in many other areas of histopathology, good communications between pathologist and clinician are vital to arrive at an accurate diagnosis, which is essential for appropriate treatment.

Types of glomerulonephritis may be described as:

- **Diffuse**: affecting all glomeruli

- **Focal**: affecting some glomeruli

- **Global**: the entire glomerulus is abnormal

- **Segmental**: only part of the glomerulus is abnormal.

Fig. 15.3 Acute proliferative ('endocapillary') glomerulonephritis (HP)

This form of global and diffuse glomerulonephritis most commonly occurs in children and often follows a streptococcal throat infection. Other possible underlying infections include bacterial endocarditis, pneumococcal pneumonia, hepatitis B or C, HIV and many others. Glomerular cellularity is markedly increased due to swelling and proliferation of endothelial and mesangial cells and infiltration by neutrophils **N**. The capillary lumina are blocked by cells but the urinary space **U** remains clear, as there has been no proliferation of epithelial cells. The obstruction of glomerular capillary lumina diminishes glomerular filtration and causes leakage of erythrocytes; hence this condition usually presents with haematuria, transient hypertension and oedema, i.e. acute nephritis.

Immunofluorescence microscopy reveals granular deposits of IgG and complement on the glomerular basement membranes and in the mesangium and, on electron microscopy, there are characteristic large subepithelial deposits known as 'humps'.

A similar pattern of glomerular damage may occur rarely in SLE without preceding infection (Class IV lupus nephritis).

Fig 15.4 Mesangial proliferative glomerulonephritis (HP)

This diffuse and global pattern of glomerular damage is characterised by increased mesangial matrix and cellularity **M**, without basement membrane abnormality **B**. This pattern of glomerular damage is typical of IgA nephropathy and the related condition Henoch–Schönlein purpura (HSP). Both may present with asymptomatic haematuria or acute nephritis. The renal changes of HSP are identical to those in IgA disease, but in HSP there is a vasculitic skin rash and gastrointestinal and joint involvement. Immunofluorescence staining reveals deposits of IgA in the mesangium and there are corresponding mesangial dense deposits by electron microscopy. Acute exacerbations of IgA nephropathy may develop segmental necrotising glomerulonephritis (Fig. 15.8) and even occasionally crescents (Fig. 15.8). Healing of these lesions leads to secondary focal segmental glomerulosclerosis (Fig. 15.8). Other conditions which have a mesangial proliferative pattern (but different immunological and electron microscopy findings) are resolving acute proliferative glomerulonephritis (Fig. 15.3) and SLE (Class II).

KEY TO FIGURES

B normal glomerular basement membrane   **D** double contour basement membrane   **M** increased mesangial matrix and cellularity   **N** neutrophils   **U** urinary space

Fig. 15.5 Mesangiocapillary (membranoproliferative) glomerulonephritis (a) (HP) (b) Methenamine silver (HP)

This diffuse and global pattern of glomerulonephritis may be either idiopathic or secondary. The clinical presentation is either nephrotic syndrome or mixed nephrotic–nephritic syndrome. *Idiopathic mesangiocapillary glomerulonephritis (MCGN)* is subdivided into *type I* and *type II*, both having a similar appearance by light microscopy. Readily visible, as in micrograph (a), is the expansion and increased cellularity of each segment of the glomerulus, producing an exaggerated lobular appearance. The characteristic feature is reduplication of the glomerular basement membranes with interposition of mesangial cells between the two layers. This is seen in micrograph (b), which is stained with a special method to demonstrate the double contour **D** of the glomerular basement membrane. There is increased mesangial cellularity and matrix **M**. White blood cells also infiltrate the glomerulus and there is often mild endothelial cell proliferation. In MCGN type I, dense deposits composed of C3 (and IgG in some cases) are found in the subendothelial position.

Type II MCGN is characterised by deposition of a ribbon of dense material of unknown composition in the glomerular basement membrane, giving rise to the alternative name of *dense deposit disease.*

Secondary MCGN is one of the patterns of renal disease in SLE (class IV lupus nephritis), where it may have additional features including immunoglobulin deposits in all parts of the glomerular basement membrane and in the mesangium, 'wire-loop lesions', a mixed pattern of immunoglobulins and complement deposition, as well as superimposed membranous or segmental patterns of glomerulonephritis. This pattern of glomerulonephritis may also occur in individuals with hepatitis B or C, cryoglobulinaemia and other conditions.

Fig. 15.6 Minimal change disease (HP)

Minimal change disease may occur at any age but is much more common in children. It presents with the nephrotic syndrome without haematuria and usually without any impairment of renal function, i.e. there is no increase in serum creatinine or urea. Some cases present after an upper respiratory tract infection and it is thought that cell-mediated immunity may be the mechanism of damage to the glomeruli. Most patients recover with no treatment, but some require immunosuppression and a few relapse after withdrawal of immunosuppression.

As the name implies, the glomeruli appear almost normal on light microscopy (as seen here). Immunofluorescence microscopy is negative. Examination of the glomeruli by electron microscopy demonstrates alterations in the structure of the podocyte foot processes, which are 'fused' or 'effaced', i.e. the foot processes form a continuous layer along the urinary side of the basement membrane. This is a non-specific change found in various types of glomerular damage, so only if it occurs in conjunction with normal light and negative immunofluorescence microscopy can it be said to confirm minimal change disease.

Fig. 15.7 **Membranous nephropathy** **(a)** H&E (HP) **(b)** IgG immunofluorescence (HP) **(c)** EM

Membranous nephropathy is a diffuse global pattern of glomerular injury where damage to the glomerular basement membrane leads to proteinuria and, often, the nephrotic syndrome. *Primary* or *idiopathic membranous nephropathy* accounts for about 85% of cases. The identical pattern of injury, known as *secondary membranous nephropathy*, may arise in individuals with malignant tumours elsewhere in the body (5–10% of cases), individuals taking certain drugs (gold, penicillamine, captopril and non-steroidal anti-inflammatory drugs) and in certain infections (hepatitis B and C, malaria). A third important category is the autoimmune disease SLE which can give rise to almost any pattern of glomerular damage (see Fig. 15.2); this pattern is known as lupus nephritis Class V.

In membranous nephropathy, immune complexes are deposited on the epithelial side of the glomerular basement membrane (subepithelial deposits). These deposits induce deposition of additional basement membrane material between the deposits, giving rise to the pathognomonic 'spikes' on the outer surface of the basement membrane which can be seen with the silver stain by light microscopy or by electron microscopy as shown in micrograph (c). By light microscopy in image (a), the glomerular basement membranes **B** appear thick, eosinophilic and sometimes slightly refractile. There is no associated endothelial or epithelial (podocyte) proliferation, although there may be a slight increase in mesangial material **M** in severe and long-standing cases. The immune complexes in most cases of membranous nephropathy consist of IgG and complement (C3). Obviously, the antigen in the immune complexes will depend on the underlying cause (e.g. DNA in SLE, viral antigens in hepatitis, probably self-antigens in the idiopathic form). Micrograph (b) shows the characteristic immunofluorescence pattern of membranous nephropathy. An antibody specific for IgG and labelled with fluorescein is incubated with a section of kidney. The antibody binds to IgG deposited in the kidney. This micrograph demonstrates IgG as bright green fluorescent granular deposits incorporated on the epithelial surface of the glomerular basement membranes. Micrograph (c) is a high-power electron micrograph of a glomerular basement membrane **B** with additional spikes **S** of basement membrane material on the epithelial side. Between the spikes, dense deposits (immune complexes) **DD** are easily identified. The presence of the immune complexes probably activates complement which, by means of the membrane attack complex, damages the glomerular basement membrane and allows leakage of protein.

KEY TO FIGURES

B glomerular basement membrane **C** crescent **DD** dense deposit **F** fibrin **M** mesangial matrix
N normal glomerular segment **R** glomerular remnant **S** spike **Sc** sclerosis

Fig. 15.8 Focal segmental glomerulonephritis (a)
Segmental necrotising glomerulonephritis (HP)
(b) Glomerular crescent (HP) **(c)** Focal segmental
glomerulosclerosis (HP)

Focal segmental glomerulonephritis affects only a
proportion of the glomeruli (focal) and only part of
each affected glomerulus (segmental).

In segmental necrotising glomerulonephritis (a), a
segment of the glomerular tuft becomes necrotic with
infiltration by neutrophils and deposition of fibrin **F**.
Adjacent segments are normal **N** or nearly normal
(depending on the underlying disease). Segmental
necrosis is often associated with proliferation of
epithelial cells of Bowman's capsule, which may
progress to frank crescent formation. An early
crescent **C** is seen here. This pattern of
glomerulonephritis is found in acute exacerbations of
IgA nephropathy, systemic vasculitis, SLE (Class III
lupus nephritis) and some cases of Goodpasture's
syndrome. Segmental necrotising lesions heal by
fibrosis, leaving a lesion very similar to focal
segmental glomerulosclerosis (FSGS) (c). As in many
cases, the immunofluorescence microscopy is vital to
make the diagnosis: in IgA nephropathy, mesangial
IgA (and usually C3) deposits are found, in
Goodpasture's there is linear deposition of IgG
around the GBM and, in SLE, all classes of
immunoglobulin and several complement components
are detected.

Continued proliferation of a crescent may
obliterate the glomerular tuft, as seen in (b), leading
to irreversible glomerular destruction and subsequent
nephron atrophy. An example is shown in (b) where
the tiny glomerular remnant **R** is surrounded by a
large crescent **C**. Large numbers of crescents are
associated with rapidly progressive renal failure, often
called *rapidly progressive glomerulonephritis* (a
clinical but not a pathological term). This is
characteristic of *Goodpasture's syndrome* where
autoantibodies are formed that react with the α3
subchain of collagen type IV found in glomerular and
alveolar basement membranes. These individuals
experience pulmonary haemorrhage as well as renal
failure. Where the renal lesion occurs in the absence
of lung disease the condition is known as
antiglomerular basement membrane disease. A large
crescent, as shown here, heals as a globally sclerosed
glomerulus. A small segmental necrotising lesion with
limited crescent formation may heal to form a
segmental sclerosing lesion as in FSGS.

FSGS (c) may occur as an idiopathic
glomerulonephritis or secondary segmental sclerosing
lesions as mentioned above. In addition, almost any
lesion that causes marked loss of nephrons may
induce secondary FSGS. The histological lesion in all
these situations is similar. Segments of some
glomeruli are replaced by fibrosis (sclerosis) **Sc**.
Hyalinosis, the deposition of plasma proteins to give
a bland eosinophilic mass, is also commonly a feature
of these lesions, although not demonstrated in this
example. Some authorities believe that idiopathic
FSGS is related to minimal change disease. Certainly
both are characterised by negative
immunofluorescence and 'fusion' of podocyte foot
processes on EM. However, the case remains to be
proven.

While focal necrotising glomerulonephritis presents
with haematuria or a nephritic syndrome, FSGS is
characterised by proteinuria and often full-blown
nephrotic syndrome. Both of these lesions may be
seen in SLE (Class III lupus nephritis).

Fig. 15.9 **Diabetic glomerulosclerosis** (*caption opposite*)

KEY TO FIGURES

BM glomerular basement membrane   **C** capsular drop   **En** endothelial cell cytoplasm   **FC** fibrin cap
H hyalinised arteriole   **K** Kimmelsteil–Wilson nodule   **P** podocyte foot process

Fig. 15.9 **Diabetic glomerulosclerosis** **(a)** Nodular glomerulosclerosis (HP) **(b)** Diffuse glomerulosclerosis (HP) **(c)** Capsular drop (PAS) (HP) **(d)** Normal glomerular basement membrane (EM) **(e)** Diabetic basement membrane (EM) *(illustrations (a), (b) and (c) opposite)*

In diabetes mellitus, renal disease may occur in several ways. Diabetics have an increased predisposition to the development of renal infections such as pyelonephritis (Fig. 15.10) and papillary necrosis (Fig. 15.12) which may cause acute renal failure. There is also a tendency to severe large vessel atherosclerosis, increasing the risk of renal ischaemia and infarction.

Long-standing diabetes mellitus may result in characteristic changes to the glomeruli (*diabetic glomerulosclerosis*). Among the early glomerular changes is a uniform and homogeneous thickening of the glomerular capillary basement membrane. This is best seen by electron microscopy as in micrograph (e), with the normal shown for comparison in micrograph (d). In both micrographs, note the glomerular capillary basement membrane **BM** invested by thin endothelial cell cytoplasm **En** on the inner aspect and by epithelial cell (podocyte) foot processes **P** externally. In diabetes, the basement membrane may be up to four or five times normal thickness.

Later, there is an increase in mesangial matrix, the latter often segmental and localised to produce characteristic acellular **Kimmelstiel–Wilson nodules K**, often with compressed mesangial cell nuclei pushed to their periphery. This is called *nodular diabetic glomerulosclerosis* and is shown in micrograph (a).

In another pattern, the mesangial matrix increase is diffuse and global, not segmental and nodular, producing the change called *diffuse diabetic*

glomerulosclerosis, illustrated in micrograph (b). Both patterns may occur in the same kidney, and nodule formation may be superimposed upon the diffuse change within the same glomerulus. In both patterns, there is escape of plasma protein across the thickened, but leaky, glomerular basement membrane into the urinary space. Occasionally, inspissated protein may be deposited on the outer surface of the glomerular tuft, forming *fibrin caps* **FC**, as seen in micrograph (b), or on the inner surface of Bowman's capsule, forming *capsular drops* **C** as seen in micrograph (c).

A characteristic feature of diabetic renal disease is *hyalinisation* of arterioles similar to that seen in hypertension (Fig. 15.13), but characteristically affecting both afferent and efferent arterioles. This arteriolar hyalinisation **H**, as seen in association with nodular diabetic glomerulosclerosis in micrograph (a), may also extend into the vascular hilum of the glomerulus. The combination of arterial atherosclerosis and arteriolar hyalinisation progressively reduces the blood flow to the glomeruli; thus chronic ischaemic changes, such as hyalinisation of glomeruli and periglomerular fibrosis, are common associated findings in diabetic renal disease.

The initial glomerular basement membrane changes result in proteinuria and even the nephrotic syndrome, but with progressive diabetic glomerulosclerosis and chronic ischaemic nephron atrophy, the features of chronic renal failure supervene.

OUTCOME OF GLOMERULAR DISORDERS

The renal disorders in which the major abnormality involves the glomerulus may subside spontaneously or with treatment. However, if they progress, glomerular blood flow is obstructed, glomerular filtration ceases and the tubules associated with affected glomeruli become involved; thus many nephrons may cease to function. When sufficient nephrons have been affected, the clinical features of the disease gradually progress to chronic renal failure.

By way of illustration, a patient with the nephrotic syndrome caused by diabetic glomerular disease may slowly develop the features of chronic renal failure as individual nephrons are destroyed. In contrast, a patient who initially presents with the acute nephritic syndrome caused by a rapidly progressive glomerulonephritis with extensive crescents (Fig. 15.8) may quickly progress to acute renal failure. As the glomeruli are rapidly destroyed by the disease process, this becomes irreversible.

Disorders of the renal tubules and interstitium

The tubules and interstitium may be primarily damaged as a result of hypovolaemic shock, by inorganic and organic toxins, or as the result of infection. In hypovolaemic states and intoxication, tubular epithelial cells may exhibit marked cytoplasmic degenerative changes or frank necrosis, leading to the pathological term *acute tubular necrosis* (Fig. 15.11) and producing the clinical syndrome of acute renal failure. Tubular epithelial cells have considerable powers of recovery and regeneration, and acute renal failure may be reversible under such circumstances if the patient can be sustained in the interim by dialysis and other supporting measures.

Another increasingly important cause of tubulointerstitial disease is drug toxicity giving rise to *interstitial nephritis*. In this condition, a large number of drugs have been implicated including certain antibiotics, non-steroidal anti-inflammatory drugs, thiazide diuretics and cimetidine. Onset may be acute or chronic. There is a mixed inflammatory infiltrate in the interstitium in which eosinophils may be prominent. Tubular damage occurs and the condition may proceed to chronic renal failure.

Infections of the kidney include acute and chronic pyelonephritis (Fig. 15.10) and tuberculosis (see Ch. 4). Acute suppurative bacterial infections of the kidney (*pyelonephritis*) usually follow ascending infection from the lower urinary tract, particularly when there is obstruction to urinary outflow such as in benign prostatic hyperplasia or pressure from the fetus in pregnancy; in such cases, coliform organisms (such as *Escherichia coli* and *Proteus* species) are the most frequent infecting agents. Infection may also spread to the kidney by the haematogenous route during episodes of bacteraemia. Acute pyelonephritis may be complicated by the development of papillary necrosis (Fig. 15.12) or pus accumulation in a dilated, obstructed pelvicalyceal system (*pyonephrosis*). Acute pyelonephritis is illustrated in Figure 15.10. Tuberculous infection of the kidneys and lower urinary tract may also arise by similar routes of spread.

Patients with urinary reflux or obstruction are prone to develop recurrent pyelonephritis; repeated attacks lead to scarring, and after many episodes the kidney becomes coarsely scarred, a phenomenon termed *chronic pyelonephritis*.

Fig. 15.10 Acute pyelonephritis (MP)

This micrograph illustrates established acute pyelonephritis. There is extensive infiltration of the kidney by small dark-staining neutrophil polymorphs **N**, which are also seen filling dilated tubules **T**. Abscess formation may ensue and, in untreated cases, multiple abscesses may merge to produce larger abscesses. These may discharge into the pelvicalyceal system to produce pyonephrosis, or through the capsule into perinephric fat to produce a perinephric abscess. Note that the glomeruli **G** are spared.

With time and repeated episodes or persisting infection, the renal parenchyma becomes permanently damaged and replaced by fibrous tissue. Eventually, the features are of end-stage kidney with loss of glomeruli as well as tubules.

KEY TO FIGURES
G glomerulus   **J** junction between normal and necrotic tissue   **N** neutrophil polymorphs   **P** renal papilla
T dilated tubules

Fig 15.11 Acute tubular necrosis (MP)

Acute tubular necrosis (ATN) is a fairly common cause of acute renal failure. One of the most common underlying causes is acute ischaemia caused by hypotension. A fairly small drop in the circulating volume in an elderly person with compromised circulation, e.g. due to dehydration after an episode of vomiting and diarrhoea, may lead to acute renal failure. A renal biopsy is sometimes necessary to determine the cause and to prevent unnecessary treatment, although the majority of cases resolve without intervention. Supportive measures are usually all that is required to allow the renal tubules to regenerate.

The term necrosis is actually a misnomer, as frank necrosis is seldom seen. The changes may be quite subtle in the early stages but in established ATN, as in this micrograph, the tubules are dilated **T** with flattening of the epithelium. This is usually most prominent in the proximal convoluted tubules, which have the highest oxygen requirement. The epithelium at higher magnification (not shown) can be seen to have lost the brush border and plasma membrane infoldings that allow the proximal convoluted tubules to perform their function. As recovery progresses, mitotic figures become apparent in the regenerating epithelium and then the specialised features of the epithelium are restored.

Fig. 15.12 Renal papillary necrosis (LP)

This low-power micrograph shows the condition known as *papillary necrosis* or *necrotising papillitis*. At the earliest stage there is coagulative necrosis of the tip of the papilla **P**, with preservation of ghost-like outlines of the papillary tubules and collecting ducts. This is followed by a neutrophil inflammatory response at the junction **J** between normal and necrotic papilla, but this largely disappears at a later stage when the necrotic papilla separates and is shed. There may also be calcification. This condition, which is probably ischaemic in nature, often occurs in association with acute infection of the urinary parenchyma and pelvicalyceal system, particularly when accompanied by an obstructive lesion in the lower urinary tract. It may also be seen with or without overt infection in diabetic nephropathy and in analgesic nephropathy. If there is sudden loss of many papillae, the patient may develop acute renal failure.

Vascular disorders

The kidney is especially vulnerable to the effects of arterial hypertension, as seen in Figures 11.1 and 11.2, and irreversible damage to nephrons may result either acutely from accelerated hypertension or progressively over a period of years in benign essential hypertension. *Hypertensive nephrosclerosis*, resulting from benign essential hypertension, is illustrated in Figure 15.13. Malignant or accelerated hypertension causes a different pattern of renal damage which is very similar to the changes seen in acute *scleroderma* and may result in acute renal failure (Fig. 15.13).

Various forms of vasculitis, including *polyarteritis nodosa* (see Fig. 11.7), *microscopic polyarteritis* (see Fig. 11.8) and Wegener's granulomatosis, also affect the kidney. Analgesic abuse nephropathy, owing to overuse of analgesic mixtures, is characterised by a chronic interstitial nephritis and papillary necrosis.

Fig. 15.13 **Hypertensive nephrosclerosis** (*caption opposite*)

Fig. 15.13 Hypertensive nephrosclerosis (a) Benign hypertensive nephrosclerosis (HP) (b) Malignant hypertensive nephrosclerosis (HP) (illustrations opposite)

The vessel changes in systemic hypertension have been discussed and illustrated in some detail in Figures 11.1 and 11.2. The kidney is particularly vulnerable to the damaging effects of these vessel changes, and renal failure is an important complication of untreated hypertension. The pathological changes in the kidney depend on the severity and rate of progression of the hypertension.

In *benign (essential) hypertension*, the hypertension is of gradual onset and progression, with only moderately elevated diastolic pressure. Large and medium-sized renal arteries show marked thickening of their walls by a combination of medial hypertrophy, elastic lamina reduplication and fibrous intimal thickening; this is shown in Figure 11.1(a). The arterioles show hyaline thickening of their walls as seen in Figure 11.1(b). These changes reduce the calibre of all renal afferent vessels and the resulting chronic ischaemia leads to progressive *sclerosis (hyalinisation)* of the glomerulus and subsequent disuse atrophy of the tubular component of the nephron.

Micrograph (a) shows a group of glomeruli, two of which have become converted into hyaline, amorphous, pink-staining masses **H** as a result of chronic ischaemia owing to hyalinisation of the walls of their afferent arterioles **Aa**; the other glomeruli are as yet unaffected. Slowly progressive loss of functioning nephrons may eventually lead to chronic renal failure and the morphological state known as end-stage kidney (Fig. 15.1).

In contrast, in *malignant (accelerated) hypertension*, where the rise in blood pressure is rapid and severe, the arterial and arteriolar changes are different. Large and medium-sized arteries may show only concentric thickening of the intima by loose, rather myxomatous, fibroblastic tissue as seen in Figure 11.2(a), and there is no elastic lamina reduplication or significant medial hypertrophy. Small arteries may show marked concentric fibroblastic intimal thickening so that the lumen is often virtually obliterated. Arterioles frequently show patchy acute necrosis of their walls with the accumulation of amorphous, brightly eosinophilic, proteinaceous material (*fibrinoid*) in the damaged walls; this is shown in Figure 11.2(b). This change is known as *fibrinoid necrosis*. In the kidney, as seen in micrograph (b), this often affects the afferent arterioles **Aa** at the glomerular hila and may extend into the glomerular tuft to affect some segments **S** of the glomerular capillary network. The onset of small vessel changes is acute and may produce an abrupt reduction in blood supply to the nephrons, often producing glomerular microinfarction and acute tubular necrosis. The effect is to produce a catastrophic reduction in glomerular filtration and the patient may develop acute oliguric or anuric renal failure. Not infrequently, the patient with long-standing benign hypertension may suddenly develop an accelerated phase, and the histological changes in the kidney may be those of mixed benign and malignant nephrosclerosis.

Pathology of renal transplantation

Renal transplantation has become a routine treatment for chronic renal failure in many countries. The transplant recipient is freed from a life of regular dialysis with a consequent improvement in quality of life. The function of the transplanted kidney may, however, be affected by a number of factors in the days, weeks and months following transplantation. The most important of these include:

■ **Acute tubular necrosis**: This is identical to acute tubular necrosis from other causes (Fig. 15.11). The major factor here is the 'cold ischaemic time', i.e. the length of time between harvesting of the kidney and re-establishment of vascular perfusion in the donor. Supportive measures may be needed in the immediate post-transplantation phase but usually this will resolve.

■ **Rejection**: See Fig. 15.14.

■ **Drug toxicity**: Routinely used immunosuppressive agents, such as ciclosporin A and related compounds (the calcineurin inhibitors), may have a range of effects on the kidney. Histologically, there may be changes in the tubules and/or the blood vessels. Exquisite control of dosage and sometimes transfer to a different agent will usually control this problem.

■ **Infection**: Transplant recipients require immunosuppression to prevent rejection of the graft and this makes them susceptible to a range of infections.

■ **Recurrent glomerulonephritis**: This is more likely to be a problem months to years after transplantation than in the early stages.

KEY TO FIGURES
Aa afferent arteriole   **H** sclerosed hyalinised glomerulus   **S** segment of glomerulus

Fig. 15.14 **Renal transplant rejection** **(a)** T-cell-mediated rejection, type I (HP) **(b)** T-cell-mediated rejection, type II (HP)

Rejection of a transplanted kidney (or other organ) depends mainly on the degree of **human leukocyte antigen (HLA)** mismatch between donor and recipient. Obviously, transplantation between identical twins has the best chance of success but this is rarely feasible. Tissue typing is routinely carried out on potential donors to identify recipients with the closest HLA match.

The **Banff classification** (designed by a panel of renal pathologists in Banff, Canada) is a semi-quantitative method for assessing rejection. Various features of rejection are graded numerically and the scores combined to classify according to the type and degree of severity of rejection. The classification is regularly reviewed and updated.

The Banff classification recognises several categories of rejection, the two most important of which are **T-cell-mediated rejection** and **antibody-mediated rejection**, both of which may have acute and chronic phases. Acute rejection occurs within days to months after transplantation while chronic rejection may last for years. Both T-cell and antibody-mediated rejection may occur at the same time and some of the histological features overlap. These micrographs illustrate the most common variant of renal transplant rejection, T-cell-mediated rejection.

Acute T-cell-mediated rejection, Banff type I, is shown in micrograph (a). The interstitium is infiltrated by lymphocytes that are also seen within the tubular epithelium (**tubulitis**) **T**. Tubulitis

represents a cell-mediated immune response directed against donor tubular epithelial cells and results in destruction of tubules. The glomeruli are generally not affected in the acute phase.

Acute T-cell-mediated rejection types II and III manifest as a T-cell immune response against vascular endothelial cells. The typical features of type II T-cell-mediated rejection shown in micrograph (b) include infiltration of the vascular endothelium by inflammatory cells and swelling and proliferation of endothelial cells, a pattern known as **intimal arteritis A**. The smooth muscle of the wall of the artery **SM** is relatively unaffected. When there is inflammation of the full thickness of the vessel wall or fibrinoid necrosis, this is classified as type III acute T-cell-mediated rejection. As the condition becomes chronic, there is intimal thickening owing to fibrosis and proliferation of myointimal cells.

Antibody-mediated rejection may show a variety of histological changes, including acute tubular, vascular and glomerular changes. Key features are the presence of the complement component C4d on the endothelium of peritubular capillaries (demonstrated by immunostaining techniques) and the presence of circulating specific antidonor antibodies in the recipient's blood.

Chronic rejection is characterised by a combination of the above changes, with tubular atrophy, interstitial fibrosis and loss of glomeruli. Unchecked, chronic rejection will inexorably proceed to end-stage kidney.

The most common malignant tumour of the kidney in adults is the *renal adenocarcinoma* (*renal cell carcinoma*) derived from the tubular epithelial cells; this is illustrated in Figure 15.17. One of its important methods of spread is by venous invasion. The kidney is also the site of an important malignant tumour of children, *nephroblastoma* or *Wilms' tumour* (Fig. 15.15); this is an example of a so-called '*small round blue cell tumour*' and is of embryological origin. Benign tumours of the kidney include *oncocytoma* (see Fig. 15.16) and *angiomyolipoma* (Fig. 15.18).

Fig. 15.15 **Nephroblastoma** (HP)

This is one of the most common malignant tumours of infants and children and is believed to originate from embryonic renal blastema. It is composed of a mixture of primitive and undifferentiated cells **C** and tubular structures **Tu**, resembling primitive renal tubules; occasionally, structures resembling immature glomeruli are also found. There are many histological variants of this tumour, some of which contain primitive tissue cells such as skeletal muscle precursors (rhabdomyoblasts).

Fig. 15.16 **Oncocytoma** (HP)

Oncocytoma is a fairly common benign renal neoplasm. Macroscopically, the tumour is a mahogany brown colour with a well-defined margin and arises in the renal cortex. There is often a central, irregular, fibrotic scar which may be identifiable radiologically. Necrosis and haemorrhage are very rare, in contrast to renal cell carcinoma. Microscopically, the tumour is composed of small, regular, round cells arranged in nests **N** as shown in this micrograph. The cell nests are separated by an oedematous stroma **S**. There is little cellular pleomorphism and minimal, if any, mitotic activity. The cells have abundant granular eosinophilic cytoplasm, resulting from the very large numbers of mitochondria that pack the cytoplasm.

BASIC SYSTEMS PATHOLOGY ■ URINARY SYSTEM

KEY TO FIGURES

A intimal arteritis   **C** undifferentiated tumour cells   **N** tumour cell nests   **S** stroma   **SM** smooth muscle
T tubulitis   **Tu** tubular structures

BASIC SYSTEMS PATHOLOGY ■ URINARY SYSTEM

Fig.15.17 **Renal cell carcinoma** (*caption opposite*)

KEY TO FIGURES
A adipose tissue   **M** foamy macrophages   **P** papillary structures   **S** smooth muscle cells   **V** blood vessels

Fig.15.17 Renal cell carcinoma (a) Clear cell carcinoma (MP) **(b)** Clear cell carcinoma (HP) **(c)** Papillary carcinoma (MP) **(d)** Chromophobe carcinoma (HP) *(illustrations opposite)*

The most common primary malignant tumour of the kidney is the *renal cell carcinoma* derived from renal tubular epithelium. Renal cell carcinoma may be subclassified according to histological and cytogenetic criteria. All types of renal cell carcinoma present with one or more of the classical triad of signs: haematuria, flank pain and a palpable mass. A few renal cell carcinomas are hereditary and some are found in *von Hippel–Lindau syndrome*, in association with cerebellar and retinal haemangioblastomas. However, the great majority of cases are sporadic. The major subtypes of renal cell carcinoma are:

■ **Clear cell carcinoma:** This is by far the most common type and generally has the worst prognosis. As seen in micrographs (a) and (b), the tumour cells are large and polygonal in shape and the cytoplasm is clear because of the accumulation of cytoplasmic glycogen and lipid. In other areas of the tumour, the cytoplasm is granular and pink-staining, more closely resembling the tubular epithelium from which these tumours are derived.

■ **Papillary (chromophil) carcinoma:** The next most common variant, this tumour is composed of papillary structures as shown in micrograph (c). The tumour is often surrounded by a thick fibrous capsule and there is typically extensive necrosis and haemorrhage. Microscopically, the tumour consists of papillary structures **P** surrounded by a

layer of cuboidal to columnar malignant epithelial cells. The papillary cores are often packed with foamy macrophages **M**. Other areas may have tubular architecture.

■ **Chromophobe carcinoma:** This tumour consists of sheets of malignant epithelial cells with pale cytoplasm (as in micrograph (d)) and prominent cell boundaries that resemble plant cells. Note the difference between this tumour and clear cell carcinoma in micrograph (b).

■ **Collecting duct carcinoma** (not illustrated): This is a rare tumour arising in the renal medulla.

■ **Sarcomatoid carcinoma** (not illustrated): This is not a separate subtype of tumour but rather a pattern that may be found in combination with any of the other types of renal cell carcinoma. As suggested by the name, the tumour cells resemble sarcoma. The presence of this pattern confers a worse prognosis.

Clear cell carcinoma tends to breach the walls of intrarenal venous tributaries and to grow as solid cords along the lumen of the renal vein towards and into the inferior vena cava. From here, venous emboli spread tumour deposits to the lung, producing typical isolated '*cannon ball secondaries*'. Renal adenocarcinoma also has a particular propensity for metastasis to bone and brain.

Fig 15.18 Angiomyolipoma (LP)

This is an uncommon but important tumour of the kidney consisting of a mixture of abnormal blood vessels **V**, sheets of smooth muscle cells **S** and adipose tissue **A**. The smooth muscle cells often have an epithelioid appearance, i.e. they are round to ovoid in shape with plentiful eosinophilic or clear cytoplasm. Most angiomyolipomas are benign but a few, usually with atypical histological features, may behave in a malignant fashion.

This tumour is very common in patients with *tuberous sclerosis* and is often multiple in these patients. Angiomyolipomas also occur in the liver and rarely at other sites.

Angiomyolipomas belong to a group of esoteric tumours called PEComas, supposedly derived from **P**erivascular **E**pithelioid **C**ells. This group includes a variety of rare tumours occurring at many anatomical sites, which are all immunoreactive for a combination of melanocyte markers (HMB45 and MelanA) and smooth muscle markers (actin and/or desmin). This group includes the clear cell 'sugar' tumour of the lung and other sites.

The most important disorders of the lower urinary tract are infection and neoplasia. Infections are common, but usually remain confined to the bladder (*cystitis*); ascending spread into the ureters and pelvicalyceal systems may result in renal parenchymal involvement (*acute pyelonephritis*) as shown in Figure 15.10. Persistent or repeated infection in the urinary tract predisposes to the development of urinary stones, particularly in the bladder and pelvicalyceal systems. Infections of the urethra (*urethritis*) are commonly sexually transmitted, involving the organisms *Gonococcus* and *Chlamydia*.

The pelvicalyceal system, ureters and bladder are lined by a specialised epithelium known as *transitional epithelium* (*urothelium*). Malignant tumours of the urothelium, known as transitional cell or urothelial carcinomas (Fig. 15.19), are common and of particular interest because of the possible role of chemical carcinogens such as aniline dyes in their pathogenesis. Urothelial carcinomas may be either invasive or non-invasive. Most of the deeply invasive tumours are high-grade carcinomas. Malignant tumours are probably preceded by the development of urothelial dysplasia and carcinoma in situ (Fig. 15.20). Benign tumours include *transitional cell papillomas* and *inverted papillomas*.

As in other areas of pathology, these tumours have recently been reclassified, with the hope that the new classification will more accurately reflect the clinical behaviour of the tumours and therefore provide a better indication of treatment requirements. At the time of writing, both old and new classifications are in use. The two classifications are outlined below.

Fig 15.19 Classification of urothelial tumours

WHO 1973 classification	WHO/ISUP consensus classification 1998
Papilloma	Papilloma
Transitional cell carcinoma Grade 1	Papillary urothelial neoplasm of uncertain malignant potential (PUNLMP)
Transitional cell carcinoma Grade 2	Low-grade urothelial carcinoma
Transitional cell carcinoma Grade 3	High-grade urothelial carcinoma

Fig. 15.20 Bladder carcinoma in situ (HP)

Carcinoma in situ of the urinary bladder is characterised by replacement of normal epithelium by cells indistinguishable from those seen in urothelial carcinoma. The epithelial cells are enlarged and crowded, with enlarged hyperchromatic nuclei and prominent mitotic figures **M**, one of which is near the epithelial surface. The epithelium is not thickened and this area might, at cystoscopy, merely appear reddened. Urothelial carcinoma in situ may be found in isolation or in association with papillary urothelial carcinoma (Fig. 15.21). These lesions are likely to progress to invasive carcinoma.

(a)

Fig. 15.21 **Urothelial (transitional cell) carcinoma** **(a)** Low grade (LP) **(b)** High grade (MP) **(c)** High grade (HP)

Urothelial (transitional cell) carcinomas (TCC) are common. All are regarded as malignant despite the fact that many show no evidence of invasion when first detected.

Micrograph (a) shows a low-grade urothelial carcinomas (TCC grade 1), with frond-like papillary outgrowths from the urothelial surface and a slender connective tissue stroma **S** supporting the layers of neoplastic cells which are enlarged and disorganised compared to normal urothelium.

In high-grade urothelial carcinomas (TCC grade 3), there may also be a surface papillary component as shown in micrograph (b). At high magnification the blood vessels **BV** in the connective tissue stroma of the papillary cores are obvious. The covering epithelium is thickened, with crowded, atypical urothelial cells, which fail to mature towards the surface. High grade urothelial carcinomas may have no papillary component but instead form a sessile ulcerated plaque. High-grade tumours, as shown in micrograph (c), may invade deeply into the bladder wall. In advanced-stage tumours, the tumour cells **T** infiltrate between smooth muscle bundles **SM** of the detrusor muscle, indicating a poor prognosis.

Urothelial carcinomas are frequently multifocal in origin, and there is a strong link between their development and exposure to certain industrial chemicals such as aniline dyes. Cigarette smoking has also been causally linked with the development of urothelial carcinomas.

The prognosis of urothelial carcinomas depends on their location, the grade of the tumour, and the extent of local invasion when the tumour is first detected. The cytology of urothelial carcinomas is shown in more detail in Figure 7.7. Occasionally, squamous carcinomas may develop in the bladder from metaplastic epithelium associated with chronic inflammation by a stone or parasitic infection (schistosomiasis). Rarely, adenocarcinoma arises from embryological urachal remnants.

(b)

(c)

KEY TO FIGURES
BV blood vessels   **M** mitotic figure   **S** stroma   **SM** smooth muscle   **T** tumour

Fig. 15.22 **Chapter review**

Site	Disorder	Main pathological features	Figure
Kidney – glomerular disorders	End-stage kidney	Sclerosed glomeruli, atrophic tubules, interstitial fibrosis	15.1
	Acute diffuse proliferative glomerulonephritis (GN)	Enlarged hypercellular glomeruli, infiltration by neutrophils, obstructed capillary loops	15.3
	Mesangial proliferative GN	Expanded mesangium with increased mesangial cells	15.4
	Mesangiocapillary (membranoproliferative) GN	Hypercellular, hyperlobular glomeruli with double contour glomerular basement membranes (GBM)	15.5
	Minimal change disease	Normal light microscopy and immunofluorescence, 'fused' podocyte foot processes on electron microscopy	15.6
	Membranous nephropathy	Thickened GBM, 'spikes' (silver stain)	15.7
	Focal segmental necrotising GN	Necrosis of glomerular segment with fibrin deposition and inflammation, may have crescent formation	15.8(a),(b)
	Focal segmental glomerulosclerosis (FSGS)	Sclerosis of a segment of the glomerular tuft	15.8(c)
	Diabetic nephropathy	Diffuse and nodular glomerulosclerosis, hyalinised arterioles, capsular drops, fibrin caps, thickened GBM	15.9
Kidney – tubulointerstitial disorders	Acute pyelonephritis	Inflammation of interstitium, prominent neutrophils, especially in tubules	15.10
	Acute tubular necrosis (ATN)	Dilated renal tubules with flattened 'simplified' epithelium, vacuolation and fragmentation of tubular cell cytoplasm	15.11
	Renal papillary necrosis	Infarction of renal papilla with inflammation at edge of infarcted area	15.12
Kidney – vascular disorders	Essential hypertension	Hypertrophied arteries with fibroelastic intimal thickening, sclerosed glomeruli	15.13(a)
	Accelerated hypertension	Fibrinoid necrosis of arterioles, 'onion-skin' intimal thickening of medium and large sized arteries, vascular thrombosis, acute ischaemia of glomeruli	15.13(b)
Kidney – transplant rejection	Acute T-cell mediated rejection	Inflammation of tubules (tubulitis) and interstitium (type I) Inflammation of arteries (intimal arteritis, transmural arteritis, fibrinoid necrosis of artery wall (types II and III))	15.14(a),(b)
Kidney – tumours	Nephroblastoma	Primitive undifferentiated cells, tubular structures	15.15
	Oncocytoma	Brown tumour macroscopically, often with central scar. Nests of bland epithelial cells with round nuclei and eosinophilic granular cytoplasm	15.16
	Renal cell carcinoma	Clear cell – cells have clear cytoplasm Papillary – papillary epithelial structures with foamy macrophages in papillary cores Chromophobe – cells with pale-stained cytoplasm and prominent cell borders	15.17
	Angiomyolipoma	Mixture of abnormal blood vessels, smooth muscle cells and adipose tissue. Most are benign	15.18
Bladder	Carcinoma in situ	Flat lesion consisting of highly atypical epithelial cells with mitotic figures and no maturation of cells towards the surface	15.20
	Urothelial carcinoma (transitional cell carcinoma (TCC))	Papillary structures covered by abnormal urothelial cells. High grade lesions may form solid ulcerated plaque. Graded as high or low (or 1, 2, 3)	15.21

16 Lymphoid and haematopoietic systems

Functions of the lymphoreticular system

The lymphoreticular system is composed of various organs and tissues which facilitate the interaction of lymphocytes with cells of monocyte–macrophage lineage in the generation of immune responses. The main organs and tissues of the system are the thymus, spleen, lymph nodes, bone marrow and mucosa-associated lymphoid tissue (MALT), such as tonsils and Peyer's patches of the gut.

Lymphocytes are produced in the bone marrow. Their number is selectively expanded, mainly in lymph nodes, in response to specific immunological requirements. Many lymphoid cells circulate through peripheral tissues via blood and lymphatic vessels in a constant search for antigens.

The monocyte–macrophage system includes tissue macrophages (histiocytes) which are found in virtually every organ. These become activated following tissue damage and, together with monocytes recruited from the blood, act as phagocytic cells in the process of organisation (see Ch. 2). These cells also process antigen for presentation to T lymphocytes. Some tissues include a population of specialised dendritic antigen-presenting cells which have a role in initiating specific immune responses.

We will consider disorders affecting some of the main organs of the haematolymphoid system as follows:

- **Lymph nodes**
  - reactive processes
  - metastatic tumours
  - primary tumours (lymphoma)
- **Bone marrow**
  - abnormalities of haematopoiesis
  - metastatic tumours
  - myeloma
  - leukaemia and lymphoma
  - myeloproliferative and myelodysplastic processes.

Reactive disorders of lymph nodes

The lymphoreticular system is remarkably labile and quickly responds to the presence of infective agents or foreign material in the activation of an immune response. There are two main patterns of immune response:

- The *cell-mediated response*: This involves the activity of T lymphocytes which are either directly or indirectly cytotoxic.

- The *humoral response*: This involves the activation of B lymphocytes which differentiate into antibody-secreting plasma cells; interaction of antibody with antigen leads to destruction or inactivation of the antigen.

Lymphadenopathy (lymph node enlargement) is a common consequence of infection and other immune reactions. Various different histological appearances can occur. These are determined by the nature of the immune stimulus and the patient's capacity to mount an immune response. In broad terms, three main patterns of non-specific lymphadenopathy are recognised which reflect reaction and expansion of different constituent areas of the lymph node (Fig. 16.1):

- follicular hyperplasia
- paracortical hyperplasia
- sinus hyperplasia/sinus histiocytosis.

Some infections and other immune stimuli give rise to more specific patterns of lymphadenopathy which can allow the pathologist to suggest a particular aetiology. Examples include the finding of multiple minute granulomas in cases of toxoplasmosis, granulomatous lymphadenitis with caseous necrosis in tuberculosis (see Ch. 4) and follicular lysis in HIV infection (see Ch. 4).

Fig. 16.1 **Reactive hyperplasia of lymph nodes** **(a)** Normal lymph node (LP) **(b)** Follicular hyperplasia (LP) **(c)** Paracortical hyperplasia (LP) **(d)** Sinus hyperplasia (LP)

Damage to or inflammation of any tissue may excite a reactive response in the draining lymph nodes. The three basic patterns of response, follicular hyperplasia, paracortical hyperplasia and sinus hyperplasia, may be seen separately or in combination, depending upon the nature of the stimulus. A low-power image of a normal lymph node is included in micrograph (a) for comparison, showing small, peripherally located follicles **F** in the cortex.

In *follicular hyperplasia*, illustrated in micrograph (b), there is an increase in number and size of cortical lymphoid follicles. This reflects a B-cell (humoral) response and results in the production and clonal expansion of antibody-secreting plasma cells.

In *paracortical (parafollicular) hyperplasia*, seen in micrograph (c), there is expansion of the T-cell parafollicular zone **P** with small, inconspicuous B-cell follicles **F** pushed to the periphery of the node beneath the capsule. This pattern is commonly seen in response to viral infection.

In *sinus hyperplasia* or *sinus histiocytosis*, shown in micrograph (d), there is no great increase in the lymphoid component of the node, but the medullary sinuses **S** are extremely prominent due to dilatation and hyperplasia of histiocytic cells lining the sinuses. This reaction is seen in nodes draining tissues from which endogenous particulate matter such as lipid is released. A common example is necrotic tumour.

KEY TO FIGURES

F follicle   **GC** germinal centre   **N** necrosis   **P** paracortex   **S** medullary sinus   **SS** subcapsular sinus
T tumour

This is less common than reactive lymphadenopathy, but is also a frequent finding in clinical practice. Although primary malignant tumours of the lymphoid system are the main focus of this section, it is important to recognise that metastatic spread of other tumours such as carcinoma and malignant melanoma to lymph nodes is a regular occurrence (see Figures 7.16 and 16.2), and so this possibility must always be considered before suggesting a diagnosis of lymphoma.

Lymphoma is a primary tumour of lymphoid tissue. This group of disorders is divided into two broad categories on the basis of the cell types present:

■ *Non-Hodgkin lymphoma (NHL)* may be derived from B or T lymphocytes.

■ *Hodgkin lymphoma (HL,* previously known as Hodgkin's disease) is characterised by the presence of *Reed–Sternberg* cells.

Lymphoma usually presents with involvement of a group of lymph nodes and may then spread to involve multiple nodal groups, as well as other haematolymphoid organs such as bone marrow and spleen. Non-Hodgkin lymphoma may arise in other organs or tissues such as skin, gut, thyroid, brain, salivary gland, lung and testis. Classification of lymphoma is complex and will be considered in the next section.

Other constituent cells of the lymph node may rarely proliferate and so give rise to lymphadenopathy. One example is a group of disorders known as *Langerhans' cell histiocytosis*. This condition has previously been known as *histiocytosis X* and by a range of eponymous designations, reflecting different patterns and severities of disease (*Letterer–Siwe, Hand–Schüller–Christian disease*, etc.). It is characterised by proliferation of histiocytic cells which resemble the Langerhans' antigen-presenting cells found in normal skin and lymph nodes. There is a spectrum of severity, ranging from benign and localised to disseminated and rapidly fatal disease which can involve skin, viscera, bone marrow and lymph nodes.

Fig. 16.2 **Metastatic colonic carcinoma in lymph node (LP)**

This micrograph shows a mesenteric lymph node from a patient with colonic adenocarcinoma (see Fig. 13.23). Carcinoma cells invade into lymphatic channels draining the primary tumour and so gain access to the regional lymph nodes through the *afferent lymphatic channels*. These malignant cells enter the *subcapsular sinus* SS of the lymph node and may settle at this site where they can proliferate to form a secondary tumour mass T. This new deposit typically resembles the primary lesion. Here, the features are those of colonic adenocarcinoma. There are areas of necrosis N with the tumour. Reactive follicles with germinal centres GC are seen within the lymph node.

LYMPH NODE SAMPLING AND EXAMINATION IN COMMON CANCERS

Examination of lymph nodes draining many malignant tumours is a routine part of the pathological assessment of tumour *stage* (the extent of disease spread, important in planning treatment and in predicting likely prognosis). The surgeon will usually excise not only the main tumour mass for examination, but also any associated groups of regional lymph nodes which drain the site of the primary mass, e.g. axillary lymph nodes in breast carcinoma, hilar and mediastinal nodes in lung cancer.

On occasion, the pathologist may receive a lymph node which contains metastatic tumour from a patient who is not already known to have pre-existing malignant disease. In this setting, examination of the metastatic deposit, often with use of special staining techniques such as immunohistochemistry, may allow the pathologist to suggest a likely site of origin of the tumour and so guide further investigation and management of the patient.

Lymphoma classification

Division of lymphomas into non-Hodgkin and Hodgkin types reflects important differences in both clinical behaviour and tumour morphology.

Non-Hodgkin lymphomas (NHL) form a large and diverse group of diseases, all of which are malignant, despite the suffix -oma. The main features common to this group are listed below:

■ Presentation is usually with painless lymphadenopathy.

■ Disease may appear to be localised to one nodal group or may be widely disseminated, with generalised lymphadenopathy and involvement of other organs.

■ Biopsy is usually performed to establish the diagnosis and to allow classification.

■ Definitive classification involves assessment of cell morphology, immunophenotype and molecular/ cytogenetic features.

■ A number of forms of non-Hodgkin lymphoma show characteristic chromosomal abnormalities which are useful in diagnosis and, in some instances, in assessing prognosis.

■ Most tumours are derived from a clonal proliferation of B or T lymphocytes and may be broadly divided into low- and high-grade types.

■ B-cell lymphomas are considerably more common than T-cell types.

■ B-cell lymphomas may arise at extranodal sites, most commonly within mucosa-associated lymphoid tissue (MALT), and these behave differently from nodal lymphomas.

■ T-cell lymphomas most frequently occur in skin and present as a disease termed *mycosis fungoides*.

Hodgkin lymphoma (HL) is less common (see Fig. 16.14)

■ Whilst most cases of NHL are widespread at the time of diagnosis, HL may be localised to a single nodal group.

■ Spread is predictable, usually by involvement of contiguous nodal groups and with dissemination to liver, spleen and bone marrow only late in disease.

■ The neoplastic cells (*Reed–Sternberg cells* and variants) often form only a small proportion of the mass, with a prominent reactive haematolymphoid cell population forming the bulk.

■ Extranodal involvement is uncommon.

THE IMPORTANCE OF TUMOUR TYPE IN CLINICAL MANAGEMENT

Hodgkin lymphoma usually spreads by orderly involvement of contiguous nodal groups and so staging of this disease is very important in planning patient management. Whilst non-Hodgkin lymphoma generally requires systemic treatment with chemotherapy, the earlier stages of Hodgkin lymphoma can often be treated effectively by localised irradiation of the affected nodal groups.

Various systems have been devised for the *classification* of haematolymphoid tumours. Classification of tumours is necessary to allow recognition of those which have similar features and facilitates improved prediction of behaviour, prognosis and response to treatment. Most earlier systems were based primarily upon the morphological appearances of the tumour cells, dividing lymphomas on the basis of architecture into *diffuse* (sheets of cells with no pattern of organisation) versus *follicular* (arranged in nodules resembling the follicles of a normal node), on the basis of cell size into small cell and large cell types (broadly reflecting low-grade or high-grade behaviour), or on the basis of similarities to normal constituent cells within the lymph node, e.g. centrocytes, centroblasts, immunoblasts, etc. Although these classification systems were useful in allowing certain subtypes of lymphoma to be described and identified, it is now recognised that morphology alone is imperfect and is insufficient to allow reliable separation of some entities which appear histologically similar but behave differently.

The development of immunohistochemical staining methods and of newer molecular techniques has revolutionised the practice of haematolymphoid pathology. The most recent internationally recognised system of classification is that of the *World Health Organization (WHO)*. This system uses a combination of clinical, morphological, immunohistochemical and molecular techniques to recognise subgroups of lymphoma with shared characteristics. The WHO classification includes a very large number of entities, but only those that are common or that illustrate an important pathophysiological concept will be considered here. A simplified classification chart which includes these disorders is shown in Fig. 16.3. In order to allow these to be placed in context more easily, an abridged version of the 2008 WHO classification system is illustrated in Figure 16.4 – but there is no need to learn this list!

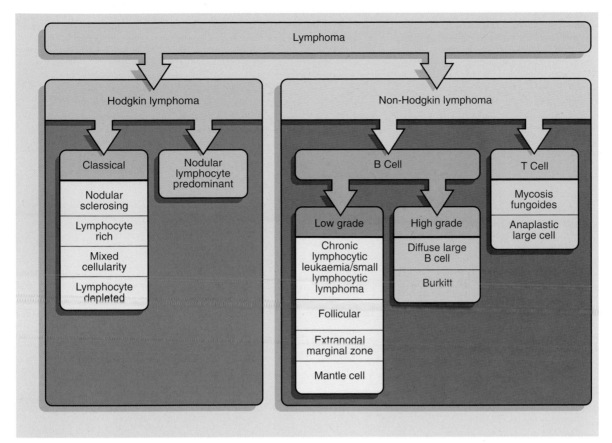

Fig. 16.3 Simplified classification chart of entities to be considered

An approach to lymph node examination in clinical practice

In clinical practice, the diagnostic pathologist first considers the **architecture** of the involved lymph node and notes the **cytological features** of the constituent cells, including cell size, nuclear shape, the presence, type and position of nucleoli and the amount and distribution of cytoplasm. This initial assessment guides the selection of appropriate immunohistochemical stains which can identify whether the tumour is of B- or T-cell lineage, as well as other markers which characterise specific subtypes of lymphoma (see Fig. 16.11).

This examination is often sufficient to achieve a diagnosis, but may be supplemented, particularly in difficult cases, by **molecular investigations**. Molecular studies can confirm **clonality** of the cell population where there is uncertainty about whether a lymphoid cell population is reactive or neoplastic (by showing that all tumour cells have the same immunoglobulin or T-cell receptor gene rearrangement) or can be used to look for non-random chromosomal translocations which characterise a particular tumour type, e.g. a t(8;14) translocation is typically present in cases of Burkitt lymphoma.

All of these findings should then be correlated with the clinical and radiological information so that an appropriate plan can be formulated for optimal patient management. From the pathologist's point of view, this may involve further staging of the tumour by sampling of tissue from other sites, e.g. bone marrow biopsy, or by the assessment of subsequent biopsies for residual disease following treatment. Some newer therapies use specific molecular targeting systems and, in some instances, pathological examination to look for immunopositivity within the tumour is needed to predict whether a certain drug will be effective, e.g. retuximab targets the CD20 antigen of B-cell tumours and so will lack efficacy in CD20-negative tumours.

CHAPTER 16

Fig. 16.4 Abridged WHO 2008 classification of non-Hodgkin and Hodgkin lymphoma

I. Precursor B-Cell Neoplasms Precursor-B lymphoblastic leukaemia/lymphoma	**IV. Peripheral T-Cell and NK-Cell Neoplasms** T-cell prolymphocytic leukaemia Large granular lymphocytic leukaemia Mycosis fungoides/Sézary syndrome

II. Peripheral B-Cell Neoplasms
Chronic lymphocytic leukaemia/small lymphocytic lymphoma
B-cell prolymphocytic leukaemia
Lymphoplasmacytic lymphoma
Splenic and nodal marginal zone lymphomas
Extranodal marginal zone lymphoma
Mantle cell lymphoma
Follicular lymphoma (and subtypes)
Marginal zone lymphoma
Hairy cell leukaemia
Plasma cell tumours (including myeloma and plasmacytoma)
Diffuse large B-cell lymphoma (and subtypes)
Burkitt lymphoma
	Peripheral T-cell lymphoma, unspecified
	Anaplastic large cell lymphoma
	Angioimmunoblastic T-cell lymphoma
	Enteropathy-associated T-cell lymphoma
	Panniculitis-like T-cell lymphoma
	Adult T-cell leukaemia/lymphoma
	NK/T-cell lymphoma, nasal type
	NK-cell leukaemia
	
	V. Hodgkin Lymphoma
	Classical subtypes
	   Nodular sclerosis
	   Mixed cellularity
	   Lymphocyte rich
	   Lymphocyte depleted
	Lymphocyte predominant

III. Precursor T-Cell Neoplasms Precursor-T lymphoblastic leukaemia/lymphoma	

B-cell non-Hodgkin lymphoma

Fig. 16.5 Chronic lymphocytic leukaemia/small lymphocytic lymphoma (a) LP (b) HP

This is a common form of non-Hodgkin lymphoma which is usually seen in older adults. As the name suggests, there is a spectrum of disease from a predominantly leukaemic form, in which there is extensive marrow involvement (see also Fig. 16.17) and the malignant cells circulate in peripheral blood, through to a lymphoma of the same morphology and immunophenotype which lacks any significant circulating component and is characterised by lymphadenopathy. Many patients have some degree of lymphadenopathy, but the term small lymphocytic lymphoma is used only in the absence of circulating atypical lymphocytes. This is a low-grade lymphoma composed of sheets of small, mature B lymphocytes with varying numbers of slightly larger prolymphocytes. These larger cells tend to be arranged in aggregates termed *proliferation centres* **PC** which give a characteristic appearance of vague nodularity on low-power examination, as illustrated in image (a). Micrograph (b) shows this at higher magnification, with small mature cells at the bottom of the field and the edge of a proliferation centre on the upper right, including many larger prolymphocytes **P**. These areas appear paler and are sometimes referred to as *pseudofollicles*.

Fig. 16.6 **Follicular lymphoma** **(a)** H&E of lymph node with follicular lymphoma (LP) **(b)** Immunohistochemical stain for bcl-2 in follicular lymphoma (LP) **(c)** Immunohistochemical stain for bcl-2 in normal reactive node (LP)

This is a common form of B-cell lymphoma which tends to occur in middle-aged and older adults and presents as painless lymphadenopathy. These tumours are derived from germinal centre B cells and usually have a nodular or *follicular* architecture **F** (a). The cells are a mixture of small centrocyte-like cells and larger centroblast-like cells. Although most tumours are low grade, an increasing proportion of centroblastic cells indicates more aggressive behaviour. The tumour cells show a similar pattern of immunopositivity to normal germinal centre B cells. Most cases are characterised by a specific chromosomal abnormality, t(14;18), which juxtaposes

the immunoglobulin heavy chain (IgH) gene on chromosome 14 with the gene for the anti-apoptotic protein bcl-2 on chromosome 18. Because IgH is expressed in normal mature B cells, this chromosomal rearrangement results in overexpression of bcl-2 protein within the tumour cells and so these cells effectively avoid the normal pathway of apoptotic destruction. In normal reactive lymph nodes, the cells of the mantle zone **MZ** are bcl-2 positive but germinal centre cells **GC** are bcl-2 negative (c). In contrast, strong bcl-2 positivity is characteristically seen within the neoplastic follicles **F** in follicular lymphoma (b).

Fig. 16.7 **Mantle cell lymphoma** (MP)

This is a relatively uncommon lymphoma but it is considered as part of the differential diagnosis in cases of small B-cell lymphoma and is important as its behaviour is significantly more aggressive than other morphologically similar tumours. Mantle cell lymphoma usually occurs at extranodal sites, particularly within the gastrointestinal tract, and may present with the clinical pattern of *lymphomatous polyposis*. Morphologically, it may have a diffuse pattern as shown here or may be vaguely nodular, occasionally adopting a mantle-zone pattern of infiltration around reactive germinal centres. The cells are slightly larger than those of the other lymphomas discussed thus far and mitotic figures **M** are more frequent. Positive nuclear staining with cyclin D1, a protein involved in regulation of cell cycle, is characteristically seen in this tumour. There is usually an associated t(11;14) translocation, juxtaposing the bcl-1 locus with the IgH gene and accounting for the overexpression of cyclin D1.

KEY TO FIGURES
F follicle   **GC** germinal centre   **M** mitotic figure   **MZ** mantle zone   **P** prolymphocytes   **PC** proliferation centre

Fig. 16.8 Gastric biopsy involved by extranodal marginal zone (MALT) lymphoma (a) H&E (MP) **(b)** H&E (HP) **(c)** Cytokeratin immunostaining (HP)

The term *MALToma* is most commonly used to refer to this group of low-grade B-cell lymphomas. These occur at *extranodal sites* such as stomach, salivary gland, thyroid gland, lacrimal gland and lung, arising from the mucosa-associated lymphoid tissue (MALT) at these sites. The cells show morphological and immunophenotypic features similar to those of a subset of mature B cells found within the normal nodal marginal zone. These are unusual, indolent tumours which, unlike most other non-Hodgkin lymphomas, tend to remain localised for long periods and may even regress in some circumstances. MALT lymphomas usually arise on a background of chronic inflammation and, in cases where the cause of this inflammatory process is remediable, such as *Helicobacter pylori*-associated gastritis, the tumour may regress following treatment of the underlying condition.

It appears that chronic antigenic stimulation initially results in polyclonal B-cell activation and proliferation as part of the normal immune response. Over time, continuing proliferation may result in accumulation of genetic aberrations and, later in the disease process, a smaller number of B-cell clones is identifiable (*oligoclonality*). Ultimately, a *monoclonal* infiltrate emerges, presumably due to selective pressures. At this point, some tumours may still regress if the initiating stimulus is removed; however, other tumours do not and, in these cases, specific chromosomal translocations are often present, particularly t(11;18). Whilst the initiating antigen is known for some forms of MALT lymphoma (e.g. *Helicobacter* gastritis, *Chlamydia* conjunctivitis), there are other chronic inflammatory disorders which are known to predispose to MALT lymphoma (e.g. Hashimoto's thyroiditis, Sjögren's syndrome) for which the initiating antigen remains elusive.

Histologically, this gastric biopsy shows an infiltrate of small lymphoid cells **L** (a) which characteristically form *lymphoepithelial lesions* **LL** by migrating into normal glandular epithelium **G**. In image (b), small lymphocytes are seen at higher magnification within the epithelium of a damaged gastric gland **G**. Immunostaining with an epithelial cell marker (c) may be used to highlight residual, partially destroyed glands and this can be helpful in diagnosis.

KEY TO FIGURES

G gastric gland   **L** lymphoid infiltrate   **LL** lymphoepithelial lesion   **M** tingible body macrophage   **MF** mitotic figure   **MP** muscularis propria   **P** peritoneal surface   **SM** submucosa   **V** villi

Fig. 16.9 Burkitt lymphoma (a) H&E of small intestine with Burkitt lymphoma (LP) **(b)** H&E of small intestine with Burkitt lymphoma (MP) **(c)** H&E of small intestine with Burkitt lymphoma (HP) **(d)** Immunostaining for cell proliferation using Ki67 (HP)

Although this is a relatively uncommon disease in industrialised countries, it is frequent in parts of Africa and illustrates certain pathophysiological concepts. The form of this disease that is typically seen in sub-Saharan Africa is known as *endemic Burkitt lymphoma*. This usually occurs in children and is closely associated with Epstein–Barr virus (EBV) infection. Sporadic and HIV-associated forms of the disease are less closely correlated with EBV. African Burkitt lymphoma typically affects the mandible or certain visceral organs, whilst the non-endemic form most frequently affects the ileocaecal area as shown here (a), and may present with symptoms of intestinal obstruction or of visceral perforation.

Histologically, the tumour is composed of sheets of intermediate-sized lymphoid cells which have an extremely high rate of proliferation. At low magnification in (a), tumour cells are seen to infiltrate through the full thickness of the wall of the terminal ileum, from the surface villi **V** of the mucosa, through the submucosa **SM**, muscularis propria **MP** and serosa to reach the peritoneal surface **P**. Characteristically, there are sheets of tumour cells with intervening *tingible body macrophages* **M** which produce a '*starry sky*' appearance (b). These cells contain apoptotic debris due to the very high rate of tumour cell turnover (c). This high proliferation rate is one of the defining features of Burkitt lymphoma. Numerous mitotic figures **MF** are seen and immunostaining to identify cells in cell cycle (using the antibody Ki67) shows that virtually 100% of tumour cells are proliferating (d). Most cases have a typical t(8;14) translocation, juxtaposing the c-MYC gene with the immunoglobulin heavy chain gene.

Fig. 16.10 Diffuse large B-cell lymphoma (HP)

This is the commonest form of high-grade B-cell lymphoma and, as the name implies, it is characterised by a *diffuse* (sheet-like) infiltrate of large B cells. The morphology of these cells is very variable, but they may resemble the centroblasts or immunoblasts seen in normal lymph nodes. Some diffuse large B-cell lymphomas arise in patients known to have a previous low-grade B-cell lymphoma such as CLL/SLL or follicular lymphoma, and can be shown by molecular methods to be clonally related to these tumours. This is termed ***high-grade transformation*** and is associated with a poor prognosis.

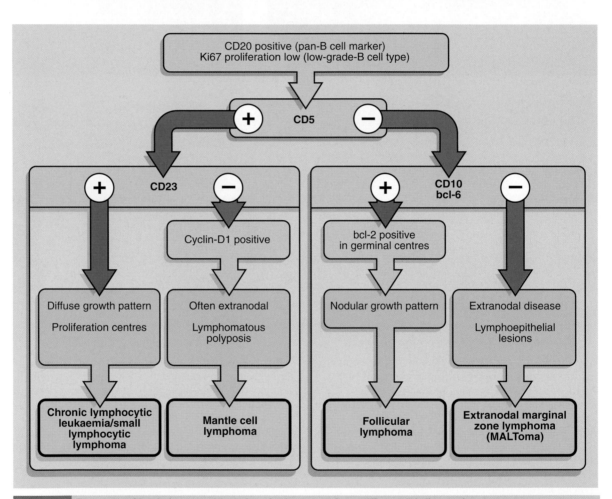

Fig. 16.11 Example of basic immunohistochemical approach to differential diagnosis

This chart illustrates a simplified scheme for use of immunohistochemistry in the differential diagnosis of low-grade B-cell non-Hodgkin lymphomas. It is important to note that these stains are never used in isolation and that their selection is guided by the morphological appearance of the lymph node. Also, occasional tumours show atypical patterns of immunoreactivity and so interpretation must always be in the context of the clinical setting, the histological appearance of the tumour and the results of ancillary investigations such as molecular testing. This chart need not be learned but aims to illustrate the general approach of the diagnostic pathologist to interpretation of immunohistochemical staining.

KEY TO FIGURES
E eosinophil   **GC** tumour giant cell   **M** atypical mitotic figure

Fig. 16.12 Mycosis fungoides (MP)

This form of T-cell lymphoma involves the skin and tends to have an indolent course. It presents as persistent, scaling, erythematous lesions which are flat initially, but gradually progress through stages described as *patch*, *plaque* and *tumour*. Systemic spread can occur late in the disease process. Early disease may mimic inflammatory disorders such as psoriasis, both clinically and pathologically. This image shows the early plaque stage of the disease. Atypical, small lymphocytes, often with complex infolding of their nuclear membranes (described as *cerebriform*) infiltrate the epidermis, but without evidence of *spongiosis* (oedema within the epidermis); this is termed *epidermotropism*.

Fig 16.13 Anaplastic large cell lymphoma (LP)

As the name suggests, this is a tumour which is composed of large, highly atypical cells. These cells usually have irregularly shaped, convoluted nuclei and tend to be of T-cell lineage. In this example, the cells have multiple large nucleoli and there is an atypical tripolar mitotic figure **M**. Fairly numerous eosinophils **E** are seen, as well as an occasional bizarre tumour giant cell **GC**.

Most cases of anaplastic large cell lymphoma are characterised by the occurrence of a specific chromosomal rearrangement which affects the *anaplastic lymphoma kinase (ALK)* gene. The effects of this abnormality can be identified by immunohistochemical staining for ALK-1. This is an important prognostic marker.

CLINICAL FEATURES OF SOME T-CELL NON-HODGKIN LYMPHOMAS

Some other types of T-cell lymphoma are of particular clinical interest. **Enteropathy-associated T-cell lymphoma** is seen in some patients who present with symptoms of **malabsorption**. Clinically, there is **steatorrhoea** (fatty diarrhoea due to failure of absorption of dietary lipid), often associated with anaemia and various vitamin deficiencies. This presentation closely resembles coeliac disease (gluten-sensitive enteropathy, see Fig. 13.15), but patients fail to respond to dietary gluten restriction and it is thought that the disorder known as **refractory coeliac disease** or **refractory sprue** is a precursor of overt lymphoma. In its earliest stages, the histological features of this disease also resemble coeliac disease, but the intraepithelial lymphocytes have an abnormal immunophenotype and sensitive molecular techniques can demonstrate clonality of the intraepithelial lymphoid cells. Over time, this may evolve into an aggressive lymphoma which often forms multiple tumour masses in the small intestine. Patients may then present with features of small intestinal obstruction or even with acute peritonitis due to perforation through a necrotic tumour mass.

A later section in this chapter deals with bone marrow disease and with leukaemias, including **acute lymphoblastic leukaemia (ALL)**. As we have previously noted, leukaemia and lymphoma are not always entirely distinct entities and the same tumour may produce either a solid tissue mass or may diffusely involve bone marrow, giving rise to a leukaemic picture. Most ALL presents as childhood leukaemia and is derived from precursor B lymphoblasts. The T-cell form of ALL is less frequent but usually occurs in adolescent boys, forming a mediastinal lymphomatous mass involving the thymus (the site of normal T-cell maturation). These patients may therefore present with symptoms related to compression of vital structures within the mediastinum such as the superior vena cava.

Hodgkin lymphoma

Fig. 16.14 Hodgkin lymphoma (*caption opposite*)

THE REED–STERNBERG CELL AND ITS VARIANTS

These large cells are essential for diagnosis of Hodgkin lymphoma. The classical form has two nuclei or a single bilobed nucleus with two prominent, inclusion-like, eosinophilic nucleoli, usually as large as normal small lymphocytes. This gives rise to the appearance of 'owl's eyes'. **Mononuclear** variants appear similar but have a single nucleus. **Lacunar cells** are associated with nodular sclerosing HL and have a folded nucleus with surrounding pale, delicate cytoplasm. This cytoplasm is often disrupted during histological processing, leaving the nucleus within a clear space (the lacuna). **Lymphohistiocytic variants (L&H cells)** are also known as 'popcorn'cells as they have abundant cytoplasm and highly convoluted nuclei, resembling popcorn kernels. These are found in nodular lymphocyte predominant HL.

Fig. 16.14 Hodgkin lymphoma (a) Nodular lymphocyte predominant pattern (HP) **(b)** Mixed cellularity pattern (HP) **(c)** Lymphocyte depleted pattern (HP) **(d)** Nodular sclerosing pattern (LP) (*illustrations opposite*)

Nodular lymphocyte predominant Hodgkin lymphoma is distinct from the classical forms of the disease. This entity was described more recently, and the Reed–Sternberg cell variants in this type are known to be activated B lymphocytes. These cells show a different pattern of immunohistochemical staining from Reed–Sternberg cells in the other (*classical*) forms of the disease and this subtype may be difficult to differentiate from some forms of B-cell non-Hodgkin lymphoma. This disease has an excellent prognosis and is illustrated in micrograph (a). Reactive lymphocytes make up the bulk of the tissue in affected nodes and form extensive sheets within which are scattered relatively few mononuclear Reed–Sternberg cells. These cells are also termed 'popcorn' cells **PC** because of the lobulated contour of their nuclei. *Classical lymphocyte rich Hodgkin lymphoma* is not illustrated but appears morphologically similar, and immunostaining is required to separate these disorders.

Mixed cellularity Hodgkin lymphoma is shown in micrograph (b). Here, classical Reed–Sternberg cells (RS cells) **RS** are mixed with a variable population of reactive cells including lymphocytes **L**, histiocytes **H**, eosinophils **E**, neutrophils **N** and plasma cells.

The type with the worst prognosis is *lymphocyte depleted Hodgkin lymphoma*. This is illustrated in micrograph (c). Affected nodes are replaced by sheets of large pleomorphic cells which are Reed–Sternberg cell variants, with only a few classical Reed–Sternberg cells **RS**. Lymphocytes **L** and other reactive cells are scanty.

Most commonly, Hodgkin lymphoma destroys the normal architecture of the lymph node completely, producing a homogeneous appearance in which no trace of the original cortico-medullary demarcation and follicular pattern remains. However, one form of Hodgkin disease, the *nodular sclerosing* pattern seen in micrograph (d), results in the deposition of broad irregular bands of pink-staining collagenous fibrous tissue **C** which separates the cellular Hodgkin tumour mass into islands, imparting a nodular appearance to the cut surface of the node. The nodular sclerosing pattern is associated with a good prognosis if diagnosed at an early stage.

Conventionally, the histological subtype of Hodgkin lymphoma has been an important indicator of prognosis, with better outcomes in variants with few Reed–Sternberg type cells and a larger proportion of reactive cells (such as lymphocyte predominant and lymphocyte rich) and therefore the worst prognosis in lymphocyte depleted disease, where Reed–Sternberg cells are very numerous. Modern management has considerably reduced these differences in outcome between histological subtypes and it is now possible to achieve complete cure of Hodgkin lymphoma. Tumour *stage* is now the primary determinant of prognosis. There is, however, a tendency for the lymphocyte predominant type to present with localised disease (excellent prognosis) while the lymphocyte depleted type typically presents with disseminated disease (poor prognosis).

Bone marrow disease

The bone marrow spaces between the trabeculae of spongy bone are occupied by adipose tissue with intervening collections of haematopoietic cells which are responsible for the production of red blood cells, white blood cells and platelets. These cell lines are derived from a reservoir of *haematopoietic stem cells* which differentiate into the various specialised cell lines in response to specific growth factors. The bone marrow is able to respond rapidly to increased demands for the various blood cells by increased proliferative activity of the precursor and stem cells.

The main diseases involving the bone marrow are:

■ abnormalities of haematopoiesis

■ metastatic tumours

■ myeloma

■ leukaemia and lymphoma

■ myeloproliferative and myelodysplastic processes.

Haematopoietic disorders

Disorders of haematopoiesis are common, but are largely outside the scope of this book. Cytological examination of smear preparations of aspirated bone marrow and histological examination of trephine biopsy specimens of bone marrow form an important method of investigating some diseases.

Most *anaemias* (lack of red cells) are the result of lack of iron, vitamin B_{12} or folate, or are due to excessive red cell breakdown (haemolytic anaemia). One type (leukoerythroblastic anaemia) is due to destruction of the haematopoietic tissue by tumour or fibrosis, and histological examination of a bone marrow biopsy is vital to establish the diagnosis.

KEY TO FIGURES
C collagen **E** eosinophil **H** histiocyte **L** lymphocyte **N** neutrophil **PC** 'popcorn' cells
RS Reed–Sternberg cell

Metastatic tumour in bone marrow

The bone marrow is a common site for blood-borne metastasis of certain malignant tumours. The tumours which most commonly spread to bone marrow are carcinomas and the most frequent primary cancers include:

■ breast carcinoma

■ lung carcinoma (see Fig. 16.15)

■ carcinoma of the kidney

■ carcinoma of the thyroid (particularly the follicular type)

■ carcinoma of the prostate (see Fig. 16.15).

In most cases, the growth of metastatic carcinoma in the bone marrow leads to destruction of trabecular bone, leading to *osteolytic* deposits which appear as lucent areas on X-ray. Carcinoma of the prostate often stimulates the active formation of new woven bone, producing *osteosclerotic* deposits which appear as increased areas of bone density on X-ray. Another tumour which frequently metastasises to bone marrow is neuroblastoma, an aggressive tumour which usually occurs in childhood.

Fig. 16.15 **Metastatic tumour in bone marrow** **(a)** H&E of bone marrow with metastatic prostatic carcinoma (MP) **(b)** Immunohistochemical staining for prostate-specific antigen (PSA) (MP) **(c)** H&E of bone marrow with metastatic lung carcinoma (MP) **(d)** Immunohistochemical staining for thyroid transcription factor 1 (TTF-1) (MP)

The bone marrow is a frequent site for deposits of metastatic carcinoma, the common primary tumours being from prostate, bronchus, breast, thyroid and kidney. Widespread replacement of bone marrow by metastatic tumour may induce *extramedullary haematopoiesis* (see Fig. 16.20) in liver and spleen.

Most metastatic deposits cause bone destruction and, when widespread, can be associated with hypercalcaemia. Metastases from carcinoma of the prostate may, however, be associated with new bone formation and result in *osteosclerosis*. This is shown in micrograph (a), where replacement of marrow by prostatic adenocarcinoma cells **C** is associated with

reactive trabecular bone formation **B**. In micrograph (b), an immunohistochemical staining method is employed to demonstrate prostate-specific antigen (PSA), a specific marker for prostatic adenocarcinoma in metastatic tumour. The clumps of tumour cells are stained dark brown.

Micrographs (c) and (d) illustrate metastatic lung carcinoma, again using an immunohistochemical stain (TTF-1) which is useful in identifying bronchogenic carcinoma cells. This antibody targets a nuclear transcription factor that is found almost exclusively in thyroid and lung tissue. The site of staining in this case is within the tumour cell nuclei.

KEY TO FIGURES
B bone   **C** carcinoma

Multiple myeloma

This group of disorders falls within the WHO category of mature B-cell neoplasms, but is considered here because its most frequent presentation is as a disseminated disease, characterised by widespread bone marrow involvement. Myeloma is characterised by neoplastic proliferation of terminally differentiated B cells that have developed the features of plasma cells and so can produce large amounts of immunoglobulin. The features of myeloma are diverse and are a product of various interrelated processes, including displacement of normal haematopoietic elements by the tumour (leading to anaemia, thrombocytopenia and immune dysfunction), bone destruction (causing pain, lytic lesions on X-ray and increased risk of fracture), renal disease and hypercalcaemia, with its associated metabolic consequences.

Fig. 16.16 Multiple myeloma (HP)

In this example from a patient with diffuse marrow involvement, the haematopoietic tissue is replaced by abnormal plasma cells which, in normal marrow, are only a very minor constituent. These have eccentric nuclei, a paranuclear hof (a pale area indicating the site of the prominent Golgi apparatus) and clock-face chromatin. Atypical, binucleate or multinucleate cell forms and more primitive plasmablasts may also be seen.

Molecular or immunohistochemical investigation reveals evidence of *light chain restriction* (i.e. all of the cells produce either κ or λ light chains, indicating monoclonality). This monoclonal immunoglobulin can be identified by *serum electrophoresis* and the light chain component can be excreted in urine, known as *Bence-Jones protein*.

Osteolytic lesions of myeloma lead to bone pain and sometimes fracture, whereas diffuse bone marrow infiltration may lead to destruction of normal haematopoietic cells, resulting in leukoerythroblastic anaemia. Solitary mass lesions in bone are termed *plasmacytomas*.

Leukaemias

Leukaemias are characterised by neoplastic proliferation of white cells within the bone marrow which then circulate within the peripheral blood. General characteristics of leukaemias include:

■ neoplastic proliferation of marrow-derived cells, forming one or more neoplastic cell lines

■ circulation of the neoplastic cells in the peripheral blood

■ suppression of normal haematopoietic activity by the expanding leukaemic cell population.

Because the neoplastic leukaemic cells circulate in the blood, the cells are usually deposited in other tissues and organs, particularly lymph nodes, liver and spleen. Leukaemias are classified according to the cell of origin, but a useful general division is into two main types: chronic leukaemias and acute leukaemias.

Chronic leukaemias are characterised by neoplastic proliferation of relatively mature white cells. Typically, the clinical course is indolent, with a long natural history. Although the neoplastic cells predominate in the marrow, other haematopoietic cells can survive alongside, and adequate numbers of red cells and platelets are produced. Chronic leukaemias are mainly seen in adults over the age of 40 but some may eventually transform into a more aggressive acute leukaemia.

Acute leukaemias are characterised by neoplastic proliferation of very immature white cells *(blast cells)*. The course of the disease is very rapid, with destruction of all other haematopoietic cell lines in the marrow. Without treatment, acute leukaemias are rapidly fatal.

■ *Chronic lymphocytic leukaemia (CLL)* is considered in the previous section owing to its overlap with small lymphocytic lymphoma (Fig. 16.5), but its appearance in the bone marrow is illustrated here (Fig. 16.17).

■ *Chronic myelogenous leukaemia (CML)* is a neoplastic proliferation of the more mature precursors of neutrophils (for example myelocytes and metamyelocytes) and occurs most commonly in adults.

■ *Acute lymphoblastic leukaemia (ALL)* is a tumour of immature lymphocyte precursors (lymphoblasts), and occurs most commonly in children (see also earlier clinical text box: T-cell ALL).

■ *Acute myeloid leukaemia (AML)* is a tumour of immature precursor cells in the myeloid series (mainly myeloblasts) and is most common in adults (Fig. 16.18). It is the most common of a group of acute leukaemias derived from various myeloid precursors, collectively called acute non-lymphoblastic leukaemias.

Some lymphomas which originate in lymph nodes may also eventually spread to involve bone marrow, and there may be enough circulating lymphoma cells in the blood to be detected in a blood film, highlighting again that there are areas of overlap between leukaemia and lymphoma.

Fig. 16.17 **Chronic lymphocytic leukaemia; bone marrow** (HP)

In chronic lymphocytic leukaemia, the marrow between bone trabeculae **B** becomes infiltrated by small lymphocytes, similar to those seen in small lymphocytic lymphoma. Very large numbers of similar cells appear in the peripheral circulation. Although occupation of the marrow is extensive, destruction of the normal haematopoietic marrow elements is not as rapid or severe as in acute lymphoblastic leukaemia and the condition runs an indolent course. This is a disease seen mainly in later life. Lymphadenopathy, splenomegaly and anaemia are commonly encountered.

Fig. 16.18 **Acute myeloid leukaemia; bone marrow** (HP)

Acute myeloid leukaemia is characterised by proliferation of primitive myeloid cells in the bone marrow. There are several subgroups, depending on degree of maturation of the neoplastic cells, from primitive *myeloblasts* through types with *promyelocyte* morphology to types with both myeloid and monocytic morphologies. The marrow is replaced by large atypical myeloid blast cells with few maturing cells (compare with Fig. 16.19). This type of leukaemia predominates in adults under 60 and presents acutely with anaemia and bleeding secondary to thrombocytopenia. Diagnosis is made on blood and marrow examination.

Myeloproliferative disorders and myelodysplastic syndromes

This complex group of disorders is now part of the World Health Organization (WHO) classification. In broad terms, ***myeloproliferative disorders*** are the result of abnormal proliferation of stem cells in the bone marrow which can differentiate into red cell (erythroid) precursors, white cell (myeloid or granulocytic) precursors, megakaryocytes or fibroblasts. As a result, the peripheral blood usually contains increased numbers of these cells, e.g. excess erythrocytes in ***polycythaemia vera*** and excess platelets in ***essential thrombocythaemia***. ***Chronic myelogenous leukaemia*** is also considered to be one of the myeloproliferative disorders. ***Myelofibrosis*** occurs due to excessive fibroblast proliferation within the marrow, obliterating the marrow cavity due to collagen deposition and so displacing normal haematopoietic progenitors (see Fig. 16.20). The myeloproliferative disorders, as well as showing frequent overlap and transition from one form to another, have a tendency to terminate in an acute leukaemic phase.

Myelodysplastic syndromes are also due to proliferation of abnormal stem cells within the marrow, but here, the maturation of cells is abnormal and so terminally differentiated blood cells are not produced. They are characterised by various ***cytopenias*** (reduced numbers of cells in the peripheral blood) and by the presence of some abnormal circulating cells. Again, there is a spectrum of disorders which overlap, including refractory anaemia, refractory anaemia with ringed sideroblasts, refractory anaemia with multilineage dysplasia, refractory anaemia with excess blasts and acute myeloid leukaemia. Morphologically, there is abnormal maturation of bone marrow cells, often involving more than one haematopoietic lineage. This is termed ***dysplasia***.

Accurate diagnosis of both myeloproliferative and myelodysplastic syndromes requires correlation of peripheral blood counts, marrow aspirates and marrow trephine biopsies, usually involving both pathologists and haematologists. There is some overlap between these two groups and this is recognised within the current WHO classification. In addition, some cases are associated with previous drug therapy with cytotoxic agents and so a comprehensive clinical history is always required. Detailed consideration of this group of disorders is outwith the scope of this text.

Fig. 16.19 Chronic myelogenous leukaemia; bone marrow (HP) (resin section)

In this disease, there is low-grade neoplastic proliferation of neutrophil precursors. Increased numbers of ***myeloblasts*** produce greatly increased numbers of ***myelocytes***, ***metamyelocytes*** and mature ***neutrophils***, all of which appear in the peripheral blood in greatly increased numbers. The marrow between bone trabeculae **B** is packed with neutrophils and late neutrophil precursors, particularly myelocytes and metamyelocytes. Increased numbers of the most primitive precursor, the myeloblast, are also present, but they are a minority population compared to acute myeloid leukaemia (Fig. 16.18). Despite the abnormal myeloid proliferation, normal haematopoietic activity continues, although at a reduced rate. Chronic myeloid leukaemia is characterised by the presence of a t(9;22) translocation known as the ***Philadelphia chromosome***.

THE PHILADELPHIA CHROMOSOME

This is a reciprocal translocation involving exchange of genetic material between chromosomes 9 and 22. It is characteristically seen in chronic myeloid leukaemia but also occurs occasionally in acute lymphoblastic leukaemia and acute myeloid leukaemia. It results in the fusion of part of the breakpoint cluster region (BCR) gene on chromosome 22 with part of the Abelson (ABL, named after a similar viral protein) gene on chromosome 9. The **chimaeric protein** formed has tyrosine kinase activity and is constitutively active, altering cell cycle proteins to promote increased proliferation, impaired DNA repair and reduced apoptotic cell death.

Clearly, this translocation is important in tumour progression, and our understanding of the molecular basis of this disease has now allowed the development of specifically targeted therapy. In recent years, drugs have been developed which act to inhibit this abnormal tyrosine kinase activity within the tumour cells. These drugs dramatically reduce proliferation of the malignant cells and reduce the risk of transformation into an acute leukaemic form (**blast crisis**). Drugs such as **imatinib** and its newer derivatives have also been used with considerable success in the treatment of other tumours such as gastrointestinal stromal tumours (see Fig. 13.14).

KEY TO FIGURES
B bone

Fig. 16.20 **Myelofibrosis** **(a)** Bone marrow, thin resin section (HP) **(b)** Liver (HP)

In this disorder, replacement of haematopoietic marrow by progressive *fibrosis* leads to loss of capacity to produce erythrocytes, leukocytes and platelets. In micrograph (a), the marrow space between bone trabeculae **B** is infiltrated by spindle-shaped fibroblastic cells **F**. This is partly compensated for by *extramedullary haematopoiesis*, when other organs of the lymphoreticular system re-acquire their fetal potential for haematopoiesis. The liver and spleen are the principal organs involved in this compensatory process and the spleen may become greatly enlarged.

Micrograph (b) shows the liver sinusoids to be distended by a population of immature erythropoietic and granulopoietic elements, as well as occasional megakaryocytes **M**. Erythroid islands are recognisable as clusters of small normoblasts **N** with densely staining nuclei.

Chapter review

This table summarises important features of the diseases discussed but is by no means comprehensive. Brief mention is made of typical patterns of immunostaining seen in some lymphomas. It is not expected that these should be memorised, but this *aide-memoire* may provide a useful basis for the reading of more advanced texts by those training in diagnostic pathology.

Fig. 16.21 **Chapter review**

Disorder	Main features	Immunostaining	Genetic change	Figure
Reactive lymphadenopathy				
Follicular hyperplasia	Enlarged reactive germinal centres Reflects humoral (B-cell) response			16.1(b)
Paracortical hyperplasia	Expansion of paracortex, small follicles Reflects cell-mediated (T-cell) response			16.1(c)
Sinus histiocytosis	Prominence of histiocytes lining sinuses Common in nodes draining carcinoma			16.1(d)
Non-Hodgkin lymphoma (NHL)				
CLL/SLL	Older adults, often leukaemic Diffuse small B-cell infiltrate Proliferation centres pathognomonic	CD5+ CD23+	Trisomy 12	16.5 16.17
Follicular lymphoma	Usually nodular (follicular) architecture Centroblasts and centrocytes but no tingible body macrophages in follicles	CD10+ bcl6+ bcl2+	t(14;18)	16.6
Mantle cell lymphoma	Often GI tract (lymphomatous polyposis) Diffuse or nodular architecture Slightly larger cells	CD5+ CD23− cyclinD1+	t(11;14)	16.7
MALT lymphoma	Extranodal sites with MALT, often gastric Associated with chronic inflammation Lymphoepithelial lesions (cytokeratin+)		t(11;18)	16.8

Fig. 16.21 Chapter review—cont'd

PART 2

CHAPTER

16

Disorder	Main features	Immunostaining	Genetic change	Figure
Diffuse large B-cell lymphoma (DLBCL)	Common, high-grade tumour Sheets of large B cells Brisk proliferation	CD20+ Ki67 high		16.10
Burkitt lymphoma	EBV associated, especially African form Sheets of intermediate-sized cells 'Starry sky' appearance	CD20+ Ki67 100%	t(8;14) c-MYC	16.9
Mycosis fungoides (MF)	Cutaneous disease, mimics psoriasis Atypical T cells infiltrate epidermis Patch, plaque and tumour stages	CD3+ CD4+		16.12
Anaplastic large cell lymphoma	Sheets of large, pleomorphic cells Irregular convoluted nuclei, mitoses ++ Usually children or young adults	ALK1+ CD30+ CD3+	t(2;5)	16.13
Hodgkin lymphoma (HL)				
Nodular lymphocyte predominant HL (nLPHL)	Vague nodularity at low power 'L+H' or 'popcorn' variant RS cells Small lymphocytes in background	CD20+ EMA+ CD30–		16.14(a)
Lymphocyte rich HL	Morphology as for nLPHL Different immunophenotype, need immunohistochemistry to distinguish– both indolent	CD20– CD30+ CD15+		Like 16.14(a)
Mixed cellularity HL	Classical RS cells Surrounding lymphocytes, histiocytes, neutrophils, eosinophils & plasma cells	CD20– CD30+ CD15+		16.14(b)
Lymphocyte depleted HL	Many RS cells and variants Few reactive cells Worse prognosis	CD20– CD30+ CD15+		16.14(c)
Nodular sclerosing HL	Nodules with bands of collagen Classical RS cells and lacunar types Mixed reactive cells, including eosinophils	CD20– CD30+ CD15+		16.14(d)
Bone marrow disorders				
Myeloma	Plasma cell tumour Production of excess immunoglobulin Bence-Jones proteinuria	CD138+ EMA+		16.16
Acute lymphoblastic leukaemia	Primitive lymphoid cell proliferation Usually in children, good prognosis Presents as a result of marrow replacement	TdT+		
Acute myeloid leukaemia	Myeloid precursor cells proliferate Various degrees of differentiation Usually adults, aggressive disease			16.18
Chronic myeloid leukaemia	Part of myeloproliferative spectrum Tumour of more mature neutrophil precursors		t(9;22) Philadelphia chromosome	16.19
Myeloproliferative disorders	Bone marrow stem cell producing excess numbers of mature cells of one or more lineage in peripheral blood			16.20(a)
Myelodysplastic syndromes	Bone marrow stem cell proliferation but failure of normal maturation and so peripheral blood cytopenias			
Other disorders				
Metastatic tumours	Mainly carcinoma and melanoma Common cancers metastatic to bone: lung, breast, prostate, kidney, thyroid			16.2 16.15
Extramedullary haematopoiesis	Response to marrow replacement or need for increased haematopoiesis Primarily spleen and liver			16.20(b)

KEY TO FIGURES
B bone   **F** fibroblast   **M** megakaryocyte   **N** normoblasts

17 Female reproductive system

Introduction

The female reproductive tract comprises the vulva, vagina, uterus, Fallopian tubes and ovaries. As in other systems, a wide range of pathological conditions may occur in these organs. Malignant tumours and their precursor conditions are of major pathological importance. An interesting feature of the female genital tract is that there is a range of epithelial malignancies that can occur at almost any site in the tract. For instance, one might imagine that endometrioid adenocarcinoma would be found only in the endometrium, but primary endometrioid adenocarcinoma also occurs in the ovary, cervix, and, very rarely, the vagina.

Disorders of the vulva

The vulva is subject to many of the conditions affecting skin elsewhere in the body, including inflammatory conditions such as **dermatitis** and **lichen planus** (see Fig. 21.7), but is also an important site for sexually transmitted infective lesions, including the chancre of primary syphilis. Many vulval inflammatory lesions lead to intense itching, so the histological features of these conditions are complicated by the effects of trauma from scratching (**lichen simplex chronicus**). In some post-menopausal women, the vulval mucosa tends to become thickened and white as a result of epithelial atrophy and subepithelial fibrosis, a condition known as **lichen sclerosus et atrophicus** (Fig. 17.1).

Many carcinomas of the vulva are preceded by epithelial dysplasia, known as **vulval intraepithelial neoplasia (VIN)** and sometimes there is associated **Human papilloma virus (HPV)** infection. Clinically, it can be difficult to differentiate these conditions from inflammatory lesions and biopsy is necessary for diagnosis. An unusual and intriguing vulval tumour is Paget's disease of the vulva, which has a similar appearance to Paget's disease of the breast (see Fig. 18.13). A small proportion of these cases are associated with an underlying adenocarcinoma, but some appear to arise as a form of carcinoma in situ of epithelial cells showing apocrine differentiation.

Most malignant tumours of the vulva are slow-growing, well-differentiated **squamous cell carcinomas**, similar to those of the skin and mucous membranes elsewhere (Figs 7.6, 17.7). They may arise in the labia majora, labia minora or clitoris and may spread deeply into the underlying connective tissue and thence via lymphatics to superficial inguinal lymph nodes. Other tumours of the vulva include benign naevi, malignant melanoma and, rarely, adenocarcinoma arising in Bartholin's glands.

Fig. 17.1 Lichen sclerosus et atrophicus (LP)

This condition of unknown aetiology presents clinically as very itchy, smooth, whitish plaques around the vulva, often with narrowing of the introitus. Histologically, there may be marked atrophy of the epidermis **E** with virtual disappearance of rete pegs **R** and skin appendages. Characteristically, the dermis contains a band of inflammatory cells **In**, mainly lymphocytes and plasma cells, the inflammatory zone being separated from the epidermis by a layer of acellular hyalinised collagen **H** in the superficial dermis. Although this condition does not exhibit epithelial dysplasia, there is an association with invasive carcinoma, with 1–4% of these patients developing invasive squamous carcinoma.

The vagina is rarely the site of important primary lesions of histopathological interest, although it is frequently the site of infections (***vaginitis***), especially by *Candida* (see Fig. 4.15), *Trichomonas* (see Fig. 4.20) and *Gardnerella vaginalis*. Primary squamous carcinoma and adenocarcinoma of the vagina do occur, but are rare.

The cervix frequently exhibits chronic inflammatory changes, described as ***chronic cervicitis*** (Fig. 17.2), which may also be associated with polypoid hyperplasia of the endocervical mucosa, sometimes with the formation of a large pedunculated ***polyp*** containing distended endocervical glands and stroma (Fig. 17.3). Clinically, the most important lesions of the cervix are ***epithelial dysplasia*** of varying degrees of severity and ***squamous cell carcinoma***, arising at the cervical squamocolumnar junction; these related conditions and their pathogenesis are considered in detail in Figures 17.4 to 17.7. ***Adenocarcinoma in situ*** and ***invasive adenocarcinoma*** of the cervix are less common than squamous cell carcinoma. Neoplastic, pre-invasive changes are termed ***cervical intraepithelial neoplasia*** or ***CIN*** and graded as 1, 2 or 3 (see Fig. 17.5). Similarly, ***vulval intraepithelial neoplasia*** is graded ***VIN 1, 2*** or ***3***, and ***vaginal intraepithelial neoplasia*** as ***VAIN 1, 2*** or ***3***. Glandular dysplasia in the cervix is less well defined and is generally reported as ***adenocarcinoma in situ (AIS)*** or ***cervical glandular intraepithelial neoplasia (CGIN)***.

Fig. 17.2 **Chronic cervicitis** (MP)

In chronic cervicitis, the ectocervical squamous epithelium **Ep** is normal except for slight thickening (acanthosis). The major changes are seen in the endocervix immediately above the squamocolumnar junction **J** where there is ***micropolyposis***, the core of each tiny polyp **P** showing a heavy chronic inflammatory cell infiltrate composed mainly of lymphocytes and plasma cells. Cervical glands may develop cystic dilatation, often termed Nabothian follicles **F**. Long-standing inflammation may lead to ***squamous metaplasia*** of the endocervical surface epithelium (see Fig. 6.5).

Fig. 17.3 **Endocervical polyp** (LP)

This micrograph shows a small benign endocervical polyp arising from the endocervical canal. The polyp is composed of cystically dilated glands **G** of varying sizes, each distended by mucin and lined by columnar endocervical mucin-secreting epithelium. As the polyp enlarges, it may develop a fibrous stroma between the cystic glands; extrusion through the external os may lead to surface ulceration. Cervical polyps are thus an important cause of abnormal vaginal bleeding.

KEY TO FIGURES

E epidermis **Ep** squamous epithelium **F** Nabothian follicle **G** gland **H** hyalinised collagen
In inflammation **J** squamocolumnar junction **P** polyp **R** rete peg

The understanding that most, if not all, invasive cervical carcinomas are preceded by a long period of pre-invasive neoplastic change in the cervix has led to a revolution in the treatment of cervical carcinomas. These changes are detectable on cytological examination of smears of the cervix, permitting early treatment and prevention of progressive disease. Cytological screening programmes in many countries have reduced the number of deaths from cervical carcinoma. Almost all cervical dysplasia and cancers (~95%) are caused by persistent infection by carcinogenic types of **Human papilloma virus (HPV)**, a very common sexually transmitted virus. Most HPV infections are self-limiting and resolve spontaneously within 2 years, but it is important to identify those most likely to progress to invasive and potentially fatal disease. Specific tests for infection with oncogenic HPV subtypes are being introduced, which may help to guide the need for treatment. In most screening programmes, a positive cytology result is followed up with direct visualisation of the cervix by colposcopy and biopsy. Correlation between cytology and histology is vital to avoid unnecessary treatment for false positives. The classification of the abnormalities seen by both modalities has undergone many modifications over the years. Figure 17.4 shows the different systems of terminology currently in use for squamous lesions. The British Cervical Screening Programme uses the British Society for Cervical Cytology (BSCC) system for classification and the WHO system for histology. The Bethesda system can be used for both. These different grading systems are not exactly equivalent and are still evolving as new information becomes available.

Fig. 17.4 Comparison of grading systems for cervical squamous dysplasia

Histological features	Traditional system	WHO system	British Society for Cervical Cytology	Bethesda system
Atypical squamous cells not meeting the criteria for dysplasia	Mild atypia	Mild atypia	Borderline nuclear abnormality	Atypical squamous cells (ASC)
Koilocytes plus mild atypia	HPV infection	HPV infection	HPV plus borderline change	Low-grade squamous intraepithelial lesion (SIL)
Dysplasia limited to lower third of epithelium	Mild dysplasia	CIN 1	Mild dyskaryosis (low-grade dyskaryosis)	Low-grade SIL
Dysplasia limited to lower two-thirds of epithelium	Moderate dysplasia	CIN 2	Moderate dyskaryosis (high-grade dyskaryosis)	High-grade SIL
Dysplasia extending into upper third of epithelium	Severe dysplasia	CIN 3	Severe dyskaryosis (high-grade dyskaryosis)	High-grade SIL
Dysplasia of full thickness of epithelium	Carcinoma in situ	CIN 3	Severe dyskaryosis (high-grade dyskaryosis)	High-grade SIL

The ectocervix is covered by stratified squamous epithelium while the endocervix has a lining of simple columnar mucin-secreting cells. The junction between the two varies during reproductive life with changes in the volume of the cervical stroma. This expands under the influence of hormones during each menstrual cycle, at menarche and during pregnancy, and this causes eversion of the vaginal end of the endocervical canal, thus exposing some of the simple columnar epithelium to the vaginal environment. This exposed epithelium appears red in relation to the surrounding stratified squamous epithelium and hence became inaccurately known as a **cervical erosion**; more appropriate is the term **cervical ectropion**. Under the influence of the vaginal environment, the ectopic columnar epithelium may undergo squamous metaplasia (see Fig. 6.5) to form stratified squamous epithelium. This metaplastic area, known as the **transformation zone**, appears to be sensitive to the oncogenic effects of HPV. Infection of the squamous epithelium of the vagina is also very common, but dysplasia and invasive carcinoma are very rare. The development of vaccines that offer good protection against oncogenic subtypes of HPV introduces the possibility of cancer prevention, if given before infection has occurred.

Infection with certain **low-risk genotypes** of HPV (6, 11, 42 and 44) results in condyloma acuminatum (genital warts) and low-grade dysplasia. The **high-risk genotypes** (most commonly 16, 18, 33, 45, 31 and 58) are more likely to result in high-grade dysplasia and to progress to invasive carcinoma. HPV 16 is the most common subtype found in patients with invasive squamous cell carcinoma, while HPV 18 is particularly associated with adenocarcinoma. The factors that influence progression from latent infection to invasive carcinoma are unknown, but may include host factors such as immune status, nutritional factors and cigarette smoking. Integration of the viral genome into the host DNA is also an important factor in progression to invasive cancer. Only a small proportion of women infected with high-risk serotypes progress to invasive carcinoma.

Fig. 17.5 **Cervical cytology**
(a) Koilocytes (HP)
(b) Mild dyskaryosis (HP)
(c) Moderate dyskaryosis (HP)
(d) Severe dyskaryosis (HP) (Papanicolaou stain)

These micrographs are from liquid-based cytology (LBC) preparations stained by the *Papanicolaou method (Pap)*. LBC technology is gradually replacing the older method of smearing the cervical cells directly onto a glass slide because of the improved preservation of the material and lower false-positive and false-negative rates. Micrograph (a) shows *koilocytes* K with mild atypia which is not enough for a diagnosis of mild dyskaryosis, referred to as borderline nuclear abnormality. Note the clearing of the cytoplasm surrounding the nucleus and compare with Figure 17.6. Micrograph (b) of *mild dyskaryosis (low-grade squamous intraepithelial lesion)* exhibits both normal cervical squamous cells S and clumps of mildly dyskaryotic cells D which have large dark-stained nuclei, a slightly irregular nuclear contour and a coarse pattern of nuclear chromatin.

As discussed in Fig. 17.4, dyskaryosis/squamous intraepithelial lesion (SIL) are terms used in cytology and, although they indicate the likelihood of finding dysplasia (CIN) on biopsy, do not correlate exactly with dysplasia.

Micrograph (c) shows *moderate dyskaryosis (high-grade squamous intraepithelial lesion (HGSIL))*. In this image, the abnormal epithelial cells D have larger nuclei and a higher nuclear to cytoplasmic ratio than in mild dyskaryosis, with coarser, more hyperchromatic nuclei.

In *severe dyskaryosis (HGSIL)* as shown in micrograph (d), the nuclear to cytoplasmic ratio is even greater although the cells overall may be smaller D. This corresponds to total lack of surface maturation so that cells resembling the basal layer cells are exfoliated at the surface.

The abnormal surface cells of dysplastic epithelium are collected when a cervical smear is taken. Most dysplasia occurs at the transformation zone, which is an area of metaplastic squamous epithelium found at the squamocolumnar junction. It is therefore important that endocervical cells are seen in the cervical smear to ensure that the correct area has been sampled.

KEY TO FIGURES
D dyskaryotic cell   **K** koilocyte   **S** normal squamous epithelial cell

Fig. 17.6 Cervical intraepithelial neoplasia (CIN) (a) Normal ectocervix (HP) **(b)** CIN 1 (HP) **(c)** CIN 2 (MP) **(d)** CIN 3 (MP)

Micrographs (a) to (d) illustrate the spectrum of cervical epithelial appearances, from normal stratified squamous epithelium through to CIN 3 (HGSIL).

As seen in micrograph (a), normal ectocervical epithelium has a typical stratified squamous form with all cell division being confined to a single basal layer of small, darkly staining cuboidal cells. As the cells undergo maturation, their eosinophilic cytoplasm expands greatly and the cells are pushed upwards into a stratum equivalent to the prickle cell layer of skin. Beyond this, the cells become flattened with further maturation, their nuclei becoming first pyknotic then undergoing karyorrhexis and karyolysis (see Fig. 1.7); the cytoplasm becomes progressively flattened until the cells are finally shed from the surface.

In CIN 1 (LGSIL), as seen in micrograph (b), the cells in the lower third of the epithelium L are enlarged, crowded and hyperchromatic and show increased mitotic activity. In this biopsy, there is also evidence of associated HPV infection with plentiful *koilocytes* K; such virus-infected cells are characteristically found in the upper layer of the epithelium and have enlarged irregular nuclei with clear cytoplasm (see also Fig. 4.14).

When dysplastic cells are seen mainly in the lower two-thirds of the epithelium as in micrograph (c), the lesion is termed CIN 2 (HGSIL). Numerous koilocytes are also seen in this example. These koilocytes represent productive infection by HPV.

In CIN 3 (HGSIL), as seen in micrograph (d), the atypical cells extend into the upper third of the epithelium. As in this example, mitotic figures **M** are common and are seen well above the basal layer; abnormal mitotic figures may also be seen.

In general, the management differs for low-grade (CIN 1) and high-grade (CIN 2 & 3) lesions. As most low-grade lesions will regress spontaneously they are generally monitored, while high-grade lesions are treated either by excision or ablation in situ, e.g. laser therapy.

A critical feature of the dysplastic examples just discussed is that the basement membrane remains sharply defined and intact. With any evidence of *microinvasion* or more extensive spread into underlying tissues, the lesion is defined as *invasive carcinoma*.

KEY TO FIGURES

E surface epithelium **K** koilocytes **L** lower third of epithelium **M** mitotic figure **N** normal vaginal mucosa
S cervical stroma **T** squamous carcinoma

Fig. 17.7 **Invasive squamous cell carcinoma of the cervix** **(a)** Microinvasive carcinoma (MP) **(b)** Invasive carcinoma (LP) **(c)** Well-differentiated carcinoma (MP)

Most cases of invasive squamous cell carcinoma of the cervix are preceded by a long premalignant phase of dysplasia (CIN). The treatment for CIN is dependent on the grade of the lesion but high-grade lesions (CIN 2 and 3/HGSIL) are generally excised, most often by loop excision biopsy. On histological examination, a few of these specimens exhibit the earliest form of invasive carcinoma with only superficial invasion of the cervical stroma. When the lesion is limited in extent (invasion less than 3 mm deep and 7 mm wide), it is termed *microinvasive carcinoma* and relatively conservative surgery such as cone biopsy or simple hysterectomy is adequate to achieve cure. As seen in micrograph (a), the surface epithelium **E** is dysplastic (CIN 3/HGSIL) (see also Fig. 17.6). Small nests of squamous carcinoma **T** are seen lying separately within the supporting stroma, the tumour cells having breached the epithelial basement membrane. Typically, the invasive component has a more squamous appearance, the cells having more plentiful eosinophilic cytoplasm than is seen in the overlying CIN 3/HGSIL.

More extensive and macroscopically obvious carcinoma of the cervix is treated by surgical removal of the uterus in toto (*radical hysterectomy*), removal of the cervix and paracervical tissues (*radical trachelectomy*) if the patient wants to preserve fertility, or by radiotherapy. Pelvic lymph nodes are also removed. Such an invasive squamous carcinoma of the cervix is illustrated at low magnification in micrograph (b). Note that purple-staining tumour **T** has replaced most of the cervical stroma and muscle, although a portion of normal vaginal mucosa **N** remains at the tumour margin. The surface of the tumour is ulcerated; this accounts for the frequent presenting feature of *post-coital bleeding*.

An area of a well-differentiated cervical squamous cell carcinoma is shown in micrograph (c). The lesion consists of sheets of mildly pleomorphic squamous cells **T** invading the cervical stroma **S**. The cells have plentiful eosinophilic cytoplasm, and are separated by a small space where intercellular bridges would be seen at higher magnification. Compare this example with well and poorly differentiated squamous cell carcinoma in Figure 7.6.

Squamous carcinomas account for about 90% of cervical malignancies, most of the remainder being adenocarcinomas arising in the endocervix. Invasive carcinomas of the cervix spread widely into local structures and become disseminated to lymph nodes in the pelvis.

Fig. 17.8 **Adenocarcinoma in situ of the endocervix** (MP)

Adenocarcinoma of the cervix is less common than squamous carcinoma and arises from the endocervical glands. It is also often preceded by dysplastic changes in the glandular epithelium. Micrograph (a) shows a small focus of *adenocarcinoma in situ (AIS)* **A** (also known as *cervical glandular intraepithelial neoplasia, CGIN*). Compare the enlarged, dysplastic columnar cells with those of the adjacent normal endocervical epithelium **E**. These glands show many of the features of adenocarcinoma but as yet have not developed the ability to invade the stroma. AIS of the cervix often occurs in association with squamous dysplasia, as in this case where the surface epithelium shows CIN 3/HGSIL **C**. AIS cells may also be detected on cervical smears. As mentioned above, adenocarcinoma of the cervix is also associated with HPV infection (80%), most often HPV 18. Invasive adenocarcinoma of the cervix is usually of mucin-producing (endocervical) type, but other types of adenocarcinoma that occur throughout the female genital tract may also occur here, e.g. endometrioid, clear cell, serous carcinoma.

Disorders of the uterus

The uterine endometrium undergoes monthly cyclical changes under the influence of hormonal stimuli during the reproductive years, except during pregnancy. Before menarche and after the menopause, the endometrial glands and stroma are compact and inactive. At menarche, around the menopause and for the first few cycles after a pregnancy, the endometrium shows a mixture of inactive and normal functional patterns. Iatrogenic factors such as oral contraceptive drugs, other hormonal treatments and intrauterine contraceptive devices may also modify the appearance of the endometrium.

Endometrial infection is uncommon, but may be associated with retained products of conception after childbirth or miscarriage, pelvic inflammatory disease or with intrauterine contraceptive devices. Endometrial tuberculosis is rare in developed countries, but much more common in countries where TB is common. Fulminant infection of the uterus by coliform organisms was once a common fatal complication following childbirth (puerperal fever) but is now uncommon in developed countries.

Excessive or uncoordinated hormonal stimulation of the endometrium may produce diffuse endometrial hyperplasia (Fig. 17.11), some variants of which are pre-malignant. Localised areas of polypoid hyperplasia forming endometrial polyps are common and benign (Fig. 17.10). The most common malignant tumour of the endometrium is *endometrioid carcinoma*, an adenocarcinoma derived from endometrial glands (Fig. 17.12). Other types of adenocarcinoma of the endometrium occur rarely, including tumours typical of the ovary such as serous, clear cell and mucinous carcinomas. Endometrial adenocarcinomas are sometimes divided into type 1 tumours (grade 1 endometroid carcinoma) which are oestrogen dependent and type 2 tumours (grade 3 endometrioid, serous carcinomas) which are usually not oestrogen dependent. The rationale for this is that type 2 tumours behave much more aggressively and require different treatment from type 1 tumours. Tumours of the endometrial stroma, *endometrial stromal sarcoma*, and mixed glandular and stromal tumours, *malignant mixed Müllerian tumours*, (*MMMT, carcinosarcoma*) are much less common but very important malignant tumours.

The myometrium is the site of one of the most common benign connective tissue tumours, the *leiomyoma* (Fig. 17.13), often known as a fibroid. Leiomyoma must be differentiated from its much rarer malignant counterpart, *leiomyosarcoma*, as well as tumours of borderline malignancy, known as smooth muscle tumours of uncertain malignant potential.

The myometrium may also contain islands of ectopic endometrium known as *adenomyosis* (Fig. 17.9), which may give rise to pain and other menstrual disturbances. Such ectopic endometrial tissue may also be found in various other sites throughout the pelvis and sometimes the abdominal cavity, where it is called *endometriosis* (Fig. 17.9). In this case, it may respond to the normal cyclical hormonal changes giving rise to bleeding into the tissues and consequent fibrosis.

Fig. 17.9 (a) **Adenomyosis of myometrium** (MP) (b) **Endometriosis of Fallopian tube** (MP)

Endometrial glands **G** and stroma **S** may be found outwith the endometrium itself. If the ectopic endometrium is found embedded deep within the myometrium **M**, the condition is known as *adenomyosis*; similar deposits at other sites are known as *endometriosis*. Adenomyosis is often associated with a symmetrical increase in myometrial volume thus enlarging the uterus; occasionally, there is a localised increase in smooth muscle to produce a leiomyoma-like mass containing endometrial islands, a lesion called an *adenomyoma*.

This ectopic endometrium represents an outgrowth of the basal endometrial layer and, in most cases, is not responsive to ovarian hormones. It is therefore not usually shed during menstruation, and thus, in contrast to endometriosis, no evidence of bleeding is seen in the tissue.

Micrograph (b) shows endometrial glands **G** and stroma **S** embedded within the wall of the Fallopian

tube. Deposits are seen within the mucosa at the top of the micrograph and the muscular wall in the bottom corners. Unlike adenomyosis, this endometrium is hormone responsive and bleeds during menstruation, causing pain. Evidence of bleeding may be seen as haemosiderin-laden macrophages in the tissue and in the lumen of the glands. The presence of free blood within the tissue often causes a marked fibrotic reaction that may cause adhesions between loops of bowel. Fibrosis of the Fallopian tubes owing to endometriosis is a common cause of infertility and of tubal ectopic pregnancy. Endometriosis of the ovary may give rise to a cyst filled with altered blood, known as a *chocolate cyst*. The most common sites for endometriosis include the Fallopian tubes, paratubal connective tissues and ovaries. It is, however, not uncommon in the abdomen and is occasionally seen within the thorax.

KEY TO FIGURES

A adenocarcinoma in situ   **C** CIN 3/HGSIL   **E** normal endocervical epithelium   **G** endometrial glands
M myometrium   **S** endometrial stroma

Fig. 17.10 Endometrial polyp (LP)

Endometrial polyps are an important but innocuous cause of abnormal uterine bleeding, usually at or near the menopause. They may have a stalk or pedicle and are often multiple. Most are composed of cystically dilated glands **C** in a fibrotic endometrial stroma **S** and covered by a layer of flattened endometrial surface cells. Thick-walled blood vessels may also be a feature. The glands and stroma in some polyps are responsive to ovarian hormones, and may thus resemble proliferative, secretory (rarely) or hyperplastic endometrium. Polyps are more common in women taking tamoxifen. Occasionally, endometrial carcinomas may arise in a polyp.

Fig. 17.11 Endometrial hyperplasia (a) Simple hyperplasia (MP) **(b)** Complex hyperplasia with atypia (HP)

Endometrial hyperplasia appears to be a response to excessive or uncoordinated oestrogen production and some variants are precursor lesions for endometrial carcinoma.

In *simple hyperplasia*, as shown in micrograph (a), the endometrial lining becomes thickened by proliferation of mildly crowded glands **G** that have a slightly irregular outline and may be dilated to form small cysts **C**. Heavy uterine bleeding is the most common presenting symptom and it is usually treated with progestogens. Features of simple hyperplasia are seen focally in *disordered proliferative endometrium*, which results from anovulatory cycles in perimenopausal women.

In *complex hyperplasia*, shown in micrograph (b), the endometrial glands **G** are more crowded, with a gland to stroma ratio of 2:1 or more. The glands are irregular in shape and size, often with papillary infoldings and more mitotic figures than in simple hyperplasia.

Marked cytological atypia **A** is rarely seen in simple hyperplasia, but is much more common in complex hyperplasia. There is nuclear and cytoplasmic pleomorphism and increased mitotic activity. All types of hyperplasia are associated with an increased risk of invasive endometrial carcinoma, which is significant only in *complex hyperplasia with atypia*; approximately 25% of these cases progress to invasive carcinoma. *Endometrial intraepithelial neoplasia (EIN)* is another terminology sometimes used to describe this condition.

Fig. 17.12 Endometrioid adenocarcinoma (MP)

Endometrioid or *endometrial adenocarcinoma* is the most common malignancy of the endometrium, so called because it resembles endometrial glands. It usually occurs in post-menopausal women and is the most important cause of post-menopausal bleeding.

Endometrioid adenocarcinoma **E** often arises in endometrium with complex hyperplasia. It may be limited to the endometrium, forming a mass bulging into the endometrial cavity, or it may invade the underlying myometrium **M** as shown in this example. Distorted, irregular, glandular patterns are typical, and focal squamous differentiation is seen frequently, known as *squamous morules* **SM**. The tumour spreads by local invasion through the myometrium and via lymphatics to iliac and para-aortic lymph nodes.

Endometrioid adenocarcinoma is graded on architectural and cytological criteria into grades 1, 2 and 3. Other factors which determine the prognosis are depth of invasion into the myometrium, involvement of the cervix, lymph node metastases and distant metastases.

Endometrial carcinomas are sometimes divided into *type 1 carcinomas*, which are epitomised by grade 1 endometrioid cancers, and *type 2*, which include grade 3 endometrioid carcinomas and other high-grade carcinomas such as the serous and clear cell types. Type 1 tumours are indolent and oestrogen dependent but type 2 tumours behave more aggressively and need more extensive treatment.

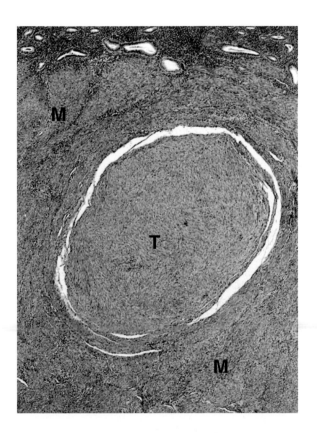

Fig. 17.13 Leiomyoma (fibroid) of myometrium (LP)

This benign tumour of myometrial smooth muscle is a common cause of abnormal or excessive uterine bleeding and pelvic discomfort. The tumour **T** is composed of fascicles (bundles) of smooth muscle cells, but larger tumours also show foci of collagen deposition, particularly towards the centre of the mass. Gradual expansion of the tumour compresses the surrounding myometrium **M** leading to atrophy of normal myometrial smooth muscle cells.

In this example, the tumour lies in the myometrium deep to the endometrium, but some arise near the endometrial cavity and may protrude into the cavity to produce a polypoid *submucosal fibroid*. Secondary changes may also occur, including extensive collagenisation, calcification (especially with increasing age) and cystic degeneration. To an extent, the growth of these tumours is hormone dependent, since they almost always shrink and partially regress after the menopause. These tumours are differentiated from *smooth muscle tumours of uncertain malignant potential* and *leiomyosarcomas* of the myometrium on the basis of the degree of mitotic activity, cellular crowding and pleomorphism and invasive margins.

KEY TO FIGURES
A cytological atypia   **C** cystic endometrial gland   **E** endometrioid adenocarcinoma   **G** endometrial gland
M myometrium   **S** endometrial stroma   **SM** squamous morule   **T** tumour

Placental disorders

Details of the various structural and functional abnormalities of the placenta, decidua, membranes and umbilical cord are generally outside the scope of this book; however, *hydatidiform mole* (Fig. 17.14) and *choriocarcinoma* (Fig. 17.15) are included as examples of disorders of placental growth. Ectopic pregnancy is discussed in Figure 17.17.

(a)

(b)

Fig. 17.14 Hydatidiform mole (a) MP **(b)** HP

The condition known as *hydatidiform mole* arises in a small proportion of pregnancies after miscarriages, terminations of pregnancy or even years after a normal pregnancy. Moles may be *partial* or *complete*. In a complete mole, as seen in micrograph (a), the chorionic villi become oedematous with central cystic spaces (*cisternae*) **S**. The cisternae are invested by a layer of hyperplastic cytotrophoblast and syncytiotrophoblast. In addition to hyperplasia of the trophoblast, there are disconnected masses of trophoblast cells **T** lying apparently free of the villi and showing mild cellular pleomorphism. Hydatidiform moles exhibit a wide spectrum of behaviours: some are eradicated by simple curettage, others persist despite repeated curettage and a small number develop into undoubtedly malignant *choriocarcinoma* (Fig. 17.15).

Complete hydatidiform mole almost always has a 46,XX karyotype but all the chromosomes are derived from the spermatozoa with none from the ovum. Partial moles have similar, but less prominent histological abnormalities, rarely develop into choriocarcinoma and have a triploid karyotype such as 69,XXY.

KEY TO FIGURES
C cytotrophoblast   **H** haemorrhage   **M** tubal mucosa   **P** purulent exudate   **S** cisterna   **Sy** syncytiotrophoblast
T trophoblast

Fig. 17.15 Choriocarcinoma (HP)

Choriocarcinoma is a malignant tumour derived from trophoblast cells, usually from abnormal gestations. The tumour consists of malignant cells resembling either cytotrophoblast cells **C** or multinucleate syncytiotrophoblast cells **Sy**. The two cell types are arranged in alternating layers, mimicking the structure of chorionic villi. No true chorionic villi are found. The tumour is typically haemorrhagic **H** because of the propensity of trophoblast cells to invade blood vessel walls. Areas of necrosis in the tumour are common. Choriocarcinoma is remarkably invasive, metastasising widely via lymphatics and the bloodstream, particularly to the lungs. Fortunately, this tumour responds well to chemotherapy.

Choriocarcinoma may also rarely occur in the ovary and in the testis, in the latter case usually as part of a mixed germ cell tumour.

Diseases of the Fallopian tubes

The Fallopian tubes may become infected by pyogenic bacteria, particularly *Gonococcus* and *Chlamydia*, and the acute inflammation, acute salpingitis (Fig. 17.16), may be complicated by obstruction of the tubal lumen, leading to chronic suppurative inflammation and abscess formation. Along with tuberculosis of the Fallopian tube, these conditions constitute an important cause of female infertility worldwide owing to obliteration of the tubal lumen. In developed countries, endometriosis (Fig. 17.9) is a relatively more common cause of infertility. Scarring of the tube and other disorders may prevent the free passage of a fertilised ovum into the endometrial cavity and implantation may occur in the tube, leading to tubal ectopic pregnancy (Fig. 17.17); this usually culminates in massive intraperitoneal haemorrhage caused by the placenta eroding through the tubal wall.

Fig. 17.16 Acute salpingitis (MP)

In *acute salpingitis*, the tubal mucosa **M** becomes hyperaemic, oedematous and infiltrated with neutrophils and the lumen becomes filled with a purulent exudate **P**. Blockage of the tubal lumen often follows, preventing drainage and leading to distension of the tube by pus (*pyosalpinx*). Sometimes the inflammation produces *adhesions* between tube, fimbriae and ovary, and extension of suppuration to these areas may produce multiple locules of pus, the *tubo-ovarian abscess*. Without the intervention of antibiotics, the combination of adhesions and suppuration rarely permits total resolution of the acute inflammation and a state of chronic inflammation generally ensues. This state, known as *chronic salpingitis*, may persist for many years, resulting in fibrosis and tubal obstruction, and is an important cause of female infertility. Chronic salpingitis may be a component of more widespread chronic inflammation involving ovaries, clinically termed *pelvic inflammatory disease (PID)*. Sometimes the inflammation dies down but the obstructed tube becomes massively distended by fluid, a condition termed *hydrosalpinx*.

Fig. 17.17 Tubal ectopic pregnancy (a) (MP) (b) (MP)

The Fallopian tube is the most frequent location for ectopic implantation of the fertilised ovum, resulting in *ectopic pregnancy*; other much rarer sites include the abdominal cavity and the ovary.

The tubal lumen becomes filled and expanded by the developing embryo (not seen in this micrograph) and the placenta. In micrograph (a), the Fallopian tube has already ruptured and chorionic villi **CV** and sheets of trophoblast **T** can be seen spilling into the peritoneal cavity **PC**. The muscular wall of the Fallopian tube **M** has been breached by trophoblast burrowing into it **B** (shown in micrograph (b)). Haemorrhage **H** is also seen within the peritoneal cavity. Haemorrhage into the lumen of the tube **H** causes *haematosalpinx*.

Ectopic pregnancies usually become dramatically apparent by severe haemorrhage into the lumen, often followed by tracking of blood into the peritoneal cavity. Thus, tubal ectopics most often present as acute abdominal emergencies; only very rarely does the pregnancy continue to near normal term.

The most common cause of tubal ectopic pregnancy is obstruction of the lumen, usually caused by infection, endometriosis and intra-abdominal adhesions. However, about 50% occur in normal Fallopian tubes.

Disorders of the ovary

Non-neoplastic cysts

Under the influence of pituitary gonadotrophins, the ovary undergoes cyclical changes providing for the development and release of a mature ovum at the midpoint of each monthly menstrual cycle and for the production of the ovarian hormones that control the menstrual cycle. During the proliferative phase of the menstrual cycle, a number of *follicles* enlarge, culminating in maturation of one follicle that discharges its single *ovum* into the Fallopian tube (ovulation). The follicle, until this time also

> **KEY TO FIGURES**
> **B** trophoblast burrowing into wall of tube   **CV** chorionic villi   **H** haemorrhage   **M** muscular wall of Fallopian tube   **PC** peritoneal cavity   **T** trophoblast

responsible for production of oestrogens, now develops into the *corpus luteum*, responsible for producing progesterone until the beginning of the next menstrual cycle when the follicle atrophies to form the redundant, collagenous *corpus albicans*. This regular sequence of changes is normally only interrupted by pregnancy, in which case the corpus luteum persists until the end of the first trimester. On occasion, however, the sequence is arrested at some stage and small *follicular* or *luteal cysts* may form. Some small cysts may also form by inclusion of islands of surface 'germinal' epithelium of the ovary; these are known as *germinal inclusion cysts*. These three types of cyst are shown in Figure 17.19.

Tumours of the ovary

Tumours may arise from each of the specialised elements that make up the ovary and may be classified into four broad groups. These groups of tumours and their major subtypes are listed in Figure 17.18 below.

- **Epithelial tumours**: Tumours of the surface ovarian epithelium are the most common. These tumours range from benign (often cystic) to frankly malignant. Intermediate between these two ends of the spectrum are tumours with a low but significant probability of metastasising. This group is called *borderline* or *atypical proliferating tumours*.

- **Stromal tumours (*sex cord–stromal tumours*)**: Tumours may develop from *granulosa cells* and *theca cells* (Fig. 17.23), as well as from spindle cells of the ovarian stroma forming *fibromas*. These may produce oestrogenic hormones and cause endocrine effects such as endometrial hyperplasia (Fig. 17.11).

- **Germ cell tumours:** The majority of ovarian germ cell tumours are benign dermoid cysts (mature cystic teratomas; see Fig. 17.24).

- **Metastatic tumours**: The ovary is a common site for metastatic carcinoma, which is frequently bilateral. A well-known example is the *Krukenberg tumour*, in which there is infiltration of the ovary by mucin-secreting adenocarcinoma of signet ring type (Figs 7.8 and 13.12); such tumours are usually derived from stomach or colon and probably reach the ovary by either transcoelomic or lymphatic spread. Tumours from other parts of the genital tract, including uterus and cervix, commonly involve the ovaries. Breast and pancreaticobiliary carcinomas also frequently metastasise to this site. The ovaries may also be involved by lymphoma.

Other disorders of the ovary

The ovary may be affected by *endometriosis* (Fig. 17.9), as well as being involved by chronic inflammation in the form of tubo-ovarian abscesses caused by primary infection of the Fallopian tube (Fig. 17.16).

Fig. 17.18 Overview of ovarian tumours

Tumour type	Subtype
Epithelial tumours	**Serous** – serous cystadenoma, borderline serous tumour, serous cystadenocarcinoma **Mucinous** – mucinous cystadenoma, borderline mucinous tumour, borderline mucinous tumour with intraepithelial carcinoma, mucinous cystadenocarcinoma **Endometrioid** – almost all are invasive carcinomas – resembles endometrioid carcinoma of the uterus – may arise from endometriosis (see Fig. 17.12) **Brenner** (transitional cell) tumour – almost all benign, rarely malignant **Clear cell** – almost all malignant and high grade – may arise from endometriosis **Undifferentiated** – too poorly differentiated to categorise **Neuroendocrine** – large cell and small cell types
Sex cord–stromal tumours	**Fibroma** **Thecoma** **Granulosa cell tumour** – adult type, juvenile type
Germ cell	**Mature teratoma** (dermoid cyst) – very common and almost always benign **Dysgerminoma** (testicular equivalent is seminoma) **Yolk sac tumour** **Choriocarcinoma**
Metastatic	From stomach, colon, breast, uterus, cervix May also be involved by lymphoma

Fig. 17.19 Non-neoplastic ovarian cysts (a) Germinal inclusion cyst (LP) (b) Follicular cyst (MP) (c) Luteal cyst (MP)

The most common type of ovarian cyst is the so-called *germinal* or *epithelial inclusion cyst*, as illustrated in micrograph (a). These cysts are commonly multiple, small and lined by a simple cuboidal epithelium **Ep**. They are thought to be derived from entrapped portions of the ovarian surface epithelium, which is erroneously but traditionally referred to as germinal epithelium.

Follicular cysts, as seen in micrograph (b), are lined internally by granulosa cells **G** which usually form a thicker layer than the flattened cells lining the germinal inclusion cyst. Continuing enlargement of the follicular cyst leads to atrophy of the lining cells so that distinction between a large follicular cyst and a germinal inclusion cyst may be difficult. Multiple follicular cysts are found in the ovaries of patients with polycystic ovary disease, frequently associated with obesity, anovulation and hirsutism.

The *luteal cyst* is probably derived from a corpus luteum that has not undergone the normal transition to a corpus albicans. The cyst is usually ovoid with a slightly irregular outline. Microscopically, it contains clear or brownish fluid and is lined by a yellow-coloured layer of variable thickness. As shown in micrograph (c), the yellow layer is composed of plump luteal cells **L** with lipid-rich cytoplasm; the inner layer is composed of granulosa cells **G**, which are also luteinised.

KEY TO FIGURES

Ep epithelium   **G** granulosa cells   **L** luteal cells   **T** tumour invading stroma

Fig. 17.20 Serous ovarian tumours (a) Serous cystadenoma (HP) **(b)** Serous papillary cystadenocarcinoma (MP) **(c)** Borderline serous tumour (LP)

Benign serous cystadenomas, which range from tiny to huge (watermelon sized), are often unilocular and are filled with a clear, watery (serous) fluid. The benign cysts are lined by columnar epithelium, resembling that of the Fallopian tube. A variant on this theme is the *serous cystadenofibroma,* which has a similar epithelium but also includes a stromal component made up of bland spindle cells in a collagenous stroma, reminiscent of *fibroadenoma* of the breast (see Fig. 18.6).

In malignant serous tumours (b), known as *serous cystadenocarcinomas,* the cystic cavity tends to be filled by complex, branching papillary structures. These are covered by columnar cells that are crowded and dysplastic. The cells are stratified and form solid sheets. Essential for the diagnosis of malignancy is evidence of invasion of the stroma by tumour **T**; indeed, the tumour may breach the capsule of the ovary, forming papillary outgrowths on the surface.

Tumours of borderline malignancy, known as *borderline* or *atypically proliferating serous tumours* (c), show many of the cytological and architectural features of serous cystadenocarcinoma but lack stromal invasion. Some papillary growths contain spherical, concentrically laminated, calcified bodies in their stroma; these *psammoma bodies* are typical of papillary tumours of the ovary, although they are also seen in papillary tumours of the thyroid and in meningiomas (see Fig. 23.14).

Fig. 17.21 **Mucinous tumours of ovary** **(a)** Benign mucinous cystadenoma (MP) **(b)** Mucinous cystadenocarcinoma (MP) **(c)** Borderline mucinous tumour (MP)

Mucinous tumours of the ovary range from benign to malignant. The *benign cystadenoma*, as shown in micrograph (a), has a characteristically smooth outer surface composed of the ovarian capsule **Cap**. The cystic locules are filled with mucin and lined by tall, columnar epithelium with uniform basal nuclei and copious, mucin-containing cytoplasm at the luminal aspect. The malignant variant, *mucinous cystadenocarcinoma*, illustrated in micrograph (b), is less common. The tumour is more solid, with smaller cystic spaces. The cells are usually recognisably columnar, but the nuclei are larger and more pleomorphic. The cells are crowded and show increased mitotic activity. Evidence of malignancy is usually demonstrated by invasion of tumour cells **T** into the supporting stroma.

Some mucinous tumours show many of the cytological features of mucinous adenocarcinoma without actual invasion of the stroma. These are called *borderline* or *atypically proliferating mucinous tumours* and their prognosis is better than for overtly malignant tumours; an example is shown in micrograph (c). These cells are thought to resemble endocervical epithelial cells. Another variant shows intestinal differentiation but, although previously these tumours were thought to be ovarian primary tumours, it has become clear that many are, in fact, metastases from the gastrointestinal tract.

KEY TO FIGURES
C cystic space   **Cap** ovarian capsule   **N** nest of transitional cells   **T** tumour cells

Fig. 17.22 Brenner tumour (LP)

Brenner tumours are almost always benign and are often incidental findings in ovaries removed for another reason. Brenner tumours consist of nests N of epithelial cells, resembling the transitional cells of the normal bladder epithelium. The epithelial cell nests may contain small cystic spaces C and are set in a stroma consisting of spindle cells which may occasionally contain lipid. Most Brenner tumours are small but they may be 20 cm or more in diameter. Rare borderline and frankly malignant variants occur. They sometimes occur in association with mucinous cystadenomas.

THE MOLECULAR BIOLOGY OF OVARIAN CARCINOMAS

The ovary gives rise to a wide range of morphological types of carcinoma which respond differently to different types of treatment. Molecular studies have begun to provide some insight into how these different tumours arise and also provide additional diagnostic techniques to help to categorise poorly differentiated examples. For instance, mucinous ovarian carcinomas tend to overexpress the k-ras oncogene. Mucinous tumours appear to develop through an orderly sequence from cystadenoma to borderline tumour to invasive carcinoma, and *k-ras* overexpression occurs early in that sequence.

Hereditary ovarian carcinoma is associated with mutations in either BRCA1 or BRCA2 (approximately 10% of all ovarian invasive carcinomas). These tumours are almost always serous carcinomas. In non-hereditary serous carcinomas, there tends to be overexpression of p53 and WT-1 (Wilms' tumour suppressor gene). Clear cell carcinomas show loss of the PTEN tumour suppressor gene.

Fig. 17.23 Sex cord–stromal tumours (a) Thecoma (MP) (b) Granulosa cell tumour (MP)

These are two of the most common of a large group of tumours known as sex cord–stromal tumours. Other tumours in this group include ovarian fibromas and Sertoli–Leydig cell tumours, which may occur in the ovary (rarely) as well as in the testis. ***Thecomas (theca cell tumours)*** are lobulated, solid tumours with a well-circumscribed margin and a bright yellow cut surface macroscopically. The tumour is composed of plump spindle cells containing fine lipid droplets, which make the cytoplasm appear foamy. This tumour usually secretes excessive amounts of oestrogens and may be associated with endometrial hyperplasia or even endometrial carcinoma. Thecomas are virtually always benign.

Most ***adult granulosa cell tumours*** occur in middle-aged to older women and are unilateral. They are composed of uniform ovoid to spindle cells resembling normal granulosa cells. The cells typically have a longitudinal nuclear groove. These may be arranged in a variety of patterns, including one mimicking follicle formation, the ***Call–Exner body*** (not illustrated here). Less well-differentiated forms may be arranged in a variety of other patterns such as the 'watered-silk pattern' as shown in (b). Most early-stage tumours have a good prognosis, but the tumour has a tendency to recur locally after many years and some are frankly malignant. The juvenile type, which is much rarer, has a distinctive histological appearance and occurs mainly, but not always, in the younger age group.

Fig. 17.24 **Benign cystic teratoma** (MP)

This tumour, formerly known as *dermoid cyst of the ovary*, is an example of a mature teratoma in which ectodermal elements usually predominate. The lesion takes the form of a unilocular cyst filled with a thick, yellowish, pasty material composed of masses of degenerating keratin **K**, often containing hair. This is produced by the lining epithelium of the cyst, which is keratinising stratified squamous epithelium resembling skin. At one end of the cyst wall, there is often a raised area within which are other teratomatous components including hair follicles **H**, sebaceous glands **S** and, occasionally, teeth. Although ectodermal derivatives predominate, particularly skin and skin appendage components, mesodermal (e.g. cartilage and smooth muscle) and endodermal (e.g. respiratory and gut epithelium) elements occur in some tumours. Neuroectodermal tissues may also be found; in this example, note the area of glial tissue **G** and a ganglion **Gan** alongside.

Cystic teratomas are most common in young women and are almost always benign. Rarely, malignant change may occur in the squamous epithelial component; this is seen in elderly patients who have harboured a cystic teratoma for many years.

In addition to benign cystic teratomas, discussed here, solid malignant ovarian teratomas occur in children and pubertal girls and are prone to widespread metastasis. Other germ cell tumours of the ovary such as dysgerminoma, choriocarcinoma and yolk sac tumour are rare and have similar histological appearances to their testicular equivalents (see Ch. 19).

KEY TO FIGURES

G glial tissue   **Gan** ganglion   **H** hair follicle   **K** keratin   **S** sebaceous gland

Fig. 17.25 Chapter review

Organ	Disorder	Main features	Figure
Vulva	Lichen sclerosus et atrophicus	Thin/thick epithelium, band of hyalinised collagen under epithelium with underlying band of chronic inflammation	17.1
	Dysplasia and carcinoma in situ (VIN)	Neoplastic epithelial cells confined to the epithelium, 3 grades (VIN 1, 2 and 3)	Like 17.6
	Invasive squamous cell carcinoma (SCC)	Similar to SCC at other sites	Like 17.7
Cervix and vagina	Chronic cervicitis	Chronic inflammation with papillary hyperplasia of the mucosa	17.2
	Endocervical polyp	Dilated endocervical glands in an inflamed fibrous stroma	17.3
	Cervical intraepithelial neoplasia (CIN)	Atypical epithelial cells confined to the epithelium, either 3 grades, (CIN 1, 2 and 3) or 2 (LGSIL and HGSIL)	17.4-17.6
	SCC	Similar to SCC at other sites	17.7
	Adenocarcinoma in situ	Dysplastic cells lining pre-existing cervical glands	17.8
	Adenocarcinoma	Adenocarcinoma – usually mucin-producing but rarely endometrioid or clear cell type	
Uterus	Adenomyosis/endometriosis	Endometrial glands in the myometrium/at other sites	17.9
	Endometrial polyp	Disorganised endometrial glands in fibrotic stroma	17.10
	Endometrial hyperplasia – simple/complex – with/without atypia	Proliferative endometrial glands with varying degrees of crowding and cytological atypia	17.11
	Endometrial carcinoma • most endometrioid • less common serous/clear cell	Adenocarcinoma invading the endometrium or myometrium	17.12
	Leiomyoma (fibroid)	Well defined nodule of smooth muscle cells in the myometrium	17.13
Placenta	Hydatidiform mole	Abnormal chorionic villi often with cystic spaces and atypical proliferating trophoblast	17.14
	Choriocarcinoma	Frankly malignant tumour consisting of layers of syncytiotrophoblast and cytotrophoblast	17.15
Fallopian tube	Acute salpingitis	Typical acute inflammation with plentiful neutrophils	17.16
	Tubal ectopic pregnancy	Chorionic villi and trophoblast invading wall of fallopian tube	17.17
Ovary	Benign, non-neoplastic cysts – epithelial inclusion cyst, follicular cyst, luteal cyst	Bland cysts lined by flattened epithelium, granulosa cells or luteinised granulosa cells	17.19
	Epithelial tumours • Serous • Endometrioid • Clear cell • Mucinous • Brenner tumour	Various types – • Fallopian tube differentiation • like uterine endometrioid carcinoma • atypical cells with clear cytoplasm • like cervical adenocarcinoma • resembles urothelial tumours	17.20 Like 17.12 17.21 17.22
	Sex cord–stromal tumours • Thecomas • Granulosa cell tumours – adult/juvenile	• Spindled cells may be luteinised • Ovoid cells froming follicular structures (Call–Exner body)	17.23(a) 17.23(b)
	Germ cell tumours • Teratoma – most are mature • Dysgerminoma • Yolk sac tumour • Choriocarinoma	• Mixture of mature (adult) tissues • Resembles seminoma	17.24 Like 19.4
	Metastatic tumours – primaries from gastric, colon, pancreas, kidney, other	Resembles primary tumour	

18 Breast

Introduction

The female breast is dependent for its normal activity on oestrogen and progestogens and thus exhibits considerable structural and functional variation throughout life. Apart from the overt changes occurring at puberty, pregnancy, lactation and menopause, more subtle changes also occur within the normal menstrual cycle. As a corollary, hormonal disturbances probably underlie various benign breast disorders and probably also play some part in the pathogenesis of more serious conditions such as **breast cancer**. Likewise, the male breast normally remains rudimentary unless breast enlargement, **gynaeco-mastia** (Fig. 18.5), is induced by exogenous or endogenous hormone imbalance; it may also result from the use of certain drugs, for example spironolactone.

Most clinically significant breast disorders present as a lump and the major imperative is to identify those that are malignant tumours so that the patient may be treated promptly. Breast cancer screening programmes use radiological techniques (**mammography** and/or **ultrasound**) to identify clinically unde-tectable, suspicious breast lesions, including abnormal calcifications. A tissue diagnosis is then made by **fine needle aspiration biopsy (FNAB)**, and/or **core biopsy** before definitive treatment is undertaken. It is expected that early removal of very small tumours will be curative.

Inflammatory disorders of the breast

Infections of the breast are uncommon and mainly occur during lactation; bacteria (usually *Staphylo-coccus aureus*) gain access through cracks and fissures in the nipple and areola. Without early antibiotic therapy, the resulting **bacterial mastitis** may be followed by the development of a **breast abscess** that may require surgical drainage. More commonly, localised areas of inflammation of the breast follow trauma, which may be of sufficient severity to produce a condition known as **fat necrosis** (Fig. 18.1).

Fig. 18.1 Fat necrosis (MP)

Trauma to the breast, sometimes quite trivial, may result in necrosis of mammary adipose tissue. The presence of necrotic adipose tissue **A** excites a chronic inflammatory cell infiltrate **In**, in which lipophages **L** (macrophages containing lipid, giving their cytoplasm a foamy appearance) and plasma cells may be present in large numbers. Fibrosis **F** of the damaged area produces a hard, often irregular, breast lump, which may resemble a breast carcinoma on palpation. Similar, more localised, changes may be seen in the breast following FNAB, core biopsy or other surgical procedures.

KEY TO FIGURES

A adipose tissue   **Ap** apocrine metaplasia   **C** cyst   **F** fibrosis   **In** inflammatory infiltrate   **L** lipophages

Non-neoplastic breast disease

Non-neoplastic breast disease includes a number of disorders that may give rise to a palpable mass or a mammographic abnormality. These conditions may include alterations to the stroma, to the glandular architecture or to the glandular epithelium; usually more than one element is involved. Calcification is not uncommon in these benign lesions and must be differentiated from calcification seen in malignant breast disease. This is not always possible using imaging techniques and biopsy may be required to determine the nature of the lesion.

Simple *fibrocystic change* involves cystic dilatation of ducts, apocrine metaplasia of the epithelium and fibrosis of stroma (Fig. 18.2). *Adenosis* refers to a benign proliferation of glands that may be combined with fibrosis (sclerosis) of the stroma to give rise to *sclerosing adenosis* (Fig. 18.3) which can be difficult to differentiate both clinically and pathologically from invasive carcinoma. Similar changes with proliferation and distortion of benign breast ducts and lobules along with fibrosis of the stroma may be seen in *radial scars* and *complex sclerosing lesions*. A third type of benign lesion is *usual ductal hyperplasia (UDH)* where there is an increase in the number of layers of cells lining the ducts, i.e. more than the normal two layers. This is generally graded as mild, moderate or florid ductal hyperplasia. *Atypical ductal hyperplasia (ADH)* (Fig. 18.4) is a condition intermediate between hyperplasia and *carcinoma in situ* and carries with it a small, but significantly increased, risk of developing carcinoma. *Columnar cell change* or *hyperplasia* is another benign lesion often associated with microcalcifications and, when there is associated epithelial atypia, it may confer a slight increase in the risk of developing cancer.

With the exception of ADH, sclerosing adenosis and atypical columnar cell lesions, the above conditions carry little or no increased risk of malignancy. Benign breast disorders may be difficult to differentiate clinically from carcinoma. Furthermore, these conditions are common and thus may occur concurrently with, but independently of, invasive carcinoma.

Fig. 18.2 Fibrocystic change (MP)

This breast lesion is so common that it is considered a normal physiological variant. It is nevertheless of great clinical importance since it may give rise to firm palpable masses and/or large cysts that require biopsy to exclude carcinoma. Calcification may also be seen in these lesions.

Typically, as in this micrograph, there is dilatation of acinar structures to form cysts **C**, accompanied by apocrine metaplasia **Ap** of epithelial cells. In apocrine metaplasia, the epithelial cells have strongly eosinophilic cytoplasm, often with apical buds and enlarged nuclei, mimicking the apocrine secretory pattern of lactation. In addition, there is variable fibrosis **F** of the stroma which may give the mass an irregular outline.

Fig. 18.3 Sclerosing adenosis (LP)

In this condition, there is fibrosis of the intralobular stroma in association with *adenosis*, i.e. proliferation of benign terminal duct–lobular units. This common lesion may give rise to a poorly defined, palpable mass in the breast or to a mammographic abnormality, including calcification. The lesion is centred on the lobules and the overall lobular pattern can still be discerned, in contrast to carcinoma in which it is usually lost. The condition is associated with a slight increase in risk of carcinoma.

As seen in this micrograph, there is a proliferation of small acinar structures **A**, which are distorted by the surrounding fibrosis **F**.

Radial scars (<10 mm) and complex sclerosing lesions (>10 mm) are related benign lesions that share some characteristics with sclerosing adenosis. As the name suggests, these lesions radiate out from a central fibrous scar.

It is most important not to mistake these benign lesions for invasive breast carcinoma. Diagnosis can be difficult on routine H&E stains, especially on a core biopsy, but immunostaining for smooth muscle actin or other muscle specific antigens will highlight the myoepithelial cells that are prominent in these lesions and absent in invasive carcinomas.

Fig. 18.4 Atypical ductal hyperplasia (MP)

Ductal hyperplasia is another common form of benign breast disease. In *usual ductal* (or *epithelial*) *hyperplasia (UDH/UEH)*, the thickness of the epithelial layer lining the ducts is increased from the normal two cells thick to three, four or more. In *atypical ductal hyperplasia (ADH)*, as illustrated in this micrograph, the ducts are distended by marked proliferation of epithelial cells, forming a swirling pattern. The cytological and architectural features show some but not all of the characteristic of low-grade *ductal carcinoma in situ (DCIS)* (see Fig. 18.9). In the new WHO classification (Fig. 18.9) this lesion is categorised as *DIN 1B (ductal intraepithelial neoplasia 1B)*.

ADH is associated with a mildly increased risk of subsequent development of invasive carcinoma, but this is less than that associated with *ductal carcinoma in situ* (Fig. 18.9). ADH is also commonly seen in breast biopsies in association with both invasive and in situ carcinoma.

KEY TO FIGURES
A acinar structures   **D** duct   **F** fibrosis

Fig. 18.5 Gynaecomastia of male breast (MP)

The male breast is normally rudimentary and inactive, consisting of fibroadipose tissue containing atrophic mammary ducts. Oestrogenic changes may result in breast hyperplasia (*gynaecomastia*). The simple mammary ducts **D** become enlarged, often with thickening of the epithelial layer and an increase in periductal fibrous tissue **F**.

Gynaecomastia may develop at puberty because of a rise in circulating oestrogens or by administration of exogenous oestrogens, for example sex change or drugs used in treatment of prostatic carcinoma. Various other drugs such as spironolactone, heroin and marijuana also cause gynaecomastia in some individuals. It may also result from alcohol abuse and, in particular, cirrhosis of the liver, which results in abnormal metabolism of androgens into oestrogens.

Neoplasms of the breast

The most common benign neoplasm of the breast is the *fibroadenoma* (Fig. 18.6), a localised proliferation of breast ducts and stroma. Such lesions occur most frequently in isolated form in women aged 25–35. The *phyllodes tumour* (Fig. 18.7) is related to the fibroadenoma except that it has a tendency to recur and some are frankly malignant. The only other benign tumour of much clinical significance is the *benign intraductal papilloma* (Fig. 18.8), usually occurring as a solitary lesion in one of the larger mammary ducts. Histologically similar papillary lesions may also be multifocal, a condition known as *intraductal papillomatosis*. These lesions tend to occur in the smaller ducts and are associated with a small but definite increase in the risk of carcinoma.

Malignant tumours of the female breast are extremely common, with a peak incidence in the decade before the menopause. Most are adenocarcinomas arising from the epithelium of the terminal duct–lobular unit, but may show features resembling lobular structures (*lobular carcinoma*) or the mammary ducts (*ductal carcinoma*); the range of histological appearances is illustrated in Figures 18.9 to 18.13. In many cases, the development of invasive breast cancer is preceded by carcinoma in situ, in which the malignant cells proliferate within the mammary ducts or lobules but do not breach the basement membrane (*ductal* or *lobular carcinoma in situ* (*DCIS* or *LCIS*)). Risk factors for breast carcinoma include younger age at menarche, later first live birth, family history of breast cancer and previous biopsy with ADH.

In addition to the main groups of lobular and ductal carcinoma, there are several subtypes of ductal carcinoma that are associated with distinct clinical and pathological features, often with a good prognosis; examples are *tubular carcinoma* and *mucinous carcinoma* of the breast (Fig. 18.10). *Medullary carcinoma* (not illustrated) is a rare variant characterised by high-grade histological features and a prominent inflammatory infiltrate.

In some cases of breast carcinoma, both in situ and invasive, malignant cells may spread along mammary and lactiferous ducts onto the surface of the nipple resulting in *Paget's disease of the nipple* (Fig. 18.13).

Sarcomas also occur in the breast, the most common being *angiosarcoma* (see Fig. 11.13). This may follow previous radiotherapy for treatment of breast carcinoma. Carcinoma of the breast does occur in males, but is extremely uncommon.

| **Fig. 18.6** | **Fibroadenoma** (LP) |

Fibroadenoma is a common, benign, solitary lesion found in the breasts of women of all ages, but most often in women under 30. It is usually considered to be a tumour, but may well represent a nodular form of benign mammary hyperplasia. The mass is well circumscribed with a pseudocapsule of connective tissue and is composed of both epithelial and stromal components. The epithelial components form glandular structures lined by mammary duct-type epithelium, whilst the stromal component is a loose, cellular form of fibrous tissue **F**. In some cases, the stroma may be myxoid.

Two patterns of growth are seen, often in the same lesion. In the *pericanalicular pattern* **P**, the epithelial component takes the form of rounded ducts that remain small and undistorted, with the stroma arranged round them in a roughly symmetrical and regular manner. By contrast, in the *intracanalicular pattern* **In**, the ducts appear elongated, but actually represent sections cut through flattened spaces compressed by nodular proliferation of the stromal component; in general, this latter pattern is more prominent in larger fibroadenomas. In both patterns of fibroadenoma, hormonal changes, such as occur in pregnancy and lactation, may induce hyperplasia of the epithelial component.

| **Fig. 18.7** | **Phyllodes tumour** (MP) |

The *phyllodes tumour* is related to the fibroadenoma, consisting of a mixture of epithelial and stromal elements. The stroma **St** is, however, more prominent in the phyllodes tumour, consisting of crowded atypical spindle cells. The stroma thus bulges into the lumen of the duct to give the characteristic leaf-like pattern **L**, seen in this micrograph, and there may be occasional mitotic figures.

These tumours have a tendency to recur locally but are usually cured by wide excision. A small proportion behave in a frankly malignant fashion with distant metastases and are thus called *malignant phyllodes tumours* (previously *cystosarcoma phyllodes*). These tumours generally have more crowded, pleomorphic stromal cells with more mitoses, stromal overgrowth and an infiltrative margin. A borderline category has also been described with features intermediate between benign and malignant phyllodes tumour.

| **Fig. 18.8** | **Intraductal papilloma** (MP) |

Papillomas of mammary duct epithelium may arise as solitary or multiple lesions. Solitary lesions, as shown here, are usually located in the larger lactiferous ducts near the nipple and present with a blood-stained discharge from the nipple. The lesions are usually small, consisting of a delicate, pink-staining supporting stroma covered by a single or double layer of cuboidal or low columnar epithelial cells, resembling the normal lining of the mammary duct; with larger lesions, the duct is often dilated. Multiple duct papillomas (*florid duct papillomatosis*) are rare, but may occur in smaller ducts in younger patients. Epithelial hyperplasia and carcinoma in situ may also arise in a breast papilloma. Malignant change is rare but carcinomas with a papillary architecture are sometimes seen.

Fig. 18.9 Ductal carcinomas of the breast (a)
Low-grade ductal carcinoma in situ (HP) **(b)** High-grade ductal carcinoma in situ (HP) **(c)** Invasive ductal carcinoma (LP)

Ductal carcinoma is divided into invasive and in situ types depending on whether the malignant cells have breached the basement membrane of the duct and invaded the stroma. Both invasive and in situ carcinomas may be associated with abnormal calcifications that may provide the only mammographic clue to the presence of small tumours.

Ductal carcinoma in situ (DCIS) is graded according to the cytological and architectural features of the lesion, with low-grade lesions conferring a moderate increase in the likelihood of invasive carcinoma while high-grade lesions are associated with a marked increase in the likelihood of invasive carcinoma. Micrograph (a) shows an example of low-grade DCIS. The epithelial cells fill and expand the ducts, forming sharply defined glandular spaces **S** separated by 'rigid' bridges **B** of cells; low-grade DCIS may form a *cribriform pattern* (as shown here), a *micropapillary* or a *solid pattern*. The cells are uniform in size and regularly placed in relation to each other.

In contrast, in high-grade DCIS, the duct is expanded by a proliferation of large, highly pleomorphic cells. As seen in micrograph (b), there is often central necrosis **Ne** (often called *comedo necrosis*), which may be calcified.

A grading system has been proposed which divides DCIS into DIN (ductal intraepithelial neoplasia) 1, 2 and 3 and attempts to incorporate atypical ductal hyperplasia, atypical columnar cell lesions and flat epithelial atypia into the classification; it has not yet been generally adopted.

Invasive ductal carcinoma (often called *ductal carcinoma, NOS*, i.e. *N*ot *O*therwise *S*pecified or ductal carcinoma, *NST*, i.e. *N*o *S*pecial *T*ype) is the most common form of invasive carcinoma and has the worst prognosis. As seen in micrograph (c), the invading malignant epithelial cells form small ductal

structures **D**, solid nests **N** and even solid sheets of cells.

The stroma **St**, as in this example, is frequently very fibrotic which gives the characteristic firm texture on palpation (see also Fig. 7.15).

Tumours are graded in an attempt to predict likely clinical behaviour and to inform the need for treatment. The most commonly used scheme assigns a numerical grade to each of three features of the tumour; namely, the degree of gland formation, the nuclear features of the tumour cells and the frequency of mitotic figures. The sum of these grades is then converted to a numerical grade 1, 2 or 3, with grade 1 being a low-grade lesion with a better prognosis and grade 3 a high-grade lesion.

BASIC SYSTEMS PATHOLOGY ■ BREAST

KEY TO FIGURES

B rigid cell bridges **D** ductal structures **F** fibrous tissue **In** intracanalicular pattern **L** leaf-like pattern
P pericanalicular pattern **N** solid cell nests **Ne** necrosis **S** glandular space **St** stroma

Fig. 18.10 **Variants of invasive ductal carcinoma** **(a)** Tubular carcinoma (MP) **(b)** Mucinous (colloid) carcinoma (MP)

Certain variants of invasive ductal carcinoma have a much better prognosis than invasive ductal carcinoma, NOS. These are much less common than invasive ductal carcinoma NOS, but two of the commoner types are invasive *tubular carcinoma* and *mucinous* or *colloid carcinoma*. Tubular carcinoma, as shown in micrograph (a), consists of malignant epithelial cells which form well-defined tubular or ductal structures **T**, with no solid nests of cells or single cell invasion. The tubules are lined by a single layer of mildly pleomorphic cells and invade into the surrounding fat with no evidence of an overall lobular architecture; this is in contrast to sclerosing adenosis (Fig. 18.3), which may be confused with tubular carcinoma.

Mucinous carcinoma, as seen in micrograph (b), is characterised by pools of mucin **Mu** in which nests of malignant cells **N** are suspended. Mucinous carcinoma is characteristically soft to palpation and has a well-defined margin of fibrous tissue **F**.

Other ductal carcinoma variants with a good prognosis that are not illustrated here include invasive *cribriform carcinoma* and *medullary carcinoma*.

Fig. 18.11 **Lobular carcinoma of the breast** (MP)

Like their ductal counterparts, lobular carcinomas are divided into in situ and invasive forms; both are often present in the same lesion. This micrograph shows *lobular carcinoma in situ (LCIS)* at the lower left, adjacent to an area of invasive carcinoma.

In LCIS, the lobules **L** are expanded and filled by small, evenly spaced epithelial cells that do not form ducts. In the rest of the micrograph, *invasive lobular carcinoma* consists of similar malignant cells **M** infiltrating the stroma in rows of cells (often described as *Indian files*) and as single cells which do not form ducts.

Lobular carcinoma in situ is often found incidentally in biopsies taken for another purpose as it usually does not give rise to a mammographic or palpable lesion. LCIS is often multifocal and is considered as a marker lesion for invasive carcinoma, rather than a premalignant lesion. Invasive lobular carcinoma is thought to imply a better prognosis than invasive ductal carcinoma, NOS, but is more likely to be bilateral and multifocal.

KEY TO FIGURES
F fibrous tissue   **L** lobular carcinoma in situ   **M** malignant cells   **Mu** mucin   **N** malignant cell nests
T tubular structures

PREDICTIVE FACTORS IN BREAST CANCER

The ideal treatment programme for each breast cancer patient is to give them exactly the right type and amount of treatment for their particular cancer. Breast cancer is not a single disease, but a group of conditions that will progress at different rates and will respond differently to different types of treatment. The difficulty for histopathologists is to identify those cancers that need extra treatment (in addition to surgery and radiotherapy) and those that will respond to hormonal therapies.

Treatment is primarily dependent on the type, grade and clinical and pathological stage of the tumour. Patient factors such as age, other health problems and patient preferences are also important. However, in addition, the presence of oestrogen and progestogen receptors (ER and PR) in breast cancer cells has been shown to confer an improved prognosis and to render the cancer susceptible to hormonal treatment. Testing cancers for ER and PR has been standard practice for many years. More recently, the presence of *human epidermal growth factor 2* (*Her-2* or *erbB2*) has been shown to confer a worse prognosis. Her-2 is a normal component of normal cells but it is overexpressed in about 20% of breast cancers, usually high-grade, high-stage, poor prognosis tumours. Tumours that overexpress Her-2 (usually because of gene amplification) are likely to respond to treatment with the drug *trastuzumab,* a humanised monoclonal antibody specifically targeted at the Her-2 protein and able to switch it off. Other Her-2 antibodies are also becoming available.

Fig. 18.12 Predictive tests in breast carcinoma (a) Oestrogen receptors IHC (MP) **(b)** Her-2 IHC (HP)

Testing for oestrogen and progestogen receptors (ER and PR) has been standard practice in pathology laboratories for many years. The usual method used is immunohistochemistry using specific monoclonal antibodies to detect the receptors. These methods, and the scoring systems used, must be carefully standardised to ensure accuracy.

Micrograph (a) shows a section of a low-grade invasive ductal carcinoma which has been stained by the immunohistochemistry method (IHC) using a monoclonal antibody specific for oestrogen receptors. Most of the malignant tumour cells **M** show strong brown staining of the nuclei, indicating oestrogen receptor positivity and thus a relatively improved prognosis. Both ER and PR are normal proteins found in the nucleus and are present in normal breast epithelial cells.

Micrograph (b) at high magnification shows a positive IHC test for Her-2. This protein is found on the cell surface and therefore strong membrane staining is required for a positive result, as seen here. Note that the cell nucleus is not stained in contrast to the ER test in (a). The test is typically validated or, in borderline cases, confirmed by in situ hybridisation to confirm gene amplification by demonstrating multiple copies of the Her-2 gene in the nucleus.

Fig. 18.13 **Paget's disease of the nipple** (HP)

Some patients with carcinoma of the breast (usually of ductal type) develop reddening and thickening of the skin of the nipple and areola, occasionally followed by ulceration. The epidermis of the nipple and areola becomes infiltrated by malignant epithelial cells with hyperchromatic nuclei and pale cytoplasm.

These cells, known as *Paget's cells* **P**, are breast carcinoma cells that have spread along the epithelium of the mammary and nipple ducts to the epidermis from an underlying in situ or invasive ductal carcinoma.

HEREDITARY BREAST CARCINOMA

Familial breast cancer constitutes about 5–10% of all breast cancers and up to 40% in women under 35. Of familial breast cancers, up to 20% occur in women with mutations in the breast cancer susceptibility genes BRCA1 and 2. Mutations in these two genes are also found in almost all women with hereditary ovarian carcinomas (see also Ch. 17). These discoveries offer the hope of genetic testing for members of affected families and the possibility of prophylactic treatment. In addition, although the histopathological appearances of these tumours are somewhat different from non-hereditary types of breast cancer, the discovery of these genes offers new insights into the mechanisms of carcinogenesis.

KEY TO FIGURES
P Paget's cells

Fig. 18.14 Chapter review

Disorder	Main features	Figure
Fat necrosis	Fat cells with loss of nuclei, inflammatory infiltrate rich in foamy histiocytes	18.1
Fibrocystic change	Dilated ducts with apocrine metaplasia of the epithelium, fibrosis of the stroma	18.2
Sclerosing adenosis	Proliferation and distortion of small benign ducts in a fibrotic stroma	18.3
Ductal hyperplasia	Increase in thickness of epithelial cell layers lining ducts	
Atypical ductal hyperplasia (ADH)	Increased epithelial cells within a duct with some, but not all, of the features of ductal carcinoma in situ	18.4
Gynaecomastia	Enlargement of ducts, increased thickness of epithelial layers, increased periductal fibrous tissue in the male breast	18.5
Fibroadenoma	Mixture of benign epithelial and stromal components forming a discrete, usually mobile mass	18.6
Phyllodes tumour	Mixture of epithelial and stromal elements with overgrowth of the stromal component giving a 'leaf-like' pattern, increased cellularity and cytologic atypia of the stroma – a few are malignant	18.7
Intraductal papilloma	Branching stromal structures covered by cuboidal or low columnar epithelial cells	18.8
Ductal carcinoma in situ (DCIS)	Atypical cells filling and expanding breast ducts – various patterns – may be high or low grade	18.9(a),(b)
Invasive ductal carcinoma	Invasive atypical cells forming ducts or solid nests – graded as 1–3 depending on architecture, cytological atypia and mitotic activity	18.9(c)
Tubular carcinoma	Invasive carcinoma consisting of well-formed small ductal structures	18.10(a)
Mucinous carcinoma	Invasive carcinoma with plentiful mucin production, often with nests of malignant cells floating in pools of mucin	18.10(b)
Lobular carcinoma in situ (LCIS)	Expanded lobular structures filled with small atypical cells showing no gland formation	18.11
Invasive lobular carcinoma	Invasive carcinoma consisting of small cells, resembling lobular cells, invades as single cells or as lines of cells known as 'Indian files'	18.11
Paget's disease of the nipple	Invasion of malignant cells into the epidermis of the nipple – usually an underlying invasive ductal carcinoma or DCIS	18.13

19 Male reproductive system

Introduction

The male reproductive system includes the testes with their related duct systems, the prostate and the penis. These organs are responsible for the production, storage and periodic emission of the male gametes, spermatozoa, as well as the production of male sex hormones, principally testosterone. The organs of this system are prone to the full range of pathological conditions seen in other organ systems. However, clinically, the most important pathological conditions are inflammation (mainly caused by infection) and tumours.

Disorders of the testis and epididymis

Inflammation of the testis *(orchitis)* may result from viral infections, for example mumps; the testis may also be the site of a gumma in the tertiary stage of syphilis (see Fig. 4.11). Other bacterial infections usually arise as a complication of infection of the lower urinary tract or following surgical instrumentation. A non-infective cause of testicular inflammation is **granulomatous orchitis**, which may follow an episode of trauma to the testis. Focal granulomatous inflammation, known as **sperm granulomas**, may also occur because of sperm retention, for example after vasectomy. Venous infarction of the testis owing to **torsion** is an important cause of testicular pain in childhood and young adulthood and is illustrated in Figure 19.1.

The most important pathological lesions of the testes are tumours, most of which are derived from germ cells; a system of classification is shown in Figure 19.2 and examples are illustrated in Figures 19.4 to 19.8.

Like the testis, the epididymis may become infected by pyogenic bacteria, associated with lower urinary tract infection and/or surgical instrumentation. When infection occurs, usually both the testis and epididymis are involved, a condition known as **acute epididymo-orchitis**. The epididymis is occasionally the site of disseminated tuberculous infection, **tuberculous epididymitis**, usually secondary to active pulmonary or renal tuberculosis.

Fig. 19.1 Torsion of the testis (LP)

The arterial supply and venous drainage of the testis pass in the long course of the spermatic cord from and to the major vessels in the abdomen and pelvis. The spermatic cord is liable to twist, leading to compression of the thin-walled veins and obstruction of venous drainage from the testis. If this state persists for several hours or more without correction, the testis **T** and epididymis **E** may become deeply congested and subsequently undergo venous infarction, in which necrosis is associated with severe congestion and extravasation of blood. Two small embryological remnants, the appendix testis and the appendix epididymis, are also liable to torsion. The histological changes are similar to those seen in venous infarction of the bowel following volvulus or strangulation (see Fig. 10.5).

Testicular tumours

Testicular tumours may arise in any of the normal components of the testis, but by far the most common are the **germ cell tumours** thought to be derived from multipotential germ cells of the seminiferous tubules. Most testicular germ cell tumours are thought to arise from a pre-malignant change in the cells lining the seminiferous tubules which is known by the term **intratubular germ cell neoplasia (ITGCN)**. Foci of ITGCN are commonly found in the testis adjacent to tumours. These (with the exception of the rare spermatocytic seminoma) are highly malignant tumours of young men, which may be cured by a combination of surgery and modern chemotherapy regimens. There are two classifications in current use: the World Health Organization (WHO) classification and the British Testicular Tumour Panel (BTTP) and the main subtypes within these are compared in Figure 19.2. Approximately two-thirds of testicular tumours contain elements of two or more different tumour types, for example *seminoma* plus *embryonal carcinoma*. There are some similarities between testicular and ovarian germ cell tumours, but it should be remembered that most ovarian germ cell tumours are mature teratomas (dermoid cysts) and behave in a benign fashion, whereas most germ cell tumours in males are malignant.

Testicular tumours are divided into two major groups and this is the important distinction as the two groups are treated differently:

■ **Seminomas**: These consist of cells resembling the normal cells lining the seminiferous tubules. This group includes *classical seminoma* (Fig. 19.4) and the rare *spermatocytic seminoma*, a relatively benign tumour that occurs in older men.

■ **Non-seminomatous germ cell tumours**: This group includes a variety of tumours that exhibit differentiation towards embryonal or extra-embryonal structures.

A small proportion of testicular tumours arise from the other cells in the testes, for example Leydig cell tumours and Sertoli cell tumours; the majority of these tumours are benign but they may secrete inappropriate sex hormones. In older men, the most common tumour of the testis is *lymphoma*, usually in association with lymphoma at other sites in the body; rarely, a testicular mass may be the first indication of lymphoma. Testicular lymphomas are almost always non-Hodgkin diffuse large B cell lymphomas (see Ch. 16).

Fig. 19.2 Classification of germ cell tumours of the testis

Tumour type	WHO (2004) classification	BTTP classification
Seminoma	Seminoma Spermatocytic seminoma	Seminoma Spermatocytic seminoma
Non-seminomatous germ cell tumours	Teratoma Embryonal carcinoma Yolk sac tumour (endodermal sinus tumour) Choriocarcinoma	Teratoma, differentiated (TD) Malignant teratoma, undifferentiated (MTU) Yolk sac tumour Malignant teratoma, trophoblastic (MTT)
Combinations of two or more non-seminomatous types	Mixed germ cell tumour	Malignant teratoma, intermediate (MTI)
Combination of two or more of any type	Mixed germ cell tumour	Combined tumour

Fig 19.3 Intratubular germ cell neoplasia (HP)

Intratubular germ cell neoplasia (ITGCN) is commonly found in testicular tissue adjacent to germ cell tumours. It is thought to be the precursor lesion of most germ cell tumours and is found also in cases of cryptorchidism and in individuals with a contralateral germ cell tumour or a strong family history.

The most common pattern, as shown here, consists of undifferentiated neoplastic cells **N**, arranged circumferentially around the basement membrane of the seminiferous tubule. The Sertoli cells **S** are pushed towards the centre to the tubule. There is no evidence of normal spermatogenesis.

KEY TO FIGURES

E epididymis **N** neoplastic germ cells **S** Sertoli cells **T** testis

Fig. 19.4 Classical seminoma (HP)

Seminoma is the most common tumour of the testis, with a peak incidence between 30 and 45 years. Macroscopically, the tumour is well circumscribed, pale, creamy-white and homogeneous, with a faint lobular pattern; necrosis and haemorrhage are rare unless the tumour is very large. Seminoma is a malignant tumour and tends to spread via lymphatics, initially to iliac and para-aortic lymph nodes.

Histologically, most seminomas show the classical appearance illustrated in this micrograph. The tumour consists of sheets of uniform polygonal cells with clear cytoplasm and a round central nucleus with a prominent nucleolus. The cells are divided into clusters by fine fibrous septa **S** which are usually infiltrated by small lymphocytes. Sometimes, the inflammation is very marked and even granulomatous and it may in these cases be difficult to identify the tumour.

In the past, attempts have been made to predict the behaviour of seminomas by grading the lesions according to a variety of criteria. The highest grade lesions under this system were called anaplastic seminomas. This grading system has little prognostic value and is no longer used. Another type of seminoma, the *spermatocytic seminoma*, occurs more often in older men than does classical seminoma; these tumours usually have a benign clinical course.

Fig. 19.5 Immature teratoma (MP)

In adults, most testicular teratomas are immature, consisting of fetal-type tissues such as cartilage **C**, poorly differentiated epithelial structures **E** and primitive mesenchyme **M**, as shown in this micrograph. These tumours tend to behave in a malignant fashion, in contrast to ovarian teratomas, which are almost always benign. Some teratomas in adults show frank malignant transformation with areas of carcinoma or sarcoma. Teratoma is a common component of mixed germ cell tumours.

Compare this to the mature teratoma of the ovary (dermoid cyst) shown in Figure 17.24, where all the tissues are fully differentiated and almost identical to the normal adult equivalents.

KEY TO FIGURES

C cartilage **D** Schiller–Duval body **E** epithelial structure **G** glandular structures **M** primitive mesenchyme **R** reticular pattern **S** septum **T** tubular structures

Fig. 19.6 Embryonal carcinoma (MP)

These tumours most often occur in men aged 20–30 and tend to be more aggressive than seminomas. Grossly, the tumour is often poorly circumscribed with areas of haemorrhage and necrosis.

The tumour at low power resembles a carcinoma. The large anaplastic tumour cells may form gland-like structures **G**, tubular structures **T** as seen in this micrograph or solid sheets of cells or papillary structures. Mitotic figures are frequent. This tumour may invade through the tunica albuginea into the epididymis.

Fig. 19.7 Yolk sac tumour (MP)

Pure *yolk sac tumour* (or *endodermal sinus tumour*) is rare in adult men but is the most common malignant germ cell tumour in male infants and young boys. Yolk sac tumour resembles the yolk sac of the developing embryo. In practice, there is a wide range of histological patterns, the most common being a lace-like (*microcystic* or *reticular*) pattern **R** of large poorly differentiated cells, as seen in this micrograph. A characteristic, but not common, feature is the *Schiller–Duval body* **D**, which resembles a fetal glomerulus. Other features include intracytoplasmic hyaline globules and extracellular deposits of basement membrane material. Often, more than one pattern will be found in an area of yolk sac tumour.

Yolk sac tumour is frequently an element of mixed germ cell tumours in adults. Yolk sac tumour secretes *α-fetoprotein (AFP)* which is easily measured in blood to monitor tumour progression.

Fig. 19.8 **Mixed testicular germ cell tumours** **(a)** Embryonal carcinoma and teratoma (MP) **(b)** Embryonal carcinoma and seminoma (HP)

Certain germ cell tumours are composed of a mixture of elements. Micrograph (a) shows a germ cell tumour consisting of immature teratoma and embryonal carcinoma (MTI). In the top left corner the embryonal carcinoma **Em** shows glandular forms as well as solid areas. In the teratoma component there is some immature cartilage **Ca**.

In micrograph (b) pale-staining cells of the seminoma component **Sem** contrast with darker-staining cells of an embryonal carcinoma **Em**. In the WHO system this tumour is classified as *embryonal carcinoma with seminoma*.

Mixed germ cell tumours may also contain foci of *choriocarcinoma* or *yolk sac tumour*. *β-hCG* is produced by trophoblastic elements and can be used as a biochemical marker for the presence of choriocarcinoma, as well as to detect tumour recurrence.

Disorders of the prostate

The prostate gland undergoes *benign nodular hyperplasia (hypertrophy)* in almost all men from middle age onwards, probably because of an alteration in hormone balance. This important lesion, shown in Figure 19.9, produces obstruction to bladder outflow as a result of pressure on the prostatic urethra; in turn, the obstruction may produce pressure effects on the proximal conducting system of the urinary tract, leading to *hydroureter* and *hydronephrosis* with pressure atrophy of the renal parenchyma. Prostatic hyperplasia also predisposes to infection and stone formation.

Invasive carcinoma of the prostate is a common and important malignant tumour in men, and is illustrated in Figure 19.11. Carcinoma of the prostate may be associated with dysplasia of the glandular epithelium. This has been named *prostatic intraepithelial neoplasia (PIN)* and is shown in Figure 19.10. The prognosis of carcinoma of the prostate can be predicted by careful grading and staging. Staging takes into consideration the size (volume) of the tumour, the degree of spread within the prostate, extension beyond the prostate and lymph node and distant metastases. Perineural and vascular invasion also contributes to assessment of prognosis. Some of these features may only be determined in radical prostatectomy specimens whereas others can be assessed on core biopsies. Imaging is also important for the detection of distant metastases, for example to bone. Small foci of low-grade tumour that are not palpable may be found in prostates removed for benign hyperplasia. Most of these tumours progress too slowly for them to cause clinically significant disease in elderly patients and, for this reason, are often called *latent carcinomas*.

KEY TO FIGURES

A acinus **C** corpora amylaceae **Ca** immature cartilage **D** high-grade PIN **E** normal epithelium
Em embryonal carcinoma **H** hyperplastic prostate nodule **M** fibromuscular connective tissue **N** compressed peripheral glands **P** papillary fold **Sem** seminoma

Fig. 19.9 Benign prostatic hyperplasia (a) LP (b) MP

Benign prostatic hyperplasia is a common condition affecting middle-aged to elderly men in which the transitional and para-urethral components of the prostate gland undergo glandular hyperplasia accompanied by hypertrophy of the intervening fibromuscular stroma of the gland. The peripheral zone of the prostate is not involved in the hyperplastic process and becomes compressed and atrophic at the outer margin.

At low magnification in micrograph (a), note the rounded nodules of hyperplastic prostatic tissue **H** in the transitional/para-urethral part of the gland and the compressed peripheral zone **N** at the periphery. Since the para-urethral component of the prostate gland is involved, compression of the urethral lumen is a frequent occurrence and is responsible for typical clinical features such as hesitancy, poor urinary

stream and urinary retention. Macroscopically, the typical hyperplastic prostate has a nodular microcystic appearance, the tiny cysts representing enormously dilated hyperplastic prostatic glandular acini which often contain small, laminated concretions known as *corpora amylaceae* **C**.

At high magnification as in micrograph (b), the acini **A** are lined by tall columnar prostatic epithelial cells with small basal nuclei. The cells have a regular arrangement but are sometimes thrown up into papillary folds **P**. Adjacent acini are separated by a variable amount of fibromuscular connective tissue **M** in which the muscular component may be hypertrophied; muscular hypertrophy is often particularly prominent in the region of the bladder neck.

Fig. 19.10 Prostatic intraepithelial neoplasia (HP)

Prostatic intraepithelial neoplasia (PIN) represents dysplasia of the tall columnar epithelium. PIN may be subclassified as high or low grade. In clinical practice, as the significance of low-grade PIN is uncertain, it is usually ignored. High-grade PIN, however, tends to occur in prostates with invasive carcinoma and therefore the finding of high-grade PIN should prompt an intensified search for invasive carcinoma.

The gland on the right, consisting of highly atypical epithelial cells **D**, is a good example of high-grade PIN. These cells, in contrast to the normal prostatic epithelium **E** (left), have enlarged pleomorphic nuclei and prominent nucleoli. The cytoplasm is more basophilic than normal. These cells are very similar to those of invasive carcinomas, but there is no evidence of stromal invasion. A layer of basal cells can be detected around the periphery of the gland, although sometimes immunostaining is required to demonstrate this.

Fig. 19.11 **Adenocarcinoma of the prostate** **(a)** Well differentiated (MP) **(b)** Poorly differentiated (MP)

This common tumour usually arises in the peripheral zone of the prostate gland, as opposed to benign prostatic hyperplasia which characteristically develops in the peri-urethral and transitional zones of the gland (Fig. 19.9). Almost all prostatic primary malignant tumours are adenocarcinomas.

Prostatic adenocarcinomas are graded by the *Gleason grading system* according to their architectural features. Gleason grade 1 lesions consist of nodules of small, well-defined glands with limited infiltration of the surrounding tissue. In contrast, grade 5 lesions consist of sheets of malignant cells with no discernible glandular differentiation and which infiltrate widely. Grades 2, 3 and 4 are intermediate. Most prostatic tumours include components of two or more of these patterns and therefore current practice gives the grade of the two most prominent components and their sum. This is known as the combined Gleason grade or score, for example combined Gleason score 3 + 5 = 8, with the

first number representing the most common component. As mentioned above, accurate grading along with staging is important to estimate the prognosis of prostatic adenocarcinoma and to guide treatment.

Micrograph (a) shows an area of Gleason grade 3 carcinoma. Small, round, malignant glands **M** lined by enlarged atypical epithelial cells are seen infiltrating between benign glands **B**. The contrast between the benign and malignant cells is particularly well demonstrated, the malignant cells being larger with prominent nucleoli and less cytoplasm. A very important feature is that the malignant glands lack the basal cell layer **E**, which is prominent in the benign glands.

Micrograph (b) shows an area of Gleason grade 5 prostatic adenocarcinoma where the malignant cells form sheets **S** of pleomorphic cells invading the stroma. No glandular structures are seen.

SCREENING FOR PROSTATE CANCER

Screening for disease is dependent on the principle that early detection increases cure rate and reduces morbidity and/or mortality. Screening is, by definition, applied to large numbers of healthy individuals. Blood testing for *prostate-specific antigen (PSA)* has been available for several years but, as yet, there is no national government-funded screening programme as there is for breast carcinoma. Although the test is cheap and has minimal side effects, the benefits of applying it to large numbers of asymptomatic men have yet to be demonstrated. The test has a significant false positive rate, thus triggering prostatic biopsies, a more expensive test with more potential side effects, in healthy men. It is also likely that the test would detect many cases of indolent, low-grade carcinoma that would be unlikely to cause appreciable problems during the lifespan of the individual. However, in clinical practice, many men are screened for prostate cancer on an individual basis, usually because they themselves have requested the test.

KEY TO FIGURES
B benign glands   **E** basal epithelial cell   **M** small malignant glands   **S** sheets of malignant cells   **T** islands of squamous cell carcinoma

Disorders of the penis

The most important pathological lesion of the penis is *squamous cell carcinoma* (Fig. 19.12) which may be preceded by a form of carcinoma in situ known as *erythroplasia of Queyrat*, histologically similar to *intraepidermal carcinoma* of skin elsewhere (see Fig. 21.14). Genital wart or *condyloma acuminatum* also occurs on the penis and are caused by infection with certain types of Human papilloma virus, as in the lower genital tract in the female. Phimosis is a common clinical condition. In some cases, this is caused by an inflammatory and fibrosing condition of the foreskin termed *balanitis xerotica obliterans*. This is histologically identical to the vulval disorder lichen sclerosus et atrophicus (see Fig. 17.1).

Fig. 19.12 Squamous carcinoma of penis (LP)

This micrograph illustrates, at low magnification, a well-differentiated keratinising squamous cell carcinoma of the glans penis, with islands of tumour **T** extending deeply into the stroma of the glans. Metastatic spread is by lymphatics to superficial inguinal nodes.

Carcinoma of the penis is usually located on the glans or prepuce and is rare in circumcised men. Chronic irritation and poor hygiene may be predisposing factors. However, evidence is accumulating that squamous carcinoma of the penis is associated with infection by Human papilloma virus (HPV) serotypes 16 and 18, the same serotypes associated with invasive carcinoma of the female cervix.

Fig. 19.13 Chapter review

Organ	Disorder	Main features	Figure
Testis	Torsion	Necrosis of tissue with extensive congestion and haemorrhage due to venous infarction	19.1
	Epididymo-orchitis	Acute inflammation, similar to acute inflammation in other tissues	Like 2.4
	Intratubular germ cell neoplasia (ITGCN)	Malignant germ cells within seminiferous tubules, usually as a single layer around the basement membrane with the Sertoli cells pushed inwards	19.3
	Seminoma	Sheets of large, undifferentiated cells separated by delicate fibrous septae usually with a lymphocytic infiltrate in the septa	19.4
	Teratoma (teratoma, differentiated)	Tumour consists of mixtures of fetal tissues e.g. cartilage, primitive mesenchyme, epithelial structures, bone etc.	19.5
	Embryonal carcinoma (malignant teratoma, undifferentiated)	Large malignant cells forming gland-like structures, solid sheets, tubular structures and papillary structures Often large necrotic areas	19.6
	Yolk sac tumour	Primitive germ cells resembling yolk sac structures Various patterns including reticular (microcystic), Schiller–Duval bodies, hyaline cytoplasmic globules	19.7
	Choriocarcinoma (malignant teratoma, trophoblastic)	Alternating layers of syncytiotrophoblast and cytotrophoblast with haemorrhage	17.15
	Mixed germ cell tumour (malignant teratoma, intermediate)	Consists of a mixture of other germ cell tumours	19.8
Prostate	Benign hyperplasia	Nodular enlargement of glandular and stromal elements of the prostate gland – usually affects the transitional and paraurethral components	19.9
	High grade prostatic intraepithelial neoplasia (PIN)	Highly atypical cells similar to those seen in invasive carcinoma confined within prostatic acini	19.10
	Adenocarcinoma	Malignant cells invading the prostate as glands, cribriform structures or sheets	19.11
Penis	Balanitis xerotica obliterans	Hyalinisation of the subepithelial collagen of the foreskin with an underlying band of inflammation	Like 17.1
	Squamous cell carcinoma	Similar to SCC elsewhere – invasion of underlying tissue by nests of atypical squamous cells, often with formation of keratin pearls	19.12

20 Endocrine system

Pituitary gland disorders

Structural defects of the pituitary gland are few, although functional abnormalities are potentially numerous, leading to under- or overproduction of one or more of the many hormones produced by the pituitary and its target endocrine glands.

The most important histopathological lesions of the pituitary gland are benign *adenomas* derived from the anterior pituitary (adenohypophysis). These commonly secrete anterior pituitary hormones and result in the development of endocrine syndromes. Adenomas may be derived from any of the normal anterior pituitary cell types and can be classified by the hormones they secrete and their pattern of staining with antibodies to pituitary hormones:

- **Prolactinomas**: secrete prolactin and may lead to infertility and, occasionally, inappropriate breast milk production

- **Corticotroph adenomas**: secrete adrenocorticotrophic hormone (ACTH) and result in *Cushing's disease* (Fig. 20.1)

- **Somatotroph adenomas**: secrete excess growth hormone and lead to *gigantism* or *acromegaly* (Fig. 20.2)

- **Thyrotroph** and **gonadotroph adenomas**: both types are rare

- **Non-secretory adenomas**: a large number of pituitary adenomas have no demonstrable hormone secretion; such tumours only become manifest by impinging on vital local structures such as the optic chiasm, causing visual disturbance, or by expanding to a size large enough to destroy the surrounding normal functioning tissue, resulting in clinical *hypopituitarism*.

Fig. 20.1 Pituitary adenoma (LP)

This image shows a pituitary gland in situ in the pituitary fossa and cut in sagittal section, showing the anterior pituitary (adenohypophysis **Ap**) and the posterior pituitary (neurohypophysis **Np**). Within the substance of the anterior pituitary lies a small *pituitary adenoma* **A** composed of cells of a uniform type. The tumour is benign, as evidenced by its well-circumscribed, non-invasive, spherical appearance, and is small enough to have caused no distortion of the pituitary outline or undue compression of adjacent normal pituitary cells.

In this particular case, the tumour cells secreted ACTH in gross excess and the patient died as a result of the metabolic and cardiac complications of Cushing's disease. In all, the illness lasted no more than 7 or 8 weeks despite its 'benign' pathogenesis.

KEY TO FIGURES

A pituitary adenoma   **Ap** adenohypophysis   **Np** neurohypophysis

Fig. 20.2 **Pituitary adenoma** **(a)** HP **(b)** Immunocytochemistry for growth hormone (HP)

As noted above, symptoms of pituitary tumours often reflect activity of the hormones they secrete. In addition, their location in the pituitary fossa can lead to compression of the optic chiasm with symptoms/signs of visual disturbance, specifically bitemporal hemianopia

As shown in micrograph (a), the typical histological appearance of a pituitary adenoma is of fields of somewhat monotonous, small to medium-sized tumour cells with moderate amounts of cytoplasm. In this case, immunocytochemistry for growth hormone is positive, shown in micrograph (b).

This patient presented with endocrine symptoms related to excess growth hormone secretion. In adults, this manifests as *acromegaly*, with abnormal growth of the viscera (including the heart), skin, soft tissues and skeleton. This last feature is particularly evident in the bones of the face, with protrusion of the jaw (*prognathism*), and in the bones of the hands and feet. In children, before the epiphyseal plates have fused, excess growth hormone secretion leads to *gigantism*, often also with features of acromegaly.

Disorders of the thyroid and parathyroid glands

A variety of pathological processes may affect the thyroid gland, leading to either diminished or excessive output of the thyroid hormone thyroxine. *Hypothyroidism* may result from dysfunction at any level of the hypothalamo–pituitary–thyroid axis and, as such, may be regarded as either primary (arising from a disorder within the thyroid gland) or secondary (as a consequence of pituitary disease). There are a number of causes of primary hypothyroidism, some of which have an autoimmune basis, for example *Hashimoto's thyroiditis* (Fig. 20.3). In cases of long-standing hypothyroidism, by the time the thyroid is examined histologically, it often shows only shrinkage, fibrosis and destruction of most of the thyroid acini, with a sparse residual infiltrate of chronic inflammatory cells. This change, known as *primary atrophic thyroiditis*, is analogous to the 'end stage' of long-standing kidney damage (see Fig. 15.1) and provides little evidence of the nature of the original thyroid abnormality.

As with hypothyroidism, *hyperthyroidism (thyrotoxicosis)* may be considered as primary (abnormality in gland) or secondary (abnormality outside of gland). In the majority of cases hyperthyroidism arises as a result of diffuse hyperplasia of the thyroid acinar cells, most commonly in the condition known as *Graves' disease* (Fig. 20.4). Sometimes the hyperplasia is confined to a single *benign thyroid adenoma*, or to one or two nodules in an otherwise inactive *multinodular goitre*. Nevertheless, the vast majority of thyroid adenomas (Fig. 20.6) and multinodular goitres (Fig. 20.5) are non-functional and do not lead to disturbances of thyroid hormone output.

Four main forms of *thyroid carcinoma* occur, namely *papillary*, *follicular*, *medullary* and *anaplastic* (in order of frequency). Medullary carcinoma of the thyroid is an uncommon malignant tumour of calcitonin-producing (parafollicular) cells and is particularly notable for its production of amyloid (see Fig. 5.8). The remaining three types arise from cuboidal follicular lining cells. Examples of papillary and follicular carcinomas are illustrated in Figure 20.7. *Lymphoma* may also arise in the thyroid gland, usually following Hashimoto's thyroiditis.

The parathyroid glands show only two important pathological abnormalities, namely *benign adenoma* and *hyperplasia* (Fig. 20.8). In both cases, there are associated primary or secondary abnormalities of parathyroid hormone and calcium metabolism leading to bone disease and hypercalcaemia. Carcinoma of the parathyroid is very rare.

Fig. 20.3 **Hashimoto's thyroiditis** (MP)

This disease is an autoimmune thyroiditis in which thyroid acini **A** are progressively destroyed by immunological processes and the gland becomes diffusely infiltrated by lymphocytes and plasma cells. In some areas, the small darkly staining lymphocytes aggregate to form typical lymphoid follicles **F**, often with germinal centres. In the early stages of the disease, the extensive lymphoid infiltrate produces a diffusely enlarged, firm thyroid gland with a pale cut surface, resembling a lymph node. Thyroid epithelial cells in this condition commonly show *oncocytic* or *Hürthle cell transformation*, the Hürthle cells **H** having strongly eosinophilic granular cytoplasm and slightly enlarged nuclei.

As thyroid follicles are progressively destroyed, the patient, who at the outset is euthyroid or even mildly hyperthyroid, becomes increasingly hypothyroid (*myxoedematous*). When almost all thyroid acini are destroyed, the lymphoid infiltrate becomes less obvious and fibrosis supervenes, with progressive reduction in size of the gland.

INVESTIGATION OF A SOLITARY THYROID NODULE

Solitary thyroid nodules (defined as palpable, discrete nodules in an otherwise unremarkable thyroid), are detectable in approximately 5% of the population, the figure increasing with age and higher in females than in males. The differential diagnosis of these solitary nodules is wide and ranges from benign disease (such as thyroiditis or adenoma) to malignant disease (metastatic or primary), though the overwhelming majority are benign. Indications of a more concerning diagnosis may be revealed through careful history taking and/or clinical examination. However, as in many fields of medicine, the clinical clues to differentiate benign from malignant disease are not foolproof and further investigations are often required.

Fine needle aspiration (FNA) is the most commonly used procedure in investigating solitary thyroid nodules, occasionally supplemented by imaging investigations such as ultrasound and radioiodine scans. A thyroid FNA is a relatively simple procedure which does not require a general anaesthetic and, in the majority of cases, can provide insight into the nature of the nodule to allow planning of further management. Thus, if the lesion is small and benign, no further action may be indicated. Alternatively, if the lesion is malignant, surgical excision can be planned, with the extent of surgery guided by the nature of the malignancy.

Fig. 20.4 Graves' disease (a) Normal thyroid (HP) **(b)** Hyperplastic thyroid (HP)

Thyroid function is normally under the control of the hypothalamic–pituitary axis via the release of thyroid-stimulating hormone (TSH) from the pituitary which stimulates thyroid acinar cells to liberate thyroxine. The resulting level of circulating thyroxine then regulates TSH production by a negative feedback mechanism.

Under certain circumstances this balance may be disrupted leading to hyperplasia and hypertrophy of thyroid acinar cells through prolonged, unchecked stimulation; this gives rise to the histological appearance known as *thyroid hyperplasia*.

Graves' disease is by far the commonest cause of pathological thyroid hyperplasia. This autoimmune disease is characterised by a triad of clinical features, namely hyperthyroidism, *exophthalmos* (protruding eyes) and non-pitting oedema of the lower limbs (*pretibial myxoedema*). In the majority of cases, circulating antibodies to the TSH receptor are produced, such as a circulating immunoglobulin called *thyroid-stimulating immunoglobulin*. This binds to TSH receptors on thyroid acinar cells, mimicking the effects of TSH and resulting in excess secretion of thyroxine. The resulting glandular appearance is described as *thyrotoxic hyperplasia* and is illustrated in image (b).

Compared to the normal thyroid in image (a), the hyperplastic acinar cells are taller and have larger nuclei, reflecting a greater degree of metabolic activity. The acini themselves are smaller than normal because of the reduced amount of colloid resulting from increased thyroxine secretion. The hyperplastic acinar cells may crowd up on one side of the acini, projecting into the lumen as papillary structures **P**. The colloid in hyperplastic follicles shows peripheral scalloping **S**, reflecting the increased utilisation of stored thyroid colloid to produce thyroxine by the hyperactive thyroid acinar cells. In addition to these features, the thyroid may sometimes contain prominent lymphocytic aggregates (not shown in this specimen).

KEY TO FIGURES

A thyroid acini **F** lymphoid follicle **H** Hürthle cells **P** papillary structure **S** scalloping

Fig. 20.5 Multinodular goitre (MP)

Goitres may be either *diffuse* or *multinodular*, depending on the pattern of involvement of the gland. In the majority of instances, deficiency of dietary iodine leads to impaired thyroid hormone synthesis. Thus, to maintain the euthyroid state, the gland becomes enlarged, driven by a compensatory rise in TSH. Initially, this is achieved through formation of larger than normal follicles, known as a *diffuse (colloid) goitre*. This may progress to *multinodular goitre*, as illustrated in this image, in which the gland

consists of multiple nodules **N** composed of follicles of varying size.

Fibrosis, haemorrhage and calcification (not illustrated) are common. Some cases of multinodular goitre have a *dominant nodule*, a single very large nodule which may be difficult to distinguish clinically from an adenoma. However, histologically, the nodular appearance of the rest of the gland will usually identify the lesion as part of multinodular goitre.

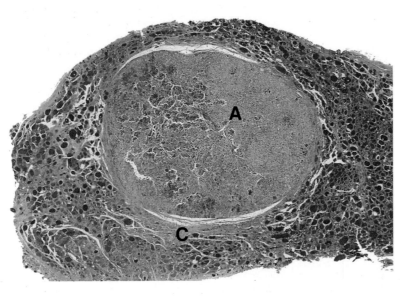

Fig. 20.6 Thyroid adenoma (LP)

Thyroid adenomas are benign tumours of follicular epithelium forming solitary, encapsulated, round nodules. In the majority of instances they are non-functional, with relatively few producing thyroid hormones (*toxic adenomas*).

This image illustrates the typical low-power appearance of a thyroid adenoma **A**, forming a readily identifiable, discrete lesion with a well-formed surrounding capsule **C**.

Occasionally, an adenoma may be difficult to differentiate from a well-differentiated *follicular carcinoma* (Fig. 20.7). In such cases thorough sampling and careful attention to the surrounding capsule is required to identify evidence of capsular or vascular invasion, features of follicular carcinoma.

KEY TO FIGURES

A adenoma **C** capsule **Co** colloid **F** follicular carcinoma **N** nodule **OA** Orphan Annie eye nuclei
S stromal core **T** surrounding thyroid gland

Fig. 20.7 **Thyroid carcinoma** **(a)** Papillary carcinoma (MP) **(b)** Papillary carcinoma (HP) **(c)** Follicular carcinoma (LP) **(d)** Follicular carcinoma (HP)

Papillary carcinomas are the most common of the thyroid malignancies, typically presenting in women under 40 years old. As illustrated in micrograph (a), the tumours form complex papillary structures, each composed of a narrow stromal core **S** covered with a layer of glandular epithelium. The stromal cores sometimes contain small, calcified, laminated bodies known as *psammoma bodies* (not shown here). At higher magnification in micrograph (b) the dispersed chromatin typical of papillary carcinoma cells can be appreciated. This imparts a characteristic, *optically clear* appearance to the nuclei, sometimes referred to as *Orphan Annie eye* nuclei **OA**. This slow-growing tumour tends to spread via lymphatics to regional nodes, but has the best prognosis of all thyroid cancers.

Follicular carcinomas are the second most common of the thyroid carcinomas. Typically, they appear as solitary lesions which may be well circumscribed (*encapsulated*) or widely invasive. Microscopically, they often display a well-structured follicular pattern and may be extremely difficult to

distinguish from a benign follicular adenoma (Fig. 20.6), particularly when encapsulated. In such cases extensive sampling of the tumour is required, in particular the capsule, looking for capsular and/or vascular invasion. Micrograph (c) shows a *minimally invasive* follicular carcinoma **F** which has breached the capsule **C** to invade the surrounding gland **T**. At higher magnification in micrograph (d), numerous small follicles containing colloid **Co** can be appreciated. In this case the tumour cells have abundant, eosinophilic cytoplasm typical of *Hürthle cells*. Bloodstream spread is the major mode of metastasis, with lung and bone as common sites of secondary tumour deposits.

Anaplastic carcinomas usually occur in the very elderly and are composed of sheets of poorly differentiated cells with little cytoplasm. These tumours grow very rapidly and extensively invade local tissues, often presenting as a bulky mass in the neck associated with symptoms of tracheal compression.

Fig. 20.8 Parathyroid hyperplasia and adenoma
(a) Normal gland (LP)
(b) Hyperplastic gland (LP)
(c) Parathyroid adenoma (LP)

The normal adult parathyroid gland contains small endocrine cells arranged in clumps or cords intermixed with adipose tissue; with increasing age, more of the gland becomes replaced by adipose tissue. Should the need arise for a greater output of parathyroid hormone, for example in cases of excessive urinary calcium loss in chronic renal failure, the endocrine cells undergo hyperplasia with loss of the adipose tissue.

Compare the hyperplastic gland in image (b) with the normal parathyroid in image (a). The hyperplastic gland is not only larger than the normal gland, but the hormonally active endocrine component has also increased, replacing the adipose tissue component. If demand for excess parathyroid hormone persists, the gland may become markedly enlarged. These hyperplastic changes usually affect all four glands uniformly. However, occasionally involvement can be asymmetrical, leading to difficulty in distinguishing hyperplasia from adenoma.

Autonomous benign tumours of the parathyroid gland, *parathyroid adenomas*, usually affect only one of the four glands, although occasionally they may be multiple. In image (c), a parathyroid adenoma replaces the whole gland. Often, a fragment of normal parathyroid tissue remains at the periphery (not seen in this example). The cellular arrangement in parathyroid adenomas is variable, with the cells arranged in sheets or in a microacinar pattern. The finding of a peripheral rim of compressed normal gland is a useful clue in distinguishing an adenoma from hyperplasia.

Where there is a parathyroid adenoma, the non-involved glands may show a suppressed parathyroid pattern, in which the endocrine component atrophies and is replaced by adipose tissue. As a result, the non-involved glands become much smaller, more adipose and difficult to find at surgery.

The adrenal gland has two distinct morphological and functional components:

- The **cortex**: This secretes three groups of steroid hormones, namely glucocorticoids (e.g. cortisol), mineralocorticoids (e.g. aldosterone) and small quantities of sex hormones. With the naked eye, the adrenal cortex appears yellow because of its high content of lipid (mainly cholesterol) which is the substrate for synthesis of steroid hormones.

- The **medulla**: This forms part of the neuroendocrine system and is responsible for the production of the catecholamines adrenaline (epinephrine) and noradrenaline (norepinephrine).

Disorders of the adrenal cortex

In response to acute stress, *atrophy of the adrenal cortex* (Fig. 20.9(b)) may arise as the normally lipid-rich cortical cells metabolise lipid in the production of steroid hormones, so becoming *lipid depleted*. This is commonly seen in adrenal glands at post-mortem, particularly when a patient has died with features of shock. It is manifest by atrophy of the gland with loss of the normal lipid vacuolation of cells of the cortex seen on microscopy. Adrenocortical atrophy may also result from steroid therapy (iatrogenic) or, occasionally, through primary autoimmune disease (*Addison's disease*). Other important, though less common, causes of adrenocortical insufficiency are mycobacterial infection and metastases.

In contrast to the picture with acute stress, with more prolonged stress the adrenal glands may become enlarged through hypertrophy and hyperplasia of cortical cells. Alternatively, *hyperplasia of the adrenal cortex* (Figs 20.9(c) and 20.9(d)) may arise as a consequence of prolonged stimulation of the adrenal cortex by pituitary-derived adrenocorticotrophic hormone (ACTH; *Cushing's disease*) or secretion of ectopic ACTH by non-pituitary tumours (*Cushing's syndrome*).

The adrenal cortex may be the site of benign *adrenocortical adenomas* (Fig. 20.10) or, rarely, malignant *adrenocortical carcinomas*. These tumours of the adrenal cortex may be functional, resulting in the following endocrine syndromes:

- **Cushing's syndrome**: caused by cortisol secreting tumours

- **Conn's syndrome**: results from aldosterone secreting tumours

- **adrenogenital syndrome**: owing to excess production of androgens.

Often, cortical hyperplasia is nodular rather than diffuse and it may be difficult to distinguish between a benign cortical adenoma and a large nodule forming part of nodular cortical hyperplasia.

Disorders of the adrenal medulla

Developmentally, the adrenal medulla arises from embryonal neural crest cells and is part of the *paraganglion system* along with a number of clusters of cells known as the *extra-adrenal paraganglia*, of which the carotid body is perhaps the best known. This paraganglion system is closely associated with the functioning of the autonomic nervous system.

The most important lesions of the adrenal medulla are tumours of the catecholamine producing (*chromaffin*) cells, known as *phaeochromocytoma*, or neuronal tumours (*neuroblastomas, ganglion cell tumours*). Phaeochromocytomas (Fig. 20.11) produce excessive adrenaline and noradrenaline and are usually benign. *Neuroblastomas* (Fig. 20.13) are highly malignant embryonal tumours of neuroblasts typically arising in childhood. Both types of adrenal medullary tumour may also arise elsewhere in the body in the extra-adrenal paraganglia.

Fig. 20.9 **Adrenal cortical atrophy and hyperplasia** **(a)** Normal gland (LP) **(b)** Atrophic gland (LP) **(c)** Diffuse hyperplasia (LP) **(d)** Nodular hyperplasia (LP)

These images, all at the same magnification, compare the normal gland (a) with adrenal atrophy and hyperplasia.

In *adrenal atrophy*, as shown in image (b), marked reduction in the size of the gland is due to atrophy of the cortex. In this example, the atrophy was caused by long-term administration of corticosteroids, resulting in suppression of pituitary ACTH.

Adrenortical hyperplasia occurs in either *diffuse* or *nodular* forms, as illustrated in images (c) and (d), respectively. In the diffuse form, the cortex **C** is

uniformly and regularly thickened, often by cells of one type. In the much more common nodular form, the cortex contains adenoma-like nodules **N** of hyperplastic cortical cells, usually of zona fasciculata type. Diffuse adrenal cortical hyperplasia is usually caused by excess stimulation by ACTH from the pituitary (*Cushing's disease*) or by ectopic ACTH secreted by a non-pituitary tumour, for example from a small cell carcinoma of lung (*Cushing's syndrome*). Nodular hyperplasia is commonly idiopathic and non-functional.

Fig. 20.10 Adrenal cortical adenoma (LP)

Hyperadrenal syndromes may result from excess secretion of hormones by a solitary benign *adrenal cortical adenoma,* the activity of which is independent of regulation by pituitary ACTH. These tumours form a circumscribed, spherical mass **A** within the cortex and may be composed of a single cell type (e.g. zona glomerulosa cells in *Conn's syndrome*), but more often contain a mixture of cortical cell types. Note how similar the adenoma is

to the nodules in nodular cortical hyperplasia in Figure 20.9d.

Cortical adenomas are a fairly frequent incidental finding at autopsy, a fact which leads to the belief that most are non-functioning and asymptomatic. Almost all cortical adenomas have a yellow cut surface, thereby distinguishing them from phaeochromocytomas which typically appear brown.

Fig. 20.11 Phaeochromocytoma (HP)

Phaeochromocytomas arise from the catecholamine producing chromaffin cells of the adrenal medulla. Most tumours are benign in their growth characteristics, but produce symptoms related to excess catecholamine secretion such as palpitations and sweating and, on occasion, may lead to potentially lethal hypertension. These tumours have a convenient association with 10%: approximately 10% are extra-adrenal (termed *paragangliomas*; Fig. 20.12), 10% are bilateral and 10% are malignant. Approximately 20% are familial, often in association with familial tumour syndromes.

Macroscopically, the cut surface of the tumour is pale brown in colour. Histologically, the tumour is composed of nests or '*zellballen*' (not seen here) of plump, irregular cells, often with pink granular cytoplasm, reflecting a high content of catecholamine-containing granules. Diagnosis of malignancy is based on evidence of invasion and spread, since purely cytological criteria are unreliable.

These tumours commonly secrete catecholamines. A diagnostic marker is *vanillyl mandelic acid (VMA)*, a metabolite which can be measured in the urine.

BASIC SYSTEMS PATHOLOGY ■ ENDOCRINE SYSTEM

KEY TO FIGURES
A adenoma   **C** cortex   **N** hyperplastic nodule

Fig. 20.12 Paraganglioma (HP)

The *paraganglion system* comprises the adrenal medulla and groups of extra-adrenal neuroendocrine cells which are widely distributed throughout the body (in or near the midline) in close association with the autonomic nervous system. Perhaps the most recognisable of these are the *carotid bodies* in the neck and the *organs of Zuckerkandl* at the bifurcation of the abdominal aorta.

Tumours may arise in these extra-adrenal paraganglia which, in all but name, are equivalent to phaeochromocytomas of the adrenal medulla (Fig. 20.11). These tumours, known as *paragangliomas*, most commonly arise in relation to the paraganglia of the abdomen and thorax, with a small number arising from paraganglia of the head and neck; those arising adjacent to the carotid arteries are referred to as *carotid body tumours*.

In this micrograph the histological similarities to adrenal phaeochromocytoma are evident, with nests (*zellballen*) **Z** of plump tumour cells with a granular cytoplasm intersected by fine vascular channels **V**. Close inspection may reveal ganglion cells **G** in some examples, as in this case.

Fig. 20.13 Adrenal embryonal tumours – neuroblastoma (HP)

Neuroblastoma is an example of a 'small round blue cell tumour' (see Fig. 7.9) believed to be derived from primitive neuroblasts in the adrenal medulla. It is highly malignant and represents the most common extracranial solid tumour of infancy.

The typical appearance of neuroblastoma is shown here. There is usually extensive haemorrhage and necrosis, but the viable areas are composed of small undifferentiated tumour cells in a pink-staining fibrillary stroma; the cells have a densely stained nucleus with scanty cytoplasm. A characteristic feature is occasional clumps of cells arranged in the form of a *Homer–Wright rosette* **R** surrounding a central zone of neurofibrils.

MULTIPLE ENDOCRINE NEOPLASIA SYNDROMES

The *multiple endocrine neoplasia (MEN)* syndromes are a group of inherited conditions characterised by tumours (benign and malignant) of multiple endocrine glands. Whilst the tumours involved may not be unique to MEN, they are distinguished from sporadic lesions by:

- a younger age at onset

- tumours preceded by hyperplasia in the gland

- presentation with multiple organs involved

- several tumours arising in one organ

- a more aggressive clinical course.

The main syndromes are *MEN-1* and *MEN-2* (further subdivided to MEN-2A, MEN-2B and familial medullary thyroid cancer), both of which are inherited in an autosomal dominant manner. In MEN-1 (*Wermer syndrome*), abnormalities of the parathyroids, pancreas and pituitary predominate, whereas in MEN-2A and -2B, phaeochromocytomas and thyroid (medullary carcinoma) tumours are typical, with mucocutaneous neuromas distinguishing MEN-2B.

KEY TO FIGURES
G ganglion cell   **R** Homer Wright rosette   **V** vascular channels   **Z** zellballen

Fig. 20.14 Chapter review

Disorder	Main features	Figure
Pituitary gland		
Pituitary adenoma	Derived from cells of anterior pituitary. May present with endocrine symptoms if hormone secreting. Typically, expanded nests of monotonous cells with moderate amounts of cytoplasm. Immunocytochemistry to identify secreted hormones	20.1 20.2
Thyroid gland		
Hashimoto's thyroiditis	Autoimmune thyroiditis with destruction of thyroid acini. Inflammatory cell infiltrate in gland with formation of lymphoid follicles	20.3
Graves' disease	Autoimmune disease. Commonest cause of pathological thyroid hyperplasia. Triad of hyperthyroidism, exophthalmos, pretibial myxoedema. Thyrotoxic hyperplasia with small acini and scalloping of colloid	20.4
Multinodular goitre	Majority as result of iodine deficiency. Nodules of varying sizes	20.5
Thyroid adenoma	Benign tumours of follicular epithelium. Encapsulated. Solitary. Majority non-functioning	20.6
Papillary carcinoma	Most common thyroid malignancy. Papillary architecture with tumour cells lining stromal cores. Optically clear nuclei (Orphan Annie eye)	20.7(a),(b)
Follicular carcinoma	Solitary, encapsulated or invasive lesions. May be difficult to differentiate from adenoma. Extensive sampling for capsular and/or vascular invasion indicated	20.7(c),(d)
Medullary carcinoma	Uncommon tumour of parafollicular cells. Notable for amyloid production	5.8
Anaplastic carcinoma	Aggressive, undifferentiated tumour arising in elderly	
Parathyroid glands		
Hyperplasia	Increased demand for parathyroid hormone results in expansion of endocrine component. Normally all four glands involved	20.8(b)
Adenoma	Benign. Usually only in one of four glands. Adenoma cells replace normal gland architecture. May be surviving rim of normal gland	20.8(c)
Adrenal glands		
Cortical atrophy	Response to stress or long-term corticosteroid administration	20.9(b)
Cortical hyperplasia	May be diffuse or, more commonly, nodular. Diffuse hyperplasia may be response to pituitary or ectopic ACTH. Nodular commonly idiopathic	20.9(c),(d)
Cortical adenoma	Independent of ACTH secretion. Solitary nodule in cortex, often of multiple cell types. Common incidental finding at autopsy	20.10
Phaeochromocytoma	Arise from medullary chromaffin cells. Symptoms of catecholamine secretion. Nests (*zellballen*) of plump cells with granular cytoplasm	20.11
Neuroblastoma	Adrenal embryonal tumour. Highly malignant. Most common childhood extracranial solid malignancy	20.13
Paraganglioma	Tumour of extra-adrenal paraganglion system. Equivalent of adrenal phaeochromocytoma. Carotid body tumour one example	20.12

21 Skin

Introduction

The skin is commonly affected by a wide range of pathologies. Some of these are cutaneous manifestations of systemic disease processes whilst others are primary disorders of the skin. Common systemic viral illnesses such as measles and chickenpox are associated with characteristic skin rashes and many autoimmune and vasculitic disorders, such as systemic lupus erythematosus, dermatomyositis, scleroderma and Henoch–Schönlein purpura, present with skin manifestations. Primary disorders of the skin are extremely common and the vast majority of these are inflammatory or neoplastic in type.

Inflammatory disorders

Skin has a limited repertoire of responses to injury. The most common of these are illustrated in Figures 21.1 to 21.4. Most stimuli result in a combination of these changes, each with varying degrees of severity. As a result, definitive diagnosis of inflammatory dermatological conditions requires careful correlation of clinical and histological findings. Few skin conditions have pathognomonic histological appearances.

Dermatitis is a common clinical term which is used to describe a wide variety of inflammatory skin conditions with diverse causes. Histologically, there are changes of acute or chronic inflammation (Figs 21.5 and 21.6). Some disorders have additional histological features which may indicate a more specific diagnosis or aetiology. Two relatively common inflammatory dermatoses with characteristic clinical and microscopic features are *lichen planus* (Fig. 21.7) and *psoriasis* (Fig. 21.8).

Systemic viral infections frequently cause skin rashes, some of which have typical histological features, e.g. Herpes simplex virus (HSV) infection (see Fig. 4.12), chickenpox and shingles. The latter two disorders are different clinical manifestations of infection by the Herpes zoster virus and the histological changes closely resemble those of HSV infection. Other viruses give rise to apparently localised skin lesions by causing proliferation of the cells of the epidermis. Common examples include *viral warts* (Fig. 21.9), which are caused by Human papilloma virus infection (see also Ch. 17), and *molluscum contagiosum* (Fig. 21.10), which is due to infection by a Pox virus.

Fig. 21.1 Abnormalities of surface keratin (MP) (a) Normal keratin (b) Hyperkeratosis (c) Parakeratosis

These images compare the appearance of normal keratin **K** of thin skin (a) with two common abnormalities of keratin. Figure (b) illustrates *hyperkeratosis* **H**. Here, the keratin layer is thickened, but otherwise histologically normal (*orthokeratosis*). This change is usually associated with thickening of the underlying granular layer **G** (stratum granulosum), termed *hypergranulosis*. Orthokeratosis is commonly seen in skin which has been chronically traumatised by scratching and, in this setting, it is usually associated with thickening of the epidermis (*acanthosis*, see Fig. 21.2).

Figure (c) shows *parakeratosis* **P**. In this case, the keratin is histologically abnormal in that it contains spindly nuclear remnants. Parakeratosis is usually associated with loss or severe thinning of the underlying granular layer. It can occur in a range of conditions but may be associated with *dysplasia* affecting the underlying epidermis (see Fig. 21.14).

Fig. 21.2 **Abnormal epidermal thickening – acanthosis** (MP)

Acanthosis is the term given to thickening of the epidermis, usually due to an increase in the depth of the stratum spinosum **S** (prickle cell layer). It is a common feature of many skin conditions, particularly chronic inflammatory conditions (Figs 21.6 and 21.7). The thickening of the epidermal layer is particularly

marked in the rete pegs **RP** which are expanded and elongated with prominent interdigitating dermal papillae **DP**. Note that there is associated thickening of the granular layer **G** (hypergranulosis) and overlying orthokeratotic hyperkeratosis **H**.

Fig. 21.3 **Intraepidermal oedema – spongiosis**
(a) MP **(b)** HP

Oedema of the epidermis causes separation of epithelial cells, particularly in the prickle cell layer, a condition known as *spongiosis*. Accumulation of oedema fluid **O** between epidermal cells causes gaps to appear. This accentuates the intercellular junctions as illustrated in micrograph (b). This oedema fluid may coalesce to form intraepidermal vesicles. Spongiosis with vesicle formation is a feature of acute dermatitis (Fig. 21.5).

KEY TO FIGURES
DP dermal papillae   **G** granular layer   **H** hyperkeratosis   **K** keratin   **O** oedema   **P** parakeratosis
RP rete peg   **S** stratum spinosum

Fig. 21.4 Other epidermal inflammatory reactions
(a) Vesicle (MP) **(b)** Bulla (LP)
(c) Pustule (MP)

Accumulations of fluid beneath or within the epidermis may cause small raised blebs on the skin. Most are due to inflammation in the epidermis. When small, such lesions are termed *vesicles*. In micrograph (a), note the small area of fluid accumulation **F**, forming a vesicle within the epidermis **E**. Some inflammatory cells **I** are present within the fluid and in the adjacent epidermis.

Larger collections of fluid are termed *bullae*. A bulla is shown in micrograph (b). The collection of fluid **F** here is larger and includes inflammatory cells and fibrin. In this case, the roof of the bulla consists of the full thickness of the epidermis and its base is the upper dermis **D**.

The term *pustule* is used to describe a collection consisting of neutrophils with some fluid, lying within or beneath the epidermis. Micrograph (c) shows a pustule **P** beneath the corneal layer of the epidermis.

Bullae and pustules are further categorised by their location, which may be *subepidermal*, *intraepidermal* or *subcorneal*.

Fig. 21.5 Acute dermatitis (MP)

In early acute dermatitis, the major changes involve the epidermis, with fluid accumulating between the prickle cells causing spongiosis **S**. As the lesion progresses, the spongiotic areas may become converted into fluid-filled vesicles **V** containing a few inflammatory cells, mainly lymphocytes and neutrophils, with variable infiltration of the epidermis by these cells. If the vesicles rupture onto the surface, crusts or scabs composed of fibrin and polymorph nuclei form. In the earlier stages, the upper dermis shows only oedema, but later there may be a mixed acute and chronic inflammatory cell infiltrate **I**, particularly around upper dermal blood vessels. This pattern is seen in the acute phase of the common inflammatory skin disease *eczema*, which is thought to have an allergic aetiology.

KEY TO FIGURES

A acanthosis   **C** chronic inflammation   **CB** Civatte bodies   **D** upper dermis   **DC** dilated capillary
DP dermal papilla   **E** epidermis   **F** fluid   **G** granular layer   **H** hyperkeratosis   **I** inflammatory cells
M microabscess   **P** pustule   **PK** parakeratosis   **R** rete peg   **S** spongiosis   **V** vesicle

Fig. 21.6 Chronic dermatitis (MP)

The histological features of chronic dermatitis are seen in many skin rashes with a variety of causes. The characteristic feature is epidermal thickening, i.e. acanthosis **A** and a variable degree of hyperkeratosis **H**. There is no infiltration of the epidermis by inflammatory cells, but the upper and mid dermis show a moderate to heavy infiltrate of chronic inflammatory cells **C**, mainly lymphocytes and plasma cells, particularly around blood vessels.

The acanthosis and hyperkeratosis may produce the clinical appearance of *lichenification*, a leather-like thickening of the skin due to chronic scratching or irritation. This feature is recognised in the term *lichen simplex chronicus*, used to describe a form of chronic, non-specific dermatitis that occurs mainly in response to scratching of skin affected by acute dermatitis. When the dermatitis is still active, the thickened epidermis will contain the same sort of spongiotic vesicles seen in Figure 21.5, for example in long-standing eczema.

Fig. 21.7 Lichen planus (a) MP (b) HP

Lichen planus is a clinically and histologically distinct type of dermatitis. In the epidermis, as seen in micrograph (a), there is hyperkeratosis **H** and thickening of the granular layer **G** (hypergranulosis). A characteristic feature is the disruption of the normally regular basal layer by vacuolar degeneration and destruction of basal cells. As seen in micrograph (b), this leaves a ragged and irregular dermo-epidermal junction in which *colloid* or *Civatte bodies* **CB** (apoptotic keratinocytes) may be seen. The dermis **D** shows a dense chronic inflammatory cell infiltrate, mainly confined to the upper third. Lichen planus may affect the mucosal surfaces of the mouth and vulva where basal cell layer damage may lead to blistering and erosion.

Fig. 21.8 Psoriasis (MP)

Psoriasis is a chronic skin disease characterised by well-demarcated, erythematous, scaly lesions. Histologically, the major feature is acanthosis with greatly elongated, narrow rete pegs **R**. Between the rete pegs, the epidermis is thinned over oedematous and expanded dermal papillae **DP** in which dilated capillaries **DC** are prominent. The alternately thick and thin epidermis is covered by a parakeratotic layer **PK** of keratin which contains small aggregations of the nuclear debris of inflammatory cells, forming *Munro microabscesses* **M**. There is a variable chronic inflammatory infiltrate in the upper dermis **D**.

Fig. 21.9 Viral wart (a) LP (b) HP

A *viral wart*, or *verruca vulgaris*, which occurs on non-traumatised skin, has an exophytic papillary form as illustrated in micrograph (a). Histologically, the epidermis **E** is irregularly thickened and covered by a thick layer of hyperkeratosis **H** in which there are *parakeratotic spires* **PS** over the tips of the more prominent papillary epidermal outgrowths.

The epidermal cells in an active viral wart usually show focal prominence of the granular layer **G** as

illustrated in image (b), with occasional areas of large, pale vacuolated cells in the upper stratum spinosum. The dermis **D** shows a chronic inflammatory cell infiltrate.

In skin areas prone to trauma, warts have a much less papillary form and may be dome-shaped (e.g. in *juvenile warts* of the hands) or inverted (e.g. *plantar warts* of the sole of the foot).

Fig. 21.10 Molluscum contagiosum (LP)

Molluscum contagiosum is a localised nodular thickening of the epidermis. This condition occurs more commonly in children and is due to infection by a Pox virus. There are lobules of epithelial proliferation with an inverted, endophytic architecture. Viral inclusion bodies **V** are easily visible, both in the proliferating epidermis, where they stain a reddish colour, and in the overlying keratin plug **K**, where they appear more darkly stained. The keratinous plug extrudes through a central pit **P** at the apex of the dome-shaped nodule which is surrounded by normal epidermis. Lesions usually resolve spontaneously.

KEY TO FIGURES

D dermis **E** epidermis **G** granular layer **H** hyperkeratosis **K** keratin plug **N** keratin nest **P** pit
PS parakeratotic spires **V** viral inclusion bodies

Neoplastic disorders

Common primary skin tumours may be divided broadly into those arising from epithelial cells, those arising from melanocytes and those arising within dermal and subcutaneous tissues. Much less commonly, skin can be involved by metastatic tumour from other sites (e.g. lung or renal cancer) or by direct invasion from an underlying neoplasm (most commonly breast cancer). Lymphoma may also affect the skin either primarily (e.g. *mycosis fungoides*, see Fig. 16.12) or in cases of systemic lymphoma.

Epithelial neoplasms

Seborrhoeic keratosis and *basal cell papilloma* are terms which are used interchangeably to describe a very common benign skin lesion which is seen predominantly in elderly patients. *Basal cell carcinoma* is a low-grade malignant tumour which resembles the basal cells of the epidermis; *squamous cell carcinoma* is a more aggressive tumour which resembles the cells of the prickle cell layer (stratum spinosum) of the epidermis. Both of these malignant tumours are strongly associated with chronic sun exposure. Chronic sun damage is also associated with premalignant change in the skin in the form of epidermal *dysplasia*, with disordered maturation of keratinocytes. Severe dysplasia, the skin equivalent of CIN 3 (see Fig. 17.6), can be described as *carcinoma in situ, intraepidermal carcinoma* or using the eponymous term *Bowen's disease*. Lesser degrees of epidermal dysplasia are termed *actinic* or *solar keratosis*.

Fig. 21.11 Seborrhoeic keratosis (a) LP (b) HP

Seborrhoeic keratosis (sometimes called *basal cell papilloma* or *seborrhoeic wart*) is a common lesion of the elderly. This is characterised by a localised proliferation of cells which resemble the normal basal cells of the epidermis, usually forming a raised warty lesion as illustrated in micrograph (a).

Such outgrowths are vulnerable to chronic trauma, leading to overlying hyperkeratosis and formation of keratin nests **N** in the lesion. These whorls of keratin (sometimes referred to as 'horn cysts') are characteristic and this is illustrated at higher magnification in micrograph (b). There is often prominent melanin pigment within the cells of the basal layer and, as a result, these lesions often appear dark brown or black in colour.

Examination of the cells at high magnification shows that the nuclei are bland and uniform and there is no evidence of significant mitotic activity. These features may be compared with those of a malignant skin tumour, basal cell carcinoma, illustrated in Figure 21.12. The aetiology of this lesion is unknown, but it is usually regarded as a benign skin tumour.

Fig. 21.12 Basal cell carcinoma (a) LP (b) HP

Basal cell carcinoma is a common tumour, composed of cells with dark-staining nuclei and sparse, poorly defined cytoplasm. Micrograph (a) shows the typical appearances of the common nodular form, with a mixture of solid nodular **N** and microcystic **MC** growth patterns. In addition to this nodular form, basal cell carcinomas show a wide range of growth patterns. The *morphoeic* variant presents as a flat, hard area of skin, and the *superficial* form as a reddish, scaly lesion. As seen in micrograph (b), the cells at the periphery of the tumour are characteristically arranged in a palisaded pattern **P**, whereas the central cells are more randomly arranged. Basal cell carcinoma arises from the basal cells of the epidermis or epidermal appendages. It behaves as a malignant tumour in that it invades dermis and any deeper underlying structures, but it almost never metastasises. Basal cell carcinomas occur most frequently on the light-exposed areas of skin, particularly the face, and usually present as nodular lesions which may undergo ragged ulceration, giving rise to the colloquial term *rodent ulcer*.

Fig. 21.13 Squamous cell carcinoma (LP)

Squamous cell carcinoma of the skin histologically resembles squamous cell carcinomas in many other sites (see Fig. 7.6). The skin tumours are usually well differentiated and highly keratinising. In this example, there is a large central plug of keratin **K** with surrounding infiltrating carcinoma.

The tumour invades through the dermis **D** and into underlying subcutaneous fat **S.** It may spread via the lymphatic channels to regional lymph nodes. Invasive squamous cell carcinoma of the skin can develop from *intraepidermal carcinoma* (*squamous cell carcinoma in situ*, see Fig. 21.14).

KEY TO FIGURES

BM basement membrane   **D** dermis   **K** keratin   **MC** microcystic pattern   **N** nodular pattern
P palisading cells   **TM** tripolar mitosis   **S** subcutaneous fat

Fig. 21.14 **Intraepidermal carcinoma** (HP)

Invasive squamous carcinoma (see Fig. 21.13) may be preceded by epidermal dysplasia. When the dysplasia is severe and involves the full thickness of the epidermis, it is termed *intraepidermal carcinoma*, *carcinoma in situ* or *Bowen's disease*. This eponymous term is reserved for lesions with a plaque-like clinical appearance.

In this micrograph, there is severe dysplasia extending through the full thickness of the epidermis, with loss of the normal organisation and stratification. The basement membrane **BM** is intact and there is no invasion of the dermis **D**. Numerous mitotic figures are seen and some of these appear atypical, with occasional tripolar forms **TM**. When the epidermal dysplasia is restricted to lower levels of the epidermis, the condition is known as *actinic (solar) keratosis*.

Melanocytic lesions

In normal skin, melanocytes are scattered in the basal layers of the epidermis, their fine cytoplasmic processes ramifying between the keratinocytes towards the skin surface. Melanocytes are responsible for the synthesis of the brown pigment melanin, which is then transferred to adjacent keratinocytes. There are significant racial and genetic differences in the melanin synthetic activity of melanocytes, resulting in the varying degrees of normal pigmentation seen in the skin. Exposure to sunlight enhances melanin synthesis and transfer into keratinocytes.

Benign pigmented skin lesions are very common and are known colloquially as 'moles'. This term encompasses a large group of benign lesions called *naevi*, which are characterised histologically by aggregates of melanocytic cells at various sites within the skin. The three main subtypes, *junctional*, *compound* and *intradermal naevi*, are shown in Figure 21.15.

Malignant melanoma is an important and highly malignant tumour of melanocytic cells. Its main features and histological variants are illustrated in Figures 21.16 to 21.19. There are also melanocytic lesions with features intermediate between a benign naevus and a malignant melanoma. These are described as *atypical* or *dysplastic naevi* and may progress to melanoma in some cases.

Benign melanocytic naevi

These are of three main types, defined according to the location of the melanocytic nests:

- **Junctional melanocytic naevus**: Nests of melanocytes are confined to the lower epidermis.

- **Compound melanocytic naevus**: Nests are located in both the lower epidermis and upper dermis.

- **Intradermal melanocytic naevus**: Nests of melanocytes are present in the dermis only.

Benign naevi have a predictable natural history and are illustrated in Figure 21.15. Most begin as flat, pigmented *junctional naevi*, with nests of pigmented melanocytes confined to the lower levels of the epidermis, sitting on the epidermal basement membrane. Purely junctional naevi are most commonly found in children. As the child grows older, some of these junctional melanocytes migrate across the basement membrane into the upper dermis where they lose most of their pigment and the cells become smaller and tightly packed together. There are some remaining pigmented junctional nests in the epidermis and smaller non-pigmented naevus cells in the dermis. At this stage, the naevus is called a *compound naevus* and the intradermal nests produce a lesion which is raised above the level of skin to form a brown, raised nodule. In early adulthood, most of the junctional nests of melanocytes migrate into the dermis until no more are present in the epidermis. At this stage, the naevus is a completely *intradermal naevus*. All of these lesions are completely benign but, rarely, a previously benign naevus will transform into a malignant melanoma. This usually occurs by a well-recognised route: the junctional nests do not completely migrate into the dermis but proliferate abnormally and show features of cytological and architectural atypia, producing a *dysplastic* or *atypical naevus*. If untreated, a proportion of these eventually become superficial spreading malignant melanoma (Figs 21.16 and 21.17).

Fig. 21.15 **Melanocytic naevi** **(a)** Junctional naevus (MP) **(b)** Compound naevus (MP) **(c)** Intradermal naevus (MP) **(d)** Dysplastic junctional naevus (HP)

In a junctional naevus (a), the melanocytes aggregate in junctional nests **J** in the lower layers of the epidermis but do not encroach into the underlying dermis. The nests are round to oval and well circumscribed and the melanocytes are pigmented.

A compound naevus (b) contains both intraepidermal junctional nests **J** and nests of naevus cells in the upper dermis **N**. The cells in the dermis become small and densely packed and are said to be '*maturing*'. As time passes, more and more naevus cells occupy the dermis and there are fewer junctional nests in the epidermis.

Eventually, all the naevus cells which formed the junctional nests have migrated into the upper dermis to form an intradermal naevus, as shown in micrograph (c).

Sometimes, the junctional melanocyte nests do not migrate completely into the dermis, but develop features of both cytological and architectural atypia, forming a dysplastic naevus. Nuclear pleomorphism is seen. Architectural atypia often takes the form of elongated nests composed of spindle-shaped melanocytes running transversely, bridging adjacent epidermal rete pegs **B**. There is usually associated fibrosis within the superficial dermis, termed *fibroplasia* **F**, and prominent *melanophages* **H** (histiocytes containing melanin pigment) may be seen.

Some pathologists use the term *atypical naevus* for lesions of this type and may then describe the degree of cytological and architectural atypia as mild, moderate or severe. This information may be helpful for clinicians when planning further patient follow-up.

KEY TO FIGURES

AM atypical melanocyte nests   **B** bridging melanocyte nests   **F** fibroplasia   **H** melanophages   **J** junctional nest
N intradermal nests   **SM** single melanocytes

Malignant melanocytic lesions (malignant melanoma)

Malignant melanoma is a malignant tumour of melanocytes, the incidence of which is increasing dramatically in white-skinned people around the world. Excessive sun exposure, particularly sunburning, is believed to be the principal cause. Neglected malignant melanomas have frequently metastasised at the time of presentation, but public awareness is leading to patients presenting earlier, such that many malignant melanomas may now be completely cured by primary excision of the lesion. Malignant melanoma spreads initially via lymphatics to regional lymph nodes and subsequently via the bloodstream, by which time control of the disease is extremely difficult.

The risk of metastasis, and therefore the prognosis, depends mainly on the following factors:

■ **Depth of tumour invasion**

– *Melanoma in situ* indicates that tumour cells have not breached the basement membrane. This indicates that the lesion lacks any metastatic potential and so excision is curative.

– *Breslow depth* is one of the main prognostic indicators in melanoma. This is measured perpendicularly from the granular cell layer of the epidermis down to the deepest invasive tumour cell. Lesions with a Breslow depth of less than 1 mm have an excellent prognosis.

– *Clark level* is an alternative means of assessing the extent of tumour invasion and is most valuable in lesions less than 1 mm in depth. This system identifies the deepest anatomical layer of the skin which is involved, e.g. Clark level 2 indicates that tumour is limited to the papillary dermis only whilst Clark level 5 describes invasion of subcutaneous tissues.

■ **Growth phase**

– *Radial growth phase* describes a lesion with predominantly horizontal (lateral) growth and without evidence of deep dermal infiltration. This pattern of growth is associated with a relatively favourable prognosis and is typically seen early in the development of the superficial spreading form of malignant melanoma. This is one of the common subtypes encountered in clinical practice (Figs 21.16 and 21.17).

– *Vertical growth phase*, in contrast, indicates that the malignant cells show predominantly vertical growth, invading deeper into the dermis. This is typical of nodular malignant melanoma and is associated with an adverse prognosis (Fig. 21.18).

■ **Lymphatic, vascular or perineural invasion**

– When present, these histological features indicate an adverse prognosis and are associated with a high risk of lymph node and distant metastases.

Other subtypes of melanoma include *lentigo maligna* (a pre-invasive form of the disease which occurs in sun-damaged skin of older patients, illustrated in Fig. 21.19), *invasive lentigo maligna melanoma* (the invasive form of the same disorder) and *acral lentiginous malignant melanoma* which, as the name suggests, occurs at acral sites (sites with thick skin such as the palms and soles). This lesion is uncommon in white-skinned populations, but occurs with relatively greater frequency in black populations owing to the presence of lesser quantities of protective melanin pigment at these sites.

Fig. 21.16 Superficial spreading malignant melanoma in situ (HP)

Here, the epidermis contains irregular nests of atypical melanocytes **AM**. Unlike in junctional naevi (see Fig. 21.15) where these are confined to the tips of rete pegs, here the nests are more randomly distributed and some extend into upper layers of the epidermis. The nests are variable in size and shape, and the melanocytes they contain are atypical and pleomorphic. Numerous single melanocytes **SM** are scattered through the upper layers of the epidermis. This is termed *Pagetoid spread* due to the resemblance to Paget's disease of the nipple (see Fig. 18.13). Some *melanophages* **H** (histiocytes containing melanin pigment) are present in the papillary dermis, but here there is no invasion of the dermis by the malignant cells (compare with Fig. 21.17).

Fig. 21.17 **Superficial spreading malignant melanoma – dermal invasion** **(a)** LP **(b)** HP

As in the superficial spreading malignant melanoma in situ shown in Figure 21.16, there are nests of atypical melanocytes in all layers of the epidermis **AM**, but in this example malignant cells have broken through the epidermal basement membrane to invade the dermis **D** in a radial/horizontal growth pattern. Again, there are prominent melanophages **M**, and some lymphocytic

inflammatory cells **I** are also present in the surrounding dermis.

In micrograph (b), the infiltrating cells show obvious nuclear pleomorphism and are seen to have prominent nucleoli. In contrast to Figure 21.16, the malignant cells lie between dermal collagen fibres and there is no basement membrane around them.

Fig. 21.18 **Malignant melanoma – nodular** (LP)

This low-power image shows the architectural pattern of a malignant melanoma with a nodular (vertical) growth phase component which invades into the deep dermis **D**.

In this case, there is no melanocyte proliferation at the dermo-epidermal junction (compare with Fig. 21.17).

The Breslow thickness of this lesion is much greater than 1 mm and the prognosis is poor, with a high chance of metastatic spread.

Fig. 21.19 **Lentigo maligna** **(a)** H&E (HP) **(b)** Immunohistochemical staining for MelanA (MP)

Lentigo maligna is a form of in situ melanoma which usually presents as an enlarging, flat, pigmented patch on the faces of elderly people. Image (a) shows an almost continuous line of single, atypical melanocytes **AM** in the basal layer. The cells show pleomorphism with enlarged, hyperchromatic nuclei. Typically, these abnormal melanocytes extend down the basal layer of skin appendages such as hair follicles **H.** This is illustrated in image (b), using an

immunohistochemical method to highlight melanocytes (stained brown). Eventually, invasion of the dermis may occur (*lentigo maligna melanoma*). In general, lentigo maligna has a prolonged period of in situ growth and invasive disease is relatively uncommon. When this occurs, it is usually manifest by the development of a nodule within the previously flat pigmented lesion.

CLINICAL ASPECTS OF MALIGNANT MELANOMA

Malignant melanoma usually presents as a new or changing pigmented lesion. On examination, the edge of the lesion is often irregular and rather ill-defined, whilst benign naevi tend to be round and uniform with a sharply defined border. Naevi also tend to be evenly pigmented whereas melanomas typically exhibit variable pigmentation, often with several different shades of black and brown. More advanced tumours can have nodular areas and sometimes show surface ulceration because the expanding mass of tumour cells destroys the overlying epidermis. Occasional lesions are not pigmented and these are termed *amelanotic melanomas*. These tumours are more difficult to recognise and may be confused with other lesions such as intradermal naevi and basal cell carcinomas. Complete excision is the initial treatment of choice in cases of melanoma.

Cysts and other skin lesions

Some common skin lesions are difficult to classify because their aetiologies are incompletely understood. Examples include the various cysts which are commonly referred to as 'sebaceous cysts' by clinicians. Common skin cysts fall into two main categories histologically, *epidermoid cysts* (Fig. 21.20) and *pilar cysts* (Fig. 21.21). Other lesions such as the *pyogenic granuloma* (Fig. 21.22) and *dermatofibroma* (Fig. 21.23) share some features with benign neoplasms, but are considered by others to be reactive proliferations, often occurring after minor injury. *Dermatofibrosarcoma protuberans* (Fig. 21.24) shows some histological similarities to dermatofibroma, but as the name suggests, this is a malignant soft tissue neoplasm (a sarcoma). Other soft tissue lesions are considered in Chapter 22.

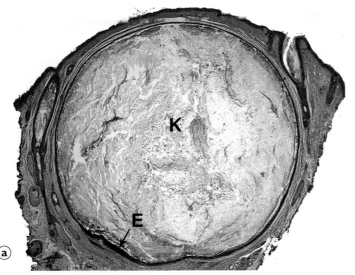

(a)

(b)

Fig. 21.20 **Epidermoid cyst**
(a) LP **(b)** HP

Epidermoid cysts (sometimes called *epidermal cysts*) are intradermal lesions which may open onto the skin surface through a punctum. The cyst contains lamellated keratin **K**, and is lined by a thin, flattened squamous epithelium **E** which, like the epidermis, has a granular layer **G**. This is illustrated at higher magnification in micrograph (b).

Trauma to the cyst may lead to rupture, associated with escape of keratin into the surrounding dermis where its presence excites a granulomatous foreign body giant cell reaction (see Fig. 3.10), with swelling, tenderness and redness around the cyst.

Clinically, these lesions are often (inaccurately) called 'sebaceous cysts', and traumatised, ruptured cysts are said to be 'infected sebaceous cysts', again inaccurately. The features of inflammation around ruptured cysts are due to the reaction to leaked keratin.

Fig. 21.21 **Pilar cyst** (HP)

Pilar cysts (sometimes called *tricholemmal cysts*) are similar to epidermoid cysts, but occur almost entirely on the scalp. They differ from epidermal cysts in the nature of the keratin **K**, which is compact and cohesive, and in the lining squamous epithelium **E** which resembles hair follicles, lacking a granular layer. These lesions are also mistakenly called 'sebaceous cysts'.

BASIC SYSTEMS PATHOLOGY ■ SKIN

KEY TO FIGURES
AM atypical melanocytes   **D** dermis   **E** epithelium   **G** granular layer   **H** hair follicle   **I** inflammatory cells
K keratin   **M** melanophages

Fig. 21.22 Pyogenic granuloma
(LP)

Pyogenic granuloma (sometimes called *lobular capillary haemangioma*) is a common lesion which may occur following a minor penetrating injury, for example by a rose thorn. It consists of a raised nodule composed of lobules of capillary-sized vessels **V**, somewhat resembling a capillary haemangioma. It may represent an abnormal overgrowth of the vascular element of normal granulation tissue. The surface of the lesion is frequently ulcerated and, in this example, there is an overlying inflammatory exudate **Ex**. A characteristic histological feature is a collarette **C** of proliferating epidermis at the base of the lesion.

Fig. 21.23 Dermatofibroma (a) LP (b) HP

Dermatofibroma (sometimes called *benign fibrous histiocytoma*) is a common skin lesion, usually occurring on the limbs of young and middle-aged people in the form of a single, firm, raised nodule, ranging in colour from white to brown.

Histologically, the lesion lies in the dermis and has ill-defined margins, being composed of irregularly arranged spindle cells resembling fibroblasts with intervening collagen fibres. The degree of cellularity seen in these lesions is variable and some forms contain abundant collagen with fewer fibroblastic cells. Scattered foamy or haemosiderin-laden histiocytes are present in some lesions, probably due to degeneration within the lesion. The overlying

epidermis **E** tends to show prominent basal layer pigmentation **P** and is often irregularly thickened, a feature described as *pseudoepitheliomatous hyperplasia*. When this change is very marked, the appearance may mimic invasive carcinoma.

Although the dermatofibroma resembles a group of soft tissue tumours which are described as '*fibrohistiocytic*' (owing to the presence of cells similar to fibroblasts and histiocytes), dermatofibromas are generally considered to be reactive lesions rather than true benign tumours. Sometimes, there is a clinical history of previous minor injury at the site of the lesion.

KEY TO FIGURES
C collarette of proliferating epidermis   **E** epidermis   **Ex** inflammatory exudate   **P** basal layer pigmentation
V vascular tissue

Fig. 21.24 Dermatofibrosarcoma protuberans (a) LP (b) HP

This is a low-grade sarcoma which usually occurs in young adults. It arises in the skin, most commonly affecting the trunk, and presents as a hard and gradually enlarging plaque. Over time, it may become raised and nodular, hence the designation 'protuberans'.

Histologically, the tumour is composed of spindle cells which show variable but usually mild pleomorphism. There are occasional mitotic figures. Although originating in the dermis, it enlarges by infiltrating laterally into adjacent dermis and deeply into subcutaneous adipose tissue, as in micrograph (b). It often infiltrates much more extensively than is apparent clinically and complete excision at first

attempt can be difficult. Incomplete excision is invariably followed by recurrence and continued local spread.

Metastasis does occur rarely and, in common with other sarcomas, this is usually blood-borne in type (rather than the pattern of lymphatic spread to local lymph nodes which is typically seen in carcinomas) and results in lung metastases.

Over time, some tumours may develop areas of higher-grade malignancy, resembling *fibrosarcoma*, a soft tissue tumour which can also occur at other sites. This transformation is manifest clinically by a rapid increase in the size of the tumour.

Fig. 21.25 Chapter review

Disorder	Main features	Figure
Responses of skin to injury		
Orthokeratosis	Thickened layer of normal keratin. No nuclear fragments. Often associated prominence of granular layer (hypergranulosis)	21.1(b)
Parakeratosis	Abnormal surface keratin with residual flecks of nuclear material. Often associated with loss or diminution of granular layer	21.1(c)
Acanthosis	Thickening of epidermis, usually associated with increased depth of the rete pegs	21.2
Spongiosis	Intraepidermal oedema due to acute inflammation, resulting in gaps between keratinocytes and highlighting intercellular junctions	21.3
Vesicle	Small accumulation of oedema fluid within epidermis due to acute inflammation, sometimes containing a few inflammatory cells	21.4(a)
Bulla	Large collection of fluid within or beneath epidermis, sometimes containing inflammatory cells and fibrin	21.4(b)
Pustule	Collection of neutrophil polymorphs and some fluid within or beneath the epidermis. May be subcorneal, intraepidermal or subepidermal	21.4(c)

Fig. 21.25 Chapter review—cont'd

Disorder	Main features	Figure
Inflammatory disorders		
Acute dermatitis	Intraepidermal oedema resulting in spongiosis and vesiculation. Some inflammatory cells in epidermis. Later, chronic inflammation in dermis	21.5
Chronic dermatitis	Acanthosis and hyperkeratosis with chronic inflammation around vessels in superficial dermis	21.6
Lichen planus	Irregular acanthosis with chronic inflammation blurring dermo-epidermal junction. Basal cell vacuolar damage and apoptotic keratinocytes	21.7
Psoriasis	Regular acanthosis with thinning of suprapapillary epidermis and dilated capillaries in oedematous papillary dermis. Munro microabscesses	21.8
Viral lesions		
Viral wart (verruca vulgaris)	Exophytic papillary lesion of epidermis with parakeratotic spires, hypergranulosis and occasional koilocytic cells. HPV infection	21.9
Molluscum contagiosum	Inverted lobules of proliferating epithelium with viral inclusions (molluscum bodies) and a central plug of keratin. Pox virus infection	21.10
Epithelial neoplasms		
Seborrhoeic keratosis (basal cell papilloma)	Benign proliferation of bland cells resembling basal cells of epidermis. Hyperkeratosis and nests of keratin. Usually exophytic	21.11
Basal cell carcinoma	Low grade malignant tumour. Small, hyperchromatic cells resembling basal cells of epidermis. Peripheral palisading. Mitotic. Various patterns	21.12
Squamous cell carcinoma	More aggressive than BCC. Larger cells with eosinophilic cytoplasm. Keratinisation. May arise from carcinoma in situ (Bowen's disease)	21.13
Intraepidermal carcinoma (carcinoma in situ, Bowen's)	Full thickness dysplasia of epidermis. Disordered architecture and cytological atypia. Basement membrane intact	21.14
Actinic keratosis (solar keratosis)	Mild to moderate epidermal dysplasia. Associated with chronic sun damage	
Melanocytic lesions		
Junctional naevus	Nests of uniform and bland pigmented melanocytic cells at dermo-epidermal junction. No naevus cells in dermis	21.15(a)
Compound naevus	Nests of naevus cells at dermo-epidermal junction and in dermis. Dermal nests smaller, less pigmented and showing maturation	21.15(b)
Intradermal naevus	No remaining junctional melanocyte nests. Mature naevus cells only within dermis	21.15(c)
Atypical naevus (dysplastic naevus)	Cytological and architectural atypia of melanocyte nests. Often more spindle-shaped cells and superficial desmoplasia	21.15(d)
Superficial spreading malignant melanoma in situ	Nests of severely atypical melanocytes with Pagetoid spread of single cells within epidermis. Basement membrane remains intact	21.16
Invasive superficial spreading malignant melanoma	Atypical melanocytes in epidermis and also invading into dermis. Breslow depth and Clark level important for prognosis	21.17
Nodular malignant melanoma	Tumour in vertical growth phase with nodule of tumour cells in dermis and minimal junctional activity. Adverse prognosis due to lesional depth	21.18
Lentigo maligna	Form of melanoma in situ found on face of elderly patients. Linear proliferation of atypical melanocytes at dermo-epidermal junction	21.19
Lentigo maligna melanoma	Invasive malignant melanoma arising from long-standing lentigo maligna. Often nodule forms within flat pigmented patch	
Other lesions		
Epidermoid cyst (epidermal cyst)	Clinical term sebaceous cyst. Cyst filled with lamellated keratin. Lined by stratified squamous epithelium. Granular layer present	21.20
Pilar cyst (tricholemmal cyst)	Clinical term sebaceous cyst. Usually scalp. Firm, amorphous keratin. Squamous lining without granular layer	21.21
Pyogenic granuloma (lobular capillary haemangioma)	Often after minor penetrating injury. Lobules of capillary size vessels. Collarette of epidermis at base	21.22
Dermatofibroma (benign fibrous histiocytoma)	Probably reactive lesion. Fibroblasts and collagen, ill-defined edge. Scattered histiocytes. Overlying epidermal hyperplasia	21.23
Dermatofibrosarcoma protuberans	Low-grade sarcoma of skin. Resembles dermatofibroma but deeply invasive and locally aggressive. May rarely metastasise	21.24

22 Bone and soft tissues

Bone

Bone is a highly specialised tissue composed of a particular type of collagen embedded in a ground substance matrix, *osteoid*. Osteoid becomes mineralised by the deposition of calcium salts in the form of *hydroxyapatite*. The osteoid is synthesised by *osteoblasts* which, in their resting state, are inactive, spindle-shaped cells lying unobtrusively on bone surfaces. When there is a need to synthesise more osteoid, osteoblasts become cuboidal and actively synthesise protein. Bone is constantly being remodelled through the removal of old bone by resorptive cells called *osteoclasts* and deposition of new osteoid by osteoblasts. Thus, the bulk and architectural arrangement of bone can be modified in response to changing functional demands and stresses. As well as its structural role, the calcified bone also provides a large calcium pool from which calcium can be withdrawn (by resorptive activity of osteoclasts) to maintain serum calcium homeostasis.

Bone fracture

Bone fracture is a common and important result of trauma. Where there is an underlying bone abnormality, for example osteoporosis, osteomalacia, Paget's disease or metastatic tumour, the trauma or extra stress required to produce bone fracture may be minimal. This is called *pathological fracture*. The healing of a bone fracture is briefly outlined in Figure 2.12 as an example of a specialised form of tissue repair.

Bone infection

Infections of the bone are now comparatively uncommon, although bacterial osteomyelitis, both pyogenic and tuberculous, were formerly important crippling diseases. Acute osteomyelitis is caused by pyogenic bacteria such as *Staphylococcus aureus* (Fig. 22.1). This usually occurs in infants and young children, the bacteria gaining access to the marrow cavity via the bloodstream. It may also follow penetrating trauma in people of any age, for example after compound (open) fracture. Pathologically, acute osteomyelitis represents abscess formation in the medullary space of the bone, but the course of the disease in bone is complicated by two factors. Firstly, increased pressure in the confined space causes infarction of further large areas of bone. Secondly, masses of dead bone (*sequestra*) behave as foreign bodies, inhibiting normal repair processes and providing a haven for bacteria which is inaccessible to body defence mechanisms. Chronic osteomyelitis may follow if treatment is delayed or inadequate. Tuberculous osteomyelitis is illustrated in Figure 4.7.

Metabolic bone disease

Osteoporosis (osteopenia) is a condition in which total bone mass is decreased due to reduction in the number or size of bone trabeculae (usually both) and thinning of cortical bone. Despite this, the bone otherwise appears structurally normal. In contrast, *osteomalacia* is a disease in which osteoid fails to undergo normal mineralisation, usually because of deficiency of vitamin D, although other causes of total body calcium depletion may also be responsible. *Rickets* is the childhood equivalent of osteomalacia. The appearances of normal bone, osteoporosis and osteomalacia are compared in Figure 22.2.

   Paget's disease of bone (Fig. 22.3) is a condition of unknown aetiology which occurs in the elderly. It is characterised by haphazard and inappropriate osteoclastic erosion of formed bone and concurrent, haphazard osteoblastic deposition of new bone. *Hyperparathyroidism*, due to excessive secretion of parathyroid hormone by a parathyroid adenoma or parathyroid hyperplasia, may cause rather similar haphazard osteoclastic erosion of bone.

Fig. 22.1 | Osteomyelitis
(a) (HP) **(b)** Necrotic bone (HP)

Micrograph (a) shows a high-power view of acute purulent osteomyelitis in the amputated toe of a diabetic patient. There is an acute inflammatory reaction in the marrow space **M** at the lower left of the field which is infiltrated by plentiful neutrophils within a fibrin meshwork. The bony trabecula is necrotic, with no viable osteocytes in the lacunae **L**. In the upper right, the marrow is fibrotic, indicating ongoing repair.

In micrograph (b), the process has progressed to a chronic phase with necrotic bone undergoing *remodelling*. The trabecula of necrotic bone **N** in the centre is surrounded by active osteoblasts **Ob** which are laying down new matrix or osteoid **Ost** on the outer surface of the dead bone. This newly formed, immature bone is termed *woven bone*, because of the haphazard arrangement of its collagen fibres. This is in contrast to the highly ordered arrangement of collagen in mature, lamellar bone. This difference can be demonstrated by viewing the specimen using polarised light.

Fig. 22.2 **Osteoporosis and osteomalacia (undecalcified resin sections, Goldner's trichrome)** (MP) **(a)** Normal bone **(b)** Osteoporosis **(c)** Osteomalacia

In the normal trabecular bone, shown in micrograph (a), the entire trabecula is fully calcified (stained green by the Goldner trichrome method).

Micrograph (b) illustrates osteoporosis, in which the bone appears qualitatively normal but its mass is diminished, with the trabeculae being reduced in both number and size. Osteoporosis is extremely common in the elderly, especially in post-menopausal women, and is exacerbated by immobility. It may also occur in an isolated limb if it is immobilised for any reason. This is a form of *disuse atrophy*. Osteoporosis is also caused by some endocrine disorders and is particularly common with corticosteroid excess (see text box).

Image (c) shows osteomalacia. Here, the trabeculae are of normal or increased thickness, but there is deficient mineralisation so that each trabecula has a central core of calcified bone (stained green) coated by an outer shell of unmineralised osteoid (stained orange-red). Osteomalacia is usually the result of vitamin D deficiency. Vitamin D deficiency in the growing child (rickets) is identical to osteomalacia pathologically. It results in gross skeletal deformity by disruption of bone mineralisation at growth plates.

KEY TO FIGURES
L lacunae **M** marrow space **N** necrotic bone **Ob** osteoblasts **Ost** osteoid

OSTEOPOROSIS IN CLINICAL PRACTICE

Loss of bone mineral density is a common clinical problem which gives rise to considerable morbidity and mortality owing to the occurrence of *pathological fractures* through the weakened bones. Such fractures occur most often in post-menopausal women and typical sites of fracture include vertebrae, femoral neck and distal radius (the so-called *Colles' type fracture*). Such injuries can result in prolonged periods of reduced mobility, exacerbating the underlying problem of reduced bone mass.

Interventions focus on trying to reduce the risk of such fractures, as well as aiming to avoid subsequent immobility if fractures do occur. Prevention of osteoporosis requires a range of interventions, aimed at maximising bone mass by promoting weight-bearing exercise and good nutrition. In higher-risk patient groups, supplementation with calcium and vitamin D may be encouraged. Drugs such as *bisphosphonates* act by preventing bone resorption by osteoclasts, and are widely used in clinical management of osteoporosis and other metabolic bone disorders.

Fig. 22.3 **Paget's disease of bone** (MP) **(a)** Active osteolytic lesion (undecalcified resin section, Goldner's trichrome) **(b)** Inactive sclerotic lesion (decalcified paraffin section, H&E)

In Paget's disease of bone, there is indiscriminate and uncontrolled osteoclastic erosion of bone followed by excessive osteoblastic activity, producing excess osteoid which subsequently becomes mineralised, leading to irregular trabecular thickening. Micrograph (a) shows abnormally large multinucleate osteoclasts **Oc** actively eroding a bone surface. Another trabecular surface shows a layer of newly deposited red-staining osteoid **Ost**, underlying rows of large active cuboidal osteoblasts **Ob**. This progressive, haphazard remodelling results in gross distortion of bone, often with marked thickening. The condition tends to be confined to a relatively small number of long bones, vertebrae or cranial bones, which may become inadequate to withstand functional stresses, leading to severe skeletal deformity (e.g. bowing of long bones) or pathological fracture.

With time, disease activity slowly diminishes. The initially highly cellular bone becomes progressively sclerotic. Usually, the bone is left thicker than before, but paradoxically weaker because much of the former strong lamellar bone is replaced by weaker woven bone. The disruption of the optimum lamellar pattern can be readily viewed by polarising microscopy, and, in old lesions as in micrograph (b), the limits of separate episodes of previous bone destruction and irregular new bone formation are marked by thin, dark mosaic lines **M.**

Bone tumours

Bone is a frequent and important site of *haematogenous metastatic spread* of malignant epithelial tumours, particularly carcinomas of bronchus, breast, kidney, thyroid and prostate (see Fig. 16.15). Metastatic tumour deposits usually destroy bone trabeculae, although carcinoma of the prostate (see Fig. 19.11) sometimes stimulates excessive new bone formation, resulting in *osteosclerotic* rather than the more usual *osteolytic* deposits.

Primary tumours of bone are much less common. These may arise from any of the cell types found in bone. The essential features of the more important of these tumours are tabulated in Figure 22.4.

■ **Osteoid osteoma** is a benign but painful tumour of bone, which is illustrated in Figure 22.5.

■ **Osteogenic sarcoma** or **osteosarcoma** is the most common malignant primary tumour of bone (Fig. 22.6). This occurs mainly in children and adolescents.

■ **Chondromas** (Fig. 22.7) are benign tumours of hyaline cartilage which may arise either on the surface of bone or within the medullary cavity where they are known as *enchondromas*. These may rarely undergo malignant transformation.

■ **Chondrosarcomas** (Fig. 22.8) are malignant cartilage tumours which mainly arise in middle-aged and elderly individuals.

As discussed in Chapter 16, malignant tumours may also arise from the haematolymphoid cells of the bone marrow, for example myeloma, lymphoma, leukaemia, etc.

In addition to true bony neoplasms, there is a miscellaneous group of tumour-like lesions which are also found in bone. The main features of these lesions are presented in Figure 22.9. The cartilage-capped *exostosis* or *osteochondroma* is the most common of these and is illustrated in Figure 22.10.

Fig. 22.4 Important primary tumours of bone				
Name of tumour	**Main pattern of cellular differentiation**	**Age and sex incidence**	**Common sites**	**Behaviour**
Osteoid osteoma (Fig. 22.5)	Osteoblast	Adolescents, M > F	Long bones, lower limb	Benign, painful, osteosclerotic
Osteosarcoma (Osteogenic sarcoma) (Fig. 22.6)	Primitive osteoblast	(i) Mainly adolescent (ii) Elderly, M > F	(i) Around knee (ii) Sites of Paget's	Highly malignant, metastasis to lungs
Chondroma (Enchondroma) (Fig. 22.7)	Chondrocyte	Common, any age	Hands and feet, long bones	Benign, very rare malignant change
Chondrosarcoma (Fig. 22.8)	Chondrocyte	Middle aged/elderly, M > F	Pelvis, ribs, vertebrae	Malignant, local spread and metastasis
Non-ossifying fibroma	Fibroblast	Mainly children and young adults	Long bones of lower limbs	Benign, osteolytic, may be multiple
Chondromyxoid fibroma	Uncertain	Young adults	Long bones, mainly tibia	Benign, osteolytic, may be painful
Giant cell tumour	Osteoclast	20–40 years, M > F	Long bones, mainly around knee	Benign, may recur locally
Chordoma	Notochord tissue	Middle aged/elderly, M > F	Sacrum, skull base	Locally aggressive bone destruction
Ewing's tumour (Fig. 7.9)	Uncertain	Children/adolescents, M > F	Shaft of long bones	Highly malignant, early metastases

KEY TO FIGURES
M mosaic lines   **Ob** osteoblast   **Oc** osteoclast   **Ost** osteoid

Fig. 22.5 **Osteoid osteoma** **(a)** Osteoid osteoma in medullary cavity (LP) **(b)** Histology of edge of lesion (MP)

Osteoid osteoma is a benign tumour of osteoblasts which usually arises in the medullary cavity of the shaft of long bones, commonly the tibia or femur. Micrograph (a) shows the typical low-power appearance of this benign tumour. Micrograph (b) shows the edge of the lesion. There is a central '*nidus*' composed of partially mineralised osteoid **Ost** in irregular masses, surrounded by a rim of actively proliferating osteoblasts **Ob**.

Fig. 22.6 **Osteogenic sarcoma (osteosarcoma)** (HP)

This relatively uncommon tumour is, nevertheless, the most frequently occurring primary malignant tumour of bone. Most cases occur in children and adolescents (usually around the knee), but it may occasionally occur in elderly patients with long-standing Paget's disease.

Histologically, there are highly pleomorphic tumour cells **T** and, towards the right of the image, these cells are producing irregular seams of delicate, pink-stained osteoid **Ost**. This osteoid is partly mineralised **MO**, producing a granular, purple appearance. There are several atypical mitotic figures **A** within this field.

These tumours are generally highly vascular and early bloodstream metastasis to the lungs is common.

SOME CLINICAL ASPECTS OF BONE TUMOURS

Primary malignant bone tumours occur mainly in children and adolescents and, traditionally, the prognosis has been extremely poor. In the past, surgical excision of the primary tumour mass was the mainstay of treatment and this normally required amputation of the affected part. With the development of newer chemotherapeutic agents, treatment and outcome in these cases has altered considerably.

Following initial biopsy for diagnosis and classification of the tumour, most patients are now treated with chemotherapy in the first instance and the tumour response is monitored closely by regular radiological imaging. After this, complete surgical excision of the residual tumour is undertaken. Amputation of limbs is avoided whenever possible by the use of new bone and/or joint prostheses which can be surgically inserted to replace the affected parts of the skeleton, leaving surrounding tissues intact. This strategy of initial treatment with systemic chemotherapy has dramatically improved the outlook for children with malignant bone tumours.

KEY TO FIGURES

A atypical mitosis **B** binucleate tumour cells **C** chondrocytes **H** hyaline matrix **MO** mineralised osteoid
Ob osteoblast **Ost** osteoid **T** tumour

Fig. 22.7 Chondroma (LP)

Chondromas are composed of well-circumscribed nodules of benign hyaline cartilage. The gross appearance is characteristic, with a semi-translucent, grey-blue appearance which is due to the hyaline matrix **H**. The neoplastic chondrocytes **C** seen within the lacunae are benign, with no dysplastic features, and are embedded in a well-formed cartilage matrix. *Enchondromas* appear identical histologically, but occur within the medullary cavity of the bone. Multiple benign cartilaginous tumours occur in rare syndromes such as *multiple enchondromatosis* or *Ollier's disease*.

Fig. 22.0 Chondrosarcoma (HP)

This malignant cartilaginous tumour usually arises in the axial skeleton at middle age and later. The tumours vary in their behaviour from indolent low-grade malignancy to very poorly differentiated and aggressive neoplasms with little obvious cartilage formation.

The tumour shown here consists of nodules of pale hyaline matrix **H**. Malignant chondrocytes **C** lie embedded within lacunae in the matrix. These cells differ from normal chondrocytes in that they are enlarged, atypical cells which may be binucleate **B** or may show crowding of two or more cells in a single lacuna. Mitotic figures may be seen in higher-grade tumours. Well-differentiated chondrosarcoma may be difficult to differentiate from benign chondroma. Careful correlation with clinical and radiological findings is essential for diagnosis.

Fig. 22.9 Tumour-like lesions of bone

Name of lesion	Age and sex	Common sites	Behaviour
Osteochondroma (exostosis)	Children/adolescents, M > F	Upper tibia, lower fibula	Non-neoplastic outgrowth of bone and cartilage, possibly derived from growth plate
Aneurysmal bone cyst	Children/adolescents, M > F	Long bones, spine	Reactive, cause unknown. Osteolytic, risk of fracture at site
Fibrous dysplasia	Children/adolescents, M > F	Long bones, facial bones	Developmental abnormality, 20% involve multiple bones. Osteolytic, risk of fracture
'Brown tumour' of hyperparathyroidism	Adults, M > F	Anywhere	Osteolytic, often multiple. Resemble giant cell tumour. Treat hyperparathyroidism

Fig. 22.10 **Osteochondroma** (LP)

Osteochondromas or *exostoses* are mushroom-shaped bony protuberances, with a cartilage cap **CC**, arising in the region of the epiphysis. It is thought that these may be derived from displacement of part of the growth plate. Endochondral ossification takes place at the deep surface of the cartilage to form cortical bone **B**. The stalk of medullary bone is continuous with the medulla of the underlying bone, without intervening cortex.

Rarely, chondrosarcoma may arise in an osteochondroma. This is much more common in individuals with the syndrome *multiple hereditary exostoses*.

In this photomicrograph, there has been artefactual separation of the perichondrium.

Diseases of the joints

The three most important disorders of joints are *osteoarthritis*, *gout* and *rheumatoid arthritis*. Osteoarthritis (Fig. 22.11) is the name given to the wear-and-tear degenerative changes that occur in some joints with increasing age. Gout is an inflammatory arthropathy caused by the deposition of urate crystals within the joints and soft tissues (illustrated in Fig. 22.12). Rheumatoid arthritis is a systemic chronic inflammatory disorder of autoimmune origin which is characterised by synovitis and arthritis (Fig. 22.13).

Fig. 22.11 **Osteoarthritis** **(a)** Early changes (MP) **(b)** Established lesion (LP)

Osteoarthritis is a degenerative disorder of articular cartilage as a result of excessive wear and tear. Secondary inflammatory changes occur in the soft tissue components of the joint.

In the earliest stages, the articular cartilage **A** loses its smooth appearance and develops surface fibrillations and flaking as shown in micrograph (a). The damaged cartilage is progressively eroded until the underlying cortical bone **B** is exposed. After prolonged articulation of naked bone with the opposing surface, the bone becomes slightly thickened, hard, dense and highly polished, a process

known as *eburnation*. At the same time, there is irregular outgrowth of new bone (*osteophytes*) at the articular margins.

In the established case shown in micrograph (b), only a small amount of articular cartilage **A** remains and the exposed bone **B** has undergone eburnation. The bone underlying the traumatised eburnated surface may undergo cystic degeneration **D**.

All of these changes lead to joint pain and progressive limitation of movement at the joint. The hips, knees and finger joints are most commonly and severely affected.

**Fig. 22.12 Gout (a) H&E
(MP) (b)** As above, viewed using
plane polarised light

Gout is an acute relapsing form of arthritis seen in individuals with **hyperuricaemia**. Gout is most often primary, i.e. of unknown cause; however, a small proportion of cases arise due to increased nucleic acid turnover, as in leukaemia or in patients with chronic renal disease who cannot excrete urate effectively.

Acute attacks of gout are precipitated by crystallisation of urate within joints, causing an acute inflammatory reaction. Over time, chronic arthritis may develop. The synovium becomes inflamed and fibrotic and this inflammatory mass or pannus may erode the underlying cartilage. *Gouty tophi* are deposits of crystalline material within the soft tissues. These have a similar histological appearance.

Micrograph (a) shows a chronic granulomatous reaction to urate crystals. The needle-shaped crystals **U** occupy the upper part of the image and there is a surrounding band of reactive histiocytes, giant cells **GC** and organising granulation tissue with numerous small vessels **V**.

The optical properties of the crystals are useful in allowing easy microscopic identification. Urate crystals exhibit strong *negative birefringence* when viewed using plane polarised light, as illustrated in micrograph (b). This concept is considered further below.

EXAMINATION OF SYNOVIAL FLUID

Joint pain is a fairly common symptom, but one which requires careful assessment. In particular, the rapid onset of severe pain in a single joint should be investigated immediately.

Gout can present in this way, as can another crystal arthritis called *pseudogout*, but acute pyogenic joint infection (*septic arthritis*) is a very important differential diagnosis since this requires urgent antibiotic treatment to prevent destruction of the joint. Other forms of arthritis, such as rheumatoid disease, tend to affect multiple joints (*polyarthropathy*), but the initial presentation is sometimes with involvement of a single joint.

Clinical examination and initial investigations such as a full blood count should be followed by aspiration of synovial fluid from the joint. Immediate examination of this specimen can be helpful in guiding treatment. Fluid can also be submitted for microbiological culture in cases of suspected joint sepsis.

Normal synovial fluid is virtually acellular but, in acute pyogenic infection, it may be transformed into pus, consisting of numerous neutrophil polymorphs. Some neutrophils are also seen in cases of acute crystal arthropathy but here, polarisation reveals the presence of crystals. As illustrated above, uric acid forms fine, needle-shaped crystals which show strong *negative birefringence*. This term refers to the physical property of rotating polarised light in a particular direction as it passes through the specimen.

In contrast, *pseudogout* is caused by precipitation of calcium pyrophosphate crystals which are rhomboid in shape and show positive birefringence. This disorder tends to affect large joints such as the knees, often in elderly patients who are being treated with diuretic drugs.

KEY TO FIGURES
A articular surface   **B** bone   **CC** cartilage cap   **D** cystic degeneration   **GC** giant cell   **U** urate crystals
V vessels

Fig. 22.13 **Rheumatoid arthritis** **(a)** Synovium (MP) **(b)** Articular cartilage (MP) **(c)** Rheumatoid skin nodule (LP) **(d)** Rheumatoid skin nodule (HP)

Rheumatoid arthritis is a systemic disorder, the predominant feature of which is chronic relapsing inflammation of articular joints, particularly the small joints of the hands. The disease affects both the synovium lining the joint capsule and the cartilage on the articular surfaces.

The earliest changes occur in the synovium which becomes thickened, excessively vascular and thrown up into papillary folds as a result of oedema and infiltration by numerous lymphocytes and plasma cells. This is illustrated in micrograph (a). This is accompanied by exudation of excess fluid into the joint space with precipitation of fibrin on the synovial surface.

The articular cartilage changes shown in micrograph (b) follow later and involve localised destruction of cartilage **C** and its replacement by fibrovascular granulation tissue known as *pannus* **P**.

Initially, joint mobility is limited by pain and swelling, then later by gross cartilage and bone destruction and fibrous ankylosis across the joint space owing to fusion of transjacent granulation tissue pannus.

Rheumatoid nodules are found in the subcutaneous tissues, most commonly in individuals with seropositive rheumatoid arthritis, i.e. those who have *rheumatoid factor* in their serum. The nodules are usually found on the extensor surfaces of the limbs and, clinically, these are firm, non-tender and mobile. Rheumatoid nodules may also occur in almost any other tissue, for example lung and spleen.

The rheumatoid nodule shown at low power in micrograph (c) consists of a central core of necrosis **N**, rimmed by a palisade of histiocytes and fibroblasts **PH**, which is in turn surrounded by fibrous tissue **F** containing lymphocytes and plasma cells.

This *palisading* or lining up of histiocytes and fibroblasts is better appreciated at high magnification in micrograph (d). An occasional giant cell **GC** can be identified. The rheumatoid nodule in fact represents a large granuloma with central necrosis.

KEY TO FIGURES
C cartilage **F** fibrous tissue **GC** giant cell **N** necrosis **NB** nerve branches **P** pannus **PH** palisading histiocytes

Soft tissue lesions

Many benign tumours and reactive tumour-like lesions commonly occur in soft tissue. Malignant soft tissue tumours (*sarcomas*) are rare and their diagnosis and classification form a highly specialist area of pathology. Here, we will illustrate some of the reactive lesions and benign tumours which are frequently encountered in clinical practice and also review the broad concepts of sarcoma pathology by consideration of a few specific tumour types.

Reactive processes and tumour-like lesions

Some soft tissue masses do not satisfy the usual criteria to be classified as true benign neoplasms and are considered to be *reactive* rather than *neoplastic*. These lesions may arise following a minor injury or in areas exposed to repetitive trauma, but such a history is not always obtained. The line between benign soft tissue tumours and reactive tumour-like lesions is not always clear and, in recent times, molecular evidence of clonality has begun to emerge for some of the entities conventionally considered to be reactive.

It is of great importance to note that some reactive soft tissue lesions may be very rapidly growing, causing clinical suspicion of malignancy. Such lesions may also appear alarming histologically, showing active proliferation with numerous mitotic figures. This possibility must always be considered before suggesting a diagnosis of soft tissue sarcoma.

A large number of soft tissue masses fall into this broad group but the majority are encountered only rarely in clinical practice. A few of the more common lesions are considered here. The *traumatic* or *amputation neuroma* is a reactive mass which may form following damage to a peripheral nerve (Fig. 22.14). A *ganglion* is a fairly common lesion which is probably related to repeated minor damage around sites of excessive tendon and joint use, e.g. around the wrists and hands of pianists and typists (Fig. 22.15). *Giant cell tumour of tendon sheath* (also known as *nodular tenosynovitis*) also tends to occur around the hands and wrists (Fig. 22.16). As the name suggests, the nature of this lesion has been the subject of considerable debate and there is increasing evidence that it may be a true benign neoplasm.

Fig. 22.14 Traumatic neuroma (MP)

This lesion typically arises following transection of a peripheral nerve, often at the time of amputation of a limb or digit. Histologically, there is a proliferation of tiny nerve branches **NB** within the fibrous connective tissue **F** of the scar.

The eponymously named *Morton's neuroma* is a similar lesion which arises on the foot from the plantar digital nerve, usually between the third and fourth toes. It is thought to be due to chronic, pressure-related nerve injury and may be exquisitely painful.

PSEUDOSARCOMA

Some reactive processes in soft tissue appear extremely alarming, both clinically and histologically, and may be described as *pseudosarcomas*. One example is *nodular fasciitis*. This typically presents as a very rapidly growing soft tissue swelling, appearing over the course of a few weeks. On close questioning, there may be a history of preceding trauma. The mass tends to be situated in the superficial fascia and usually has ill-defined margins (unlike most benign tumours which tend to be encapsulated). Histologically, this is a proliferation of spindle cells, often with very numerous mitotic figures. There is a high risk of over-diagnosing malignancy in this setting and great care is required to recognise that this is a reactive process, rather than a sarcoma.

Fig. 22.15 Ganglion (LP)

Ganglia most commonly affect the hands and wrists, presenting as a firm and mobile mass in the vicinity of tendons and synovial joints. The size of these lesions may fluctuate and, historically, treatment involved striking the affected part with a heavy book! This simple intervention often causes the lump to disappear by dispersing fluid contents, but most lesions recur over time and surgical excision provides a more definitive solution.

Histologically, there is usually a cystic space **C** with a fibrous wall **W** and no discernable lining. Foci of myxoid change **M** are present in the surrounding connective tissue. Sometimes, the cystic spaces may be lined by histiocytic cells resembling synovial lining cells.

Most lesions appear to arise from the sheath of synovium which invests the tendons, although some can be shown to connect with an adjacent synovial joint.

Fig. 22.16 Giant cell tumour of tendon sheath (nodular tenosynovitis) (a) LP **(b)** HP

This is a common lesion which typically occurs around the fingers. It is usually a firm nodule with a lobulated surface.

Histologically, there is a proliferation of bland polygonal cells with eosinophilic cytoplasm, as well as a scattering of multinucleate, osteoclast-like giant cells **GC**. Some lesions show areas of haemosiderin **H** deposition within macrophages, and collections of foamy macrophages **FM** containing lipid may also be prominent.

It is closely related to another soft tissue lesion with the highly descriptive name *pigmented villonodular synovitis*. This disorder usually affects the synovium of the knee joint and typically presents with swelling, joint pain and reduced joint mobility. Although the histological features are extremely similar, this process diffusely affects the joint and frequently recurs following treatment.

KEY TO FIGURES

C cystic space   **FM** foamy macrophages   **GC** giant cells   **H** haemosiderin   **M** myxoid change   **T** fibrin thrombus   **W** fibrous wall

Benign tumours

One of the commonest of all soft tissue lesions is the *lipoma*, a benign tumour which resembles normal adipose tissue (Fig. 22.17). Other benign soft tissue tumours may show patterns of differentiation resembling smooth muscle (*leiomyoma*, see Figs 17.13 and 7.15), blood vessels (*haemangioma*, see Fig. 11.9), peripheral nerves (*Schwannoma*, see Fig. 23.15 and *neurofibroma*, see Fig. 23.16), striated muscle (*rhabdomyoma*) or fibrous tissue (*fibroma*).

Fig. 22.17 Lipoma (a) Lipoma (LP) **(b)** Lipoma (HP) **(c)** Angiolipoma (HP)

The lipoma is a very common tumour which usually occurs within the subcutaneous fatty tissue of the trunk or limbs. They are soft, fairly well-defined lesions which are usually painless. Micrograph (a) shows a low power view of a benign lipoma with a well-defined edge. The lesion is composed of sheets of uniform adipocytes. These cells have a very small nucleus which is displaced to the periphery of the cell by a large globule of lipid, illustrated at higher magnification in image (b). In some patients, multiple tender lesions occur and, histologically, these differ from usual lipomas in that they contain multiple small blood vessels, some of which contain fibrin thrombi **T**. These lesions are called *angiolipomas* and an example is shown in image (c).

Malignant tumours

Primary malignant tumours of soft tissue or *sarcomas* are rare and form a highly specialist area of practice. The approach to diagnosis is rather similar to that used in haematolymphoid pathology and typically requires careful correlation of the clinical and radiological findings with the histological appearance and pattern of immunohistochemical staining. Molecular studies may also be of value because many soft tissue tumours have characteristic non-random chromosomal rearrangements.

Classification of soft tissue tumours is complex and is currently based upon the *World Health Organization (WHO)* system. This uses a combination of clinical, histological, immunohistochemical and molecular features. In the past, sarcomas were often considered to arise from the tissue type which they resembled, e.g. *liposarcomas* were thought to develop due to malignant transformation of normal or benign adipose tissue. It is now accepted that most sarcomas do not arise from benign precursor lesions. Classification is therefore based upon the concept that tumour cells may *differentiate* so that they resemble normal tissues to a lesser or greater degree. This allows the description of groups of tumours which resemble tissues such as fat (*liposarcoma*, see Fig. 22.18), smooth muscle (*leiomyosarcoma*, illustrated in Fig. 7.9), striated muscle (*rhabdomyosarcoma*), blood vessels (*angiosarcoma*, illustrated in Fig. 11.13), nerves (*malignant peripheral nerve sheath tumour*), fibrous tissue (*fibrosarcoma*), etc.

Some sarcomas lack any resemblance to normal tissues or structures but have sufficiently distinctive clinical, histological, immunohistochemical and molecular features to allow reliable identification. These are described within the WHO classification as *tumours of uncertain histogenesis*. The entity *synovial sarcoma*, despite its rather misleading name, is included within this group.

The term *pleomorphic sarcoma* is used for very aggressive and highly malignant tumours which do not resemble any normal tissues. By definition, these sarcomas show no immunohistochemical evidence of a particular pattern of differentiation and, as the name suggests, they are composed of highly pleomorphic malignant cells. An older term for these tumours which is still seen in some textbooks is *malignant fibrous histiocytoma*, based upon the supposed resemblance of the large and often multinucleate tumour cells to histiocytes. Pleomorphic sarcoma is one of the more common forms of soft tissue sarcoma in adults. An example is shown in Figure 22.19.

SOME FEATURES OF SOFT TISSUE SARCOMAS

Soft tissue sarcomas occur over a wide age range and are one of the most common forms of malignancy in childhood. Benign soft tissue tumours usually occur in superficial sites whereas sarcomas are more likely to form deep-seated masses. Sarcomas are typically larger than benign tumours and, unlike carcinomas (which tend to spread through lymphatic channels to regional lymph nodes in the first instance), sarcomas typically metastasise via the bloodstream, giving rise to lung and bony metastases.

Fig. 22.18 **Liposarcoma** (HP)

Liposarcomas tend to occur in older adults and usually arise at deep soft tissue sites in the extremities or retroperitoneum. Most are characterised by the presence of *lipoblasts*, tumour cells with multiple cytoplasmic vacuoles which typically indent the nucleus of the cell **L**. In contrast, normal adipocytes have a single, large vacuole in the cytoplasm which displaces the nucleus to the periphery of the cell. This example is a pleomorphic tumour which includes many lipoblasts. There is evidence of mitotic activity **M**. There are several different morphological subtypes of liposarcoma, including myxoid, round cell, well-differentiated and de-differentiated variants. In common with many other sarcomas, molecular methods are useful in diagnosis (see below).

MOLECULAR METHODS IN SARCOMA PATHOLOGY

Most malignant tumours, such as the common carcinomas, exhibit a wide range of genetic abnormalities, but these are rarely helpful in clinical diagnosis. In contrast, many soft tissue tumours exhibit highly characteristic non-random chromosomal rearrangements.

These are diagnostically useful in many cases and their recognition has also brought about advances in the understanding of tumour classification and in the development of some targeted drug therapies for the management of malignant disease (e.g. use of imatinib in treatment of gastrointestinal stromal tumours as discussed in Ch. 13).

Liposarcomas are interesting because molecular biology has contributed to the understanding of tumour classification. Myxoid liposarcomas and round cell liposarcomas typically exhibit a t(12;16) translocation, whilst well-differentiated and de-differentiated variants usually show evidence of a supernumerary giant 'ring' or 'marker' chromosome (formed of amplified genetic material from chromosome 12). If fresh tumour tissue is available, classical cytogenetic techniques can be used to demonstrate these abnormalities, helping to confirm the diagnosis.

Fig. 22.19 **Pleomorphic sarcoma (malignant fibrous histiocytoma)** **(a)** MP **(b)** HP

Micrograph (a) shows a highly pleomorphic tumour composed of plump, spindle-shaped cells and very large, histiocyte-like cells. There is no resemblance to any normal tissue.

At high magnification in image (b), the nuclei are large, irregular and have prominent nucleoli. Some giant cell forms are present **GC** and there are several mitotic figures **M**, including an atypical form **AM**.

In the past, the term 'malignant fibrous histiocytoma' was used to describe a large number of sarcomas with pleomorphic morphology and with no clear evidence of any specific pattern of differentiation. With increasing application of immunohistochemical and molecular techniques, many of these tumours can now be assigned to more specific diagnostic categories.

KEY TO FIGURES
AM atypical mitosis   **GC** tumour giant cells   **L** lipoblast   **M** mitotic figure

Fig. 22.20 **Chapter review**

Disorder	Main features	Figure
Non-neoplastic bone disorders		
Fracture	Common following trauma. Specialised form of repair with callus. Pathological fracture occurs through bone weakened by disease	2.12
Osteomyelitis	Pyogenic organisms such as *Staphylococcus aureus*, TB now rare. Haematogenous spread or after penetrating injury, e.g. open fracture. Sequestrum of dead bone inhibits resolution	22.1
Osteoporosis	Reduction in bone mass. Qualitatively normal bone mineralisation. Common cause of pathological fracture in postmenopausal women	22.2(b)
Osteomalacia/rickets	Incomplete mineralisation of normal sized trabeculae. Due to vitamin D deficiency. Called rickets in children and associated with deformity	22.2(c)
Paget's disease of bone	Uncontrolled osteoblastic and osteoclastic activity. Thickened but weakened bone. Mosaic cement lines. Risk secondary osteosarcoma	22.3
Benign and tumour-like lesions of bone		
Osteochondroma (exostosis)	Non-neoplastic outgrowth of bone with cartilage cap at epiphysis. Hereditary form with multiple lesions. Small risk of chondrosarcoma	22.10
Osteoid osteoma	Benign bone-forming tumour in medullary cavity of long bones. Central nidus. Typically painful and relieved by aspirin	22.5
Chondroma (enchondroma)	Benign cartilage-forming tumour. Enchondroma in medullary cavity. Rare syndromes with multiple lesions, e.g. Ollier's disease	22.7
Malignant bone tumours		
Metastatic carcinoma	Commonest form of malignant tumour in bone. Typically from lung, breast, prostatic, renal and thyroid carcinomas. Usually lytic on X-ray	16.15
Osteosarcoma	Malignant bone-forming tumour. Children/adolescents or secondary to Paget's in elderly. Long bones, early haematogenous spread	22.6
Chondrosarcoma	Malignant cartilage-forming tumour. Axial skeleton, usually older adults	22.8
Ewing's sarcoma	Small round blue cell tumour. Usually children, typically shaft of long bones. Highly aggressive behaviour	7.9(b)
Joint disease		
Osteoarthritis	Common degenerative disease. Fibrillation of hyaline cartilage, eburnation, subchondral cysts and osteophyte formation	22.11
Gout	Crystal arthropathy. Deposition of uric acid crystals in synovial fluid and/or forming tophi. Needle-shaped, strong negative birefringence	22.12
Pseudogout	Crystal arthropathy. Deposition of calcium pyrophosphate crystals in large joints. Rhomboid crystals, weak positive birefringence	
Septic arthritis	Pyogenic and tuberculous types. Usually single acutely painful joint. Needs urgent antibiotic treatment to limit joint damage	
Rheumatoid arthritis	Systemic inflammatory disease with symmetrical small joint polyarthropathy. Inflamed synovium, sometimes rheumatoid nodules	22.13
Benign and reactive soft tissue lesions		
Traumatic neuroma (amputation neuroma)	Reactive proliferation of small nerve branches in scar following transaction of peripheral nerve. Morton's neuroma on foot similar	22.14
Ganglion	Reactive cystic lesion, usually hands or wrists. Myxoid degeneration and cysts associated with tendon sheath or near joint	22.15
Giant cell tumour of tendon sheath (nodular tenosynovitis)	Common, typically fingers. Localised firm nodule. Mixture of giant cells and mononuclear cells with haemosiderin and foamy histiocytes	22.16
Pigmented villonodular synovitis	Similar to giant cell tumour but diffusely affects single joint. Commonly knee, often locally recurrent after treatment	Like 22.16
Lipoma	Common benign tumour of fat. Soft swelling, usually in subcutaneous tissues. Mature adipose tissue	22.17(a)
Angiolipoma	Similar to lipoma but often painful due to small, capillary vessels with fibrin thrombi. Often multiple	22.17(b)
Leiomyoma	Benign smooth muscle tumour. In skin, well-defined and derived from vessels (angioleiomyoma) or with irregular edge (from pilar muscle)	7.15(a) 17.13
Haemangioma	Benign proliferation of blood vessels. Common in skin. In liver, association with contraceptives. Capillary or cavernous sized channels	11.9

Fig. 22.20 Chapter review—cont'd

Disorder	Main features	Figure
Benign and reactive soft tissue lesions (continued)		
Schwannoma	Benign tumour of Schwann cells. Encapsulated. Spindle-shaped cells with cellular Antoni A (nuclear palisading) and myxoid Antoni B areas	23.15
Neurofibroma	Benign tumour of peripheral nerves. Ill-defined edges. Spindle cells. Multiple in von Recklinghausen's disease (neurofibromatosis)	23.16
Rhabdomyoma	Rare benign tumour of striated muscle. Cardiac rhabdomyomas typically occur in young children	
Malignant soft tissue tumours		
Liposarcoma	Malignant fatty tumour. Adults, deep soft tissue sites. Lipoblasts typical. Various types, cytogenetics helpful	22.18
Leiomyosarcoma	Malignant tumour of smooth muscle. Pleomorphic spindle-shaped cells with eosinophilic cytoplasm	7.9(a)
Angiosarcoma	Malignant tumour forming vessels. Aggressive behaviour. May complicate chronic lymphoedema or follow irradiation	11.13
Malignant peripheral nerve sheath tumour	Malignant tumour derived from peripheral nerves. Association with neurofibromatosis	
Fibrosarcoma	Malignant proliferation of fibroblasts. Typically, fascicles of spindle cells with 'herringbone' architecture	
Synovial sarcoma	Sarcoma of uncertain histogenesis. Typical combination of spindle cells and epithelioid areas (biphasic). Cytogenetics shows t(X;18)	
Pleomorphic sarcoma (malignant fibrous histiocytoma)	Pleomorphic, high grade tumour with no clear evidence of differentiation. Older adults, aggressive behaviour	22.19

23 Nervous system

Introduction

Although, in common with any other organ system, the central nervous system (CNS) is susceptible to infection, trauma and the processes of infarction, inflammation and neoplasia, the anatomy and metabolic requirements of the CNS modify its response to common injurious agents and render it prone to unique pathological processes.

Tissues of the CNS

■ **Neurons** are the functional units of the nervous system. A typical neuron is composed of a cell body (*soma*) rich in rough endoplasmic reticulum (*Nissl substance*), short afferent cell processes (*dendrites*) and a main efferent cell process (the *axon*). Except in development, neurons are not capable of replication and hence, once a neuronal cell body dies, regeneration is not possible. Damage to the axon with preservation of the soma can, however, be repaired by regeneration of the axon.

■ **Specialised support cells (glial cells)** are of four types: astrocytes, oligodendrocytes, microglia and ependymal cells. *Astrocytes*, with their delicate cytoplasmic processes, form a 'fibrillary' supporting framework for neurons and other cells of the CNS, participate in maintenance of the blood–brain barrier and proliferate following damage. *Oligodendrocytes* form myelin sheaths around axons in the CNS. Their counterparts in the peripheral nervous system are the *Schwann cells*. *Microglia* are cells with short processes and are the CNS equivalent of quiescent macrophages. *Ependymal cells* provide a lining to the ventricles and central canal of the spinal cord.

■ **Blood vessels** in the brain have a specialised structure for maintenance of the *blood–brain barrier*. This limits transport and diffusion from the vascular compartment into the CNS. Connective tissues in the CNS are limited to the meninges, choroid plexuses and around blood vessels. The relative paucity of fibroblastic cells means that healing in the CNS is generally not marked by fibrous scarring. In the peripheral nervous system, connective tissue and associated blood vessels are found in association with individual axons (*endoneurium*), bundles of axons (*perineurium*) and peripheral nerves (*epineurium*).

Response of CNS tissues to injury

Neurons have a limited ability to survive significant changes in their metabolic or physical environment and are said to be *selectively vulnerable* compared to the more robust astrocytes or microglial cells. Neurons may undergo reversible cell damage which is recognisable histologically by swelling of the cell body associated with loss of Nissl substance, a process termed *chromatolysis*. This process is particularly seen in the cell body of a neuron after damage to the axonal process. As discussed in Chapter 1, necrosis of brain tissue usually results in liquefaction, leaving a fluid-filled space.

Following injury or necrosis, healing through granulation tissue and fibrous scarring is an uncommon event in the CNS, a result of a relative lack of fibroblasts. Initially, there is an exudative response with activation of local microglia and recruitment of phagocytic monocytes to phagocytose dead tissue. This is followed by proliferation of astrocytes to form an *astrocytic scar*. This process is generally termed *gliosis* and is a common end product of damage to the specialised structures of the CNS. If there is extensive tissue necrosis, for example following infarction, the gliotic response is insufficient to repair the whole defect and a fluid-filled space lined by gliosis (*glia limitans*) remains.

Where healing through granulation tissue and collagenous fibrosis occurs, it is in relation to healing of inflammatory processes such as around a cerebral abscess. It also occurs in disease involving the meninges, such as acute bacterial meningitis and tuberculous meningitis (see Fig. 4.7).

Fig. 23.1 **Neuronal death and astrocytic response** (a) Normal (HP) **(b)** Early hypoxic/ischaemic response (HP) **(c)** Later response (HP)

Neurons are especially vulnerable to hypoxia such as may occur following cardiac or respiratory arrest. At an early stage, dead neurons become shrunken and eosinophilic with pyknosis of the nuclei. This change particularly affects large neurons and is shown in micrograph (b) where recently dead neurons **I** in the thalamus are present. Compare the neurons in this field with the normal neurons **N** in the adjacent image (a) of a normal thalamus. Note that surrounding cells such as oligodendrocytes and astrocytes are unaffected.

Following such damage, dead neurons will be removed by phagocytic cells and there is associated proliferation of astrocytes in the damaged area. This is seen in micrograph (c) which is a similar area of the thalamus to that shown in (a) and (b), but subject to an episode of hypoxia several weeks earlier. No neurons are seen in this field where a large number of pink-stained astrocytes **A** are noted. This process, termed gliosis, is a common end result of damage to the central nervous system.

KEY TO FIGURES
A astrocytes **I** ischaemic neuron **N** normal neuron

Vascular disorders of the CNS

The brain is responsible for approximately 20% of total body oxygen consumption at rest. Under normal circumstances cerebral blood flow is maintained through the process of *cerebral autoregulation* such that delivery of oxygen to the brain is not compromised. Where this process fails, the consequence is the *ischaemic cell process*, with decreasing vulnerability from neurons through glia to microglia and blood vessels. Hence, brief interruptions in blood flow are reflected in *selective neuronal necrosis*, whilst longer interruptions or cessation of flow result in *cerebral infarction* or *stroke*, a term used to describe the sudden onset of a persistent focal neurological deficit such as paralysis, disturbance of speech, coordination or sensation. The majority of strokes arise as a consequence of atheroma, thrombosis or embolism. *Cerebral haemorrhage* is also an important cause of stroke and may arise following reperfusion of a vessel occluded by thrombus or through rupture of small intracerebral vessels.

Cerebral infarction may follow thrombosis of a cerebral artery, often superimposed on atheroma of cerebral vessels. This is commonly seen in the vertebrobasilar territory, resulting in brainstem infarction. Cerebral infarction may also result from occlusion of a vessel by embolus. Such emboli most commonly arise from complicated atheroma of the carotid arteries (usually at the bifurcation), from the left side of the heart (frequently from mural thrombus after myocardial infarction), from atrial thrombosis in atrial fibrillation or from thrombotic vegetations on the aortic or mitral valves. More insidious disease results from progressive arteriosclerosis of small vessels in the brain causing degeneration of white matter with small areas of micro-infarction in the cerebral cortex. This is a common cause of dementia (progressive intellectual deterioration) in the elderly and is termed *multi-infarct dementia*.

Primary intracerebral haemorrhage is most often a complication of hypertension. The muscular walls of small vessels in the brain are replaced by collagenous tissue which leaves the vessels prone to rupture. Typically, hypertension-related intracerebral haemorrhages occur in or around the basal ganglia. Where intracerebral haemorrhage arises elsewhere in the brain (lobar haematomas), other aetiologies should be considered. Accumulation of β-amyloid in the walls of small vessels in the superficial cerebral cortex and adjacent meninges, *cerebral amyloid angiopathy*, represents a further important pathology which may predispose to intracerebral haemorrhage. Less common causes of primary intracerebral haemorrhage include congenital abnormalities of cerebral vessels forming *arteriovenous malformations*, saccular aneurysms, vasculitis and haemorrhage into primary or secondary brain tumours.

Intracranial haemorrhage may also occur from vessels outside the brain. *Subarachnoid haemorrhage* arises as a result of rupture of vessels in the subarachnoid space. The most common reason is rupture of a small aneurysm arising on one of the main cerebral arteries, descriptively termed a *saccular (berry) aneurysm* (see Fig. 11.5). *Subdural haemorrhage* results from bleeding from fragile veins which traverse the subdural space. This most commonly occurs in the elderly as a result of trauma which may be relatively trivial. *Extradural haemorrhage* is a result of bleeding from arterial vessels outside the dura, a common complication of trauma to the head, especially with skull fracture. The middle meningeal vessels are most vulnerable.

Fig. 23.2 **Infarction** (*caption opposite*)

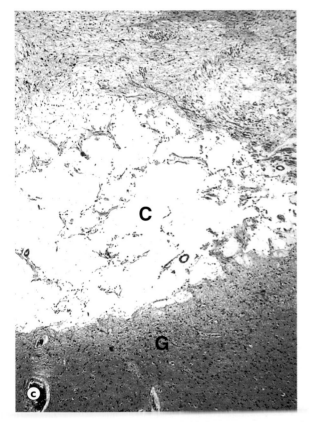

Fig. 23.2 **Infarction**
(a) Early infarct (LP) *(illustration opposite)*
(b) Later infarct (MP)
(c) Old (cystic) infarct (LP)

These three micrographs illustrate histological features of cerebral infarction at a variety of stages in evolution.

The earliest histological manifestations involve neurons, which become shrunken, eosinophilic and exhibit nuclear pyknosis. These changes are detectable within hours of infarction and established by 6 to 12 hours. Typically, microscopic disruption of small capillary vessels with extravasation of red cells is also present at this stage. Unlike other tissues, in cerebral infarction a neutrophilic response is only transient and macrophage infiltration dominates the cellular reaction from about 2 days post-infarction. This is accompanied by proliferation of small vessels at the margin of the infarcted territory.

Macroscopically, cerebral infarcts can be either haemorrhagic or 'anaemic' (pale). The haemorrhagic pattern is thought to be a result of reperfusion of capillaries damaged by the initial ischaemic episode.

Micrograph (a) illustrates an area of infarction in the cerebellum of a patient dying 2 days after infarction. The infarcted area on the left exhibits loss of basophilia because of necrosis **N** of the small neurons of the granular layer and extravasation of erythrocytes **E**.

Following infarction, organisation and repair take place. The dead tissue becomes infiltrated by macrophages recruited from blood monocytes which phagocytose lipid-rich myelin and take on a foamy appearance. By about 7 to 10 days post infarction, the infarct has become liquefied and partly cystic. Micrograph (b) shows this phase in a cerebral infarct. The infarcted area **Inf** consists of a homogeneous mass of necrotic tissue with remnants of karyorrhectic nuclei. Surrounding this area is a zone of lipid-containing macrophages **M** and beyond this is a peripheral zone of proliferating astrocytes and blood vessels **V**. Glial proliferation (*gliosis*) is the equivalent of granulation tissue in infarcts elsewhere in the body and is intended to fill the infarcted territory. The resulting glial scar is formed not of fibrous tissue but of the cell bodies and processes of astrocytes. This phase lasts up to 2 months post infarction.

When an infarct is large, the process of gliosis does not completely fill the defect and a cyst-like cavity remains, lined by dense astrocytic tissue. Micrograph (c) shows an old cystic infarct in the internal capsule with the central cavity **C** surrounded by glial tissue **G**. There is no neuronal regeneration following a cerebral infarct. Some of the early clinical manifestations of cerebral infarction may be due to oedema occurring in relatively undamaged tissue at the margins of the infarcted territory. This oedema resolves and explains some of the clinical improvement which a patient may experience with time.

KEY TO FIGURES
C cystic cavity **E** erythrocytes **G** glial tissue **Inf** infarcted area **M** macrophages **N** necrosis
V proliferating astrocytes and blood vessels

Degenerative diseases of the CNS

Certain diseases of the CNS are characterised by progressive degeneration of neurons and/or white matter:

- **Alzheimer's disease** is a common cause of irreversible cognitive impairment (dementia), mainly in the elderly. The aetiology is unknown, but there are distinct histological abnormalities (Fig. 23.3) which distinguish the condition from dementia with Lewy bodies (see below) and vascular dementia.

- **Parkinson's disease** (Fig. 23.4) causes clinical features of tremor, slow movement and rigidity as a result of degeneration of nerve cells in the substantia nigra. The cause is unknown.

- **Dementia with Lewy bodies** (Fig. 23.5) is clinically similar to Alzheimer's disease, though there are some key differences with fluctuating cognition, visual hallucinations and parkinsonism often encountered in this type of dementia. It has brainstem pathology identical to that seen in Parkinson's disease but, in addition, similar neuronal pathology is present in cortical neurons and serves as the substrate for cognitive impairment.

- **Vascular dementia** typically manifests clinically with a stepwise deterioration in cognitive function and focal neurological signs. A number of possible pathologies may be encountered in association with vascular dementias, reflecting whether the disease involves small or large vessels.

- **Motor neuron disease** is the result of specific degeneration of motor neurons in the cerebral cortex, brainstem and spinal cord. Cells degenerate over a period of a few years resulting in progressive denervation of muscle with insidious paralysis and death. The cause of this disease is unknown.

- **Creutzfeldt–Jakob disease (CJD)** is a cause of rapid onset, progressive dementia resulting from extensive death of neurons in the cerebral cortex (Fig. 23.6). It is unique among degenerative diseases of the CNS in that a transmissible cause has been demonstrated (*variant CJD*) although poorly characterised. The infective agent, known as *prion protein*, is closely related to that which causes scrapie in sheep and bovine spongiform encephalopathy in cattle.

Fig. 23.3 **Alzheimer's disease** **(a)** LP **(b)** Amyloid immunocytochemistry (LP) **(c)** Tau immunocytochemistry (HP)

Alzheimer's disease (AD) is the commonest neurodegenerative disease, with an incidence which increases with age. The typical presentation is in the seventh decade with symptoms of memory failure, progressing steadily to involve motor skills, speech and sensation. The cause is unknown, though in a small proportion of cases a genetic association has been identified.

Macroscopically there may be striking thinning of gyri, particularly those of the frontal and temporal lobes. Histologically, plaques, neurofibrillary tangles and neuronal loss are identified. *Plaques* **P** are accumulations of a peptide (*amyloid β*) and appear as amorphous, pink masses in the cortex (a) which may be revealed with immunocytochemistry (b). *Neurofibrillary tangles* appear as flame-shaped skeins formed by the abnormal accumulation of cytoskeletal filaments, in particular the microtubule associated protein tau, which can be demonstrated using immunocytochemical techniques, as in micgrograph (c).

Fig. 23.4 Parkinson's disease (HP)

Parkinson's disease is caused by idiopathic destruction of neurons in the substantia nigra resulting in loss of the neurotransmitter dopamine. Histologically, distinctive inclusions are seen in the remaining neurons.

This specimen, from the substantia nigra of a patient with Parkinson's disease, shows a typical neuromelanin-containing neuron within which is a *classical Lewy body* L. These are rounded, pink-staining inclusions often with a surrounding pale halo. These inclusions are composed of aggregates of the protein *α-synuclein* together with a number of other proteins.

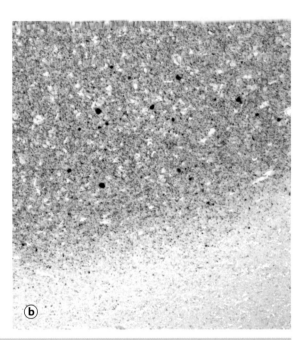

Fig. 23.5 Dementia with Lewy bodies (a) HP (b) α-Synuclein immunocytochemistry (MP)

Dementia with Lewy bodies (DLB) is the second commonest neurodegenerative disease and shares clinical similarities with AD. However, in contrast to AD, patients with DLB often present with visual hallucinations, prominent fluctuations in cognition and parkinsonian motor symptoms, in particular rigidity and slowness of movement (*bradykinesia*). Patients may also be highly sensitive to certain antipsychotic medications.

Macroscopically, there may be thinning of the gyri of the frontal and temporal lobes, perhaps not as marked as in AD. Pallor of the substantia nigra is typically present.

In contrast to the classical Lewy bodies of the substantia nigra, *cortical Lewy bodies* CL appear as ill-defined, pink, cytoplasmic inclusions, most readily identified in the neurons of the deeper layers of the temporal and frontal cortex (a). They are perhaps best demonstrated by immunocytochemistry for α-synuclein, as in micrograph (b).

KEY TO FIGURES
CL cortical Lewy body   **L** classical Lewy body   **P** senile plaque

Fig. 23.6 **Prion diseases** **(a)** Spongiform change in cerebral cortex (LP) **(b)** Amyloid plaque in variant Creutzfeldt-Jakob disease (HP)

The prion diseases are also known as the *spongiform encephalopathies* and have a common molecular pathological basis. Prion diseases occur in several species in addition to man, the most notable being scrapie in sheep and bovine spongiform encephalopathy (BSE) in cattle.

These diseases are biologically unique as they can be transmitted by a protein-only agent. Prion protein is a normal cellular protein associated with the cell membrane. In disease, the three-dimensional configuration of the protein becomes altered such that it aggregates in cells and is resistant to degradation. Importantly, it is believed that the abnormal configuration of the protein is able to bring about conversion of normal prion protein to a pathological form, such that disease can be transmitted.

Most human prion diseases occur sporadically (*sporadic Creutzfeldt–Jakob disease*). They can, however, be transmitted by inoculation, both to other species and also from person to person iatrogenically by corneal transplantation, use of cadaveric dural grafts, neurosurgery with contaminated instruments and treatment with human growth hormone or gonadotrophins obtained from cadavers (*iatrogenic Creutzfeldt–Jakob disease*). *Variant Creutzfeldt–Jakob disease (vCJD)* is believed to have been transmitted to man from BSE-infected cattle through consumption of contaminated beef. In addition,

several human prion diseases can be inherited in an autosomal dominant fashion if there are mutations in the prion gene that give rise to an abnormal protein configuration (*Gerstmann–Sträussler–Sheinker syndrome* and *fatal familial insomnia*). Importantly, protein derived from a genetic cause can transmit disease by inoculation.

In a healthcare setting, prion diseases represent a potential biological hazard, mainly from inoculation, and so autopsy and histological procedures have to be carried out to appropriate health and safety standards.

The main pathological changes seen in the nervous system are neuronal loss, vacuolation (termed *spongiform change*) and astrocytic gliosis. These features can be seen in micrograph (a) where the cerebral cortex shows loss of neurons and is largely replaced by rounded vacuoles. Astrocytic gliosis is best seen if special stains are used to detect astrocyte proliferation. In some cases accumulated prion protein forms plaques of amyloid. This is particularly seen in vCJD as shown in micrograph (b), where plaques of amyloid **A** are surrounded by spongiform change. In vCJD, but not other forms, prion protein accumulates in lymphoid tissues, such as tonsil, where it can be demonstrated using immunohistochemical techniques.

KEY TO FIGURES
A amyloid plaque

Infections in the CNS may arise as a consequence of bacterial, viral or fungal agents and result in inflammatory processes which may be divided into those involving the meninges (*meningitis*) or the CNS parenchyma (*encephalitis* in the brain; *myelitis* in the spinal cord). *Encephalomyelitis* and *meningo-encephalitis* describe conditions where a mixed pattern of involvement occurs.

Bacterial pathogens

Bacterial meningitis may be a severe life-threatening disease. Survivors are commonly left with brain damage. The common infective agents are the meningococcus (*Neisseria meningitidis*), the pneumococcus (*Streptococcus pneumoniae*) and *Haemophilus influenzae*.

Histologically, there is an acute, purulent, neutrophilic response in the meninges with secondary thrombosis of many of the blood vessels supplying the CNS. Treatment with antibiotics may allow recovery. However, healing may be complicated by fibrosis in the meninges.

In the majority of cases CNS infections arise as a consequence of haematogenous spread. In the remaining, small proportion of cases infection may arise as a complication of a surgical procedure (including lumbar puncture) or as a consequence of local spread such as from an infected air sinus.

Where there is impairment in cell-mediated immunity, such as encountered in AIDS, organ transplantation, chemotherapy or haematolymphoid malignancy, there is an increased incidence of tuberculous meningitis. Typically, this takes the form of **granulomatous meningitis** (see Fig. 4.7), though the cellular response may be minimal in situations of severe immunological compromise.

Viral pathogens

Viral meningitis is commonly due to an *enterovirus* and is rarely fatal. Typically, it results in a transient lymphocytic response in the meninges.

Encephalitis and myelitis are usually caused by viral infections, some having a particular propensity to affect specific types of neuron. In viral encephalitis or myelitis, there are three main histological features:

■ focal neuronal loss and phagocytosis as a direct result of viral infection

■ lymphocytic 'cuffing' of vessels with increase in microglial cells; this is because of a local immune response

■ astrocytic reaction with increase in number and size of astrocytes in response to loss of neurons.

The commonest acute necrotising encephalitis is Herpes simplex type 1 (HSV-1) infection. Typically, the history is one of fever, confusion, headache and frontotemporal localising signs. This latter feature reflects the preferential involvement of the frontal and temporal lobes, which can be detected as an asymmetrical imaging abnormality on CT scanning. HSV-1 causes a severe form of generalised encephalitis with extensive necrosis of brain tissue (Fig. 23.7).

In contrast, the Polio virus tends to attack motor cells of the anterior horn of the spinal cord causing **poliomyelitis** and, for this reason, is termed a **neurotropic virus**. Rabies virus is also neurotropic and results in a meningo-encephalitis with virus inclusions visible in neuronal cells. Papovavirus infection of the CNS occurs in immunosuppressed patients and particularly affects oligodendroglial cells resulting in loss of myelin in white matter. The disease is termed **progressive multifocal leukoencephalopathy**. The Human immunodeficiency virus (HIV-1), which causes AIDS, also affects the CNS and can result in **HIV encephalitis** (Fig. 23.8). Persistent viral infection of the brain occurs in some cases with Measles virus and results in a chronic degeneration of nerve cells in a disease termed **subacute sclerosing panencephalitis**.

Fungal/protozoal pathogens

Fungal infections of the CNS are rare and are mainly confined to immunosuppressed patients. The most common causative organisms are *Aspergillus*, *Zygomycosis* and *Cryptococcus* species (see Fig. 4.18). Lesions usually take the form of abscesses.

Brain abscesses

Typical cerebral abscesses may develop as a consequence of meningitis or may be the result of direct spread of infection from the skull (such as complicating middle ear infection) or of blood-borne spread from an infection elsewhere in the body, such as the lung. There is commonly a mixed infection including anaerobic organisms. Histologically, there is a pus-filled cavity walled off by fibrosis generated through granulation tissue derived from local blood vessels. Around this fibrous cavity wall, there is a reactive astrocytic response.

Fig. 23.7 Herpes simplex encephalitis (MP)

Viral encephalitis may be caused by *Herpes simplex type 1*, the same virus which causes 'cold sores'. The virus spreads to involve the frontal lobes, limbic system and temporal lobes of the brain. The typical histological features of an encephalitis are seen, namely neuronal death, lymphocytic cuffing of vessels and astrocyte proliferation. There is, however, severe necrosis of the affected areas of brain, which become semi-liquid as macrophages phagocytose dead tissue.

This micrograph shows an area of cortex replaced by a mixture of macrophages and astrocytes with a small vessel cuffed by lymphocytes **L**. Careful examination of tissue may reveal eosinophilic viral inclusion bodies in nuclei of remaining neurons. Immunocytochemistry tests can detect herpes viral antigen and are used diagnostically. Electron microscopy is another method used to detect the virus. Prompt treatment with antiviral drugs may halt progression of the disease. However, late presentation commonly results in death or severe neurological deficit.

Fig. 23.8 HIV encephalitis (HP)

Neurological dysfunction is common in AIDS, including opportunistic infections, primary central nervous system lymphoma and direct or indirect effects of the HIV virus itself.

One such condition, *HIV encephalitis*, is shown here. The characteristic feature is inflammation of white matter with aggregates of mononuclear cells **M** and associated multinucleate giant cells **G**. These are found throughout the central nervous system, usually close to a small blood vessel, and may be associated with foci of necrosis and reactive gliosis. Virus can be detected within cells in these areas. The clinical features are of insidious dementia, mood disorders and motor abnormalities.

KEY TO FIGURES

D demyelinated area   **G** multinucleated giant cell   **L** lymphocytes   **M** mononuclear cells   **W** white matter

Primary demyelinating diseases

Primary demyelinating diseases result in selective loss of myelin sheaths with (relative) preservation of axons. Commonest of these is ***multiple sclerosis*** (MS), where episodes of demyelination occur in multiple different sites in the CNS and at different times (i.e. separated in place and time). The typical lesions of MS are well-defined foci of demyelination, ***plaques***, distributed throughout the cerebral hemispheres, brainstem and spinal cord. It is postulated there is an abnormal immunological reaction, possibly triggered by a viral infection, resulting in focal myelin destruction.

There are three histological stages in the demyelinating process. First, during an acute episode, myelin breakdown occurs associated with lymphocyte and macrophage infiltration of the affected area, termed a *plaque*. At this stage there is clinical evidence of focal neurological dysfunction. Although the primary damage is against myelin, secondary damage to axons also occurs. In the second phase, astrocytes proliferate and gradually infiltrate the demyelinated area which exhibits a continued lymphocytic infiltration. In the final phase of evolution of the plaque, cellularity is reduced, astrocytes shrink in size and the process becomes 'burnt out'.

Fig. 23.9 **Multiple sclerosis** **(a)** H&E (LP) **(b)** H&E (MP) **(c)** Myelin stain (LP) **(d)** Myelin stain (MP)

Micrographs (a) and (b) show the typical H&E appearance of demyelination. The pale-staining demyelinated area **D** is easily distinguished from the normal-staining white matter **W**. In the medium power image (b) the increase in cellularity in these regions is a result of macrophages and reactive astrocytes. Another typical feature is cuffing of small blood vessels by lymphocytes **L**. Micrographs (c) and (d) illustrate the same fields stained by a method to demonstrate myelin. Normal myelin stains dark blue, with areas of demyelination **D** appearing pale-stained. Note the well-defined boundary between demyelinated plaque and normal white matter.

BASIC SYSTEMS PATHOLOGY ■ NERVOUS SYSTEM

Tumours of the CNS

Primary tumours of the CNS are uncommon, accounting for approximately 2% of cancer deaths in adults and 10% in children, though metastases to the brain from extracranial malignancies are, by contrast, relatively common. Despite their rarity, there are numerous different types of tumours arising from the CNS or its coverings with origins in **neuroepithelial tissue** (glia, neurons, embryonal tissues), meninges and lymphoid cells.

Unlike tumours elsewhere in the body, the distinction between benign and malignant CNS tumours is less apparent. As such, a unique system of classification and grading of tumours of the CNS exists which is based on light microscopy assessment supplemented by immunocytochemistry stains and, increasingly, molecular diagnostic techniques. This system is regularly revised and updated (currently WHO 2007) and grades CNS tumours from slow-growing (**WHO grade I**) to rapidly growing and highly aggressive (**WHO grade IV**). Figure 23.10 lists the more common examples and their corresponding WHO grades.

Over and above growth rate and tumour grade, any CNS tumour may exert harmful effects by growing into vital structures or by causing swelling of the brain around the tumour. Hence a small, WHO grade 1 (low-grade) tumour may have serious consequences if it is located in or adjacent to the cardiorespiratory control centres of the brainstem.

Fig. 23.10 **Common examples of tumours of the CNS and its coverings**

Presumed cell of origin	WHO grade	Presumed cell of origin	WHO grade
Oligodendroglial		**Embryonal**	
Oligodendroglioma	II	Medulloblastoma	IV
Anaplastic oligiodendroglioma	III		
		Neuronal and mixed glioneuronal	
Astroglial		Ganglioglioma	I or III
Pilocytic astrocytoma	I	Central neurocytoma	II
Diffuse astrocytoma	II		
Anaplastic astrocytoma	III	**Nerve sheath**	
Glioblastoma	IV	Schwannoma	I
		Neurofibroma	I
Mixed glial		Malignant peripheral nerve sheath tumour	II, III or IV
Oligoastrocytoma	II		
Anaplastic oligoastrocytoma	III	**Meningeal**	
		Meningioma (various subtypes)	I
Ependymal		Atypical meningioma	II
Ependymoma	II	Anaplastic meningioma	III
Anaplastic ependymoma	III		

Fig. 23.11 **Tumours of astroglial origin** (*caption opposite*)

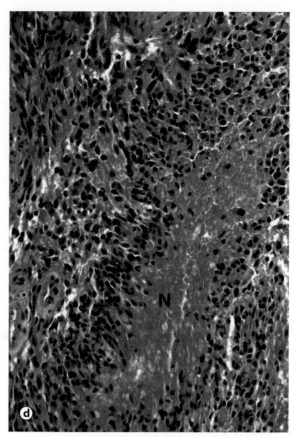

Fig. 23.11 **Tumours of astroglial origin** **(a)** Pilocytic astrocytoma (MP) **(b)** Pilocytic astrocytoma (HP) **(c)** Diffuse astrocytoma (HP) **(d)** Glioblastoma (MP) ((a) and (b) *illustrations opposite*)

Astrocytomas may arise anywhere in the cerebral hemispheres, brainstem, cerebellum or spinal cord and can present in all age groups from young children to the elderly. They range from the low-grade, slow-growing, well-circumscribed *pilocytic astrocytoma (WHO grade I)* to the high-grade, aggressive, widely infiltrative *glioblastoma (WHO grade IV)*.

Micrograph (a) shows an example of a pilocytic astrocytoma composed of mildly pleomorphic cells with round to spindle-shaped nuclei, fine, 'hair-like' cellular processes and typically thick-walled blood vessels **V**. At higher magnification in micrograph (b) another distinctive feature is readily appreciated, the *eosinophilic granular body* **E**. These are characteristic of many of the low-grade glial tumours. Pilocytic astrocytomas most commonly present in children and young adults as cerebellar tumours, though they can occur at other sites, including the optic nerves where they are known as *optic glioma*s.

A *diffuse astrocytoma (WHO grade II)* is illustrated in micrograph (c). Tumour cells have pink cytoplasm and fine cellular processes imparting a 'fibrillary' appearance to the background. Low-grade astrocytomas may show a degree of pleomorphism, but do not contain vascular proliferation or necrosis.

Glioblastoma (WHO grade IV) is a tumour composed of highly atypical glial cells of varying sizes. As seen in micrograph (d), these vary from small cells which exhibit little tendency to differentiation, to cells exhibiting astrocytic morphology, through to large, bizarre, giant tumour cells. Necrosis **N** is a typical feature of this type of tumour, together with high cellularity and vascular proliferation. These tumours have a very poor prognosis.

Intermediate between diffuse astrocytomas and glioblastomas are astrocytomas which exhibit cytological pleomorphism and readily identified mitotic activity. These are termed *anaplastic astrocytomas (WHO grade III)*.

Management of astrocytomas is based on a balance of need for intervention, likely growth rate and risk of surgery. Surgical intervention in low-grade gliomas is often delayed until symptoms are such that decompression of the tumour is indicated. Where possible, in the higher-grade tumours, surgery to excise as much tumour as possible is performed while preserving brain function. This may then be followed by radiotherapy and, increasingly, chemotherapy.

BASIC SYSTEMS PATHOLOGY ■ NERVOUS SYSTEM

KEY TO FIGURES
E eosinophilic granular body   **N** Necrosis   **V** thick-walled blood vessel

Fig. 23.12 **Oligodendroglioma** (HP)

Oligodendrogliomas most commonly arise in the cerebral hemispheres, often in the frontal lobes, and are composed of cells resembling oligodendrocytes. The typical *oligodendroglioma (WHO grade II)* is composed of a homogeneous sheets of cells with uniform rounded nuclei, a clear cytoplasm forming a 'halo' around the nucleus and a network of finely branching small blood vessels **V**. Microscopic foci of calcification are frequently seen.

The presence of a high mitotic count, nuclear pleomorphism, necrosis and vascular proliferation may be associated with more aggressive behaviour. Tumours exhibiting such features are termed *anaplastic oligodendrogliomas (WHO grade III)*.

Molecular diagnostics has proved of great value in the management of oligodendrogliomas, with certain molecular signatures associated with a considerably more favourable outcome (see below).

MOLECULAR NEUROPATHOLOGY

Surgical diagnostic neuropathology is increasingly employing molecular techniques in a quest to improve the diagnosis and management of patients with brain tumours. This is particularly evident in oligodendrogliomas and mixed gliomas which have an oligodendroglial component. In such tumours, it had been accepted for some time that two patients with similar presentations and, to all intents and purposes, morphologically identical tumours by light microscopy could have remarkably different responses to therapy and, with that, quite different outcomes. Frustratingly, predicting which cases might respond best to treatment proved difficult until a specific molecular signature was identified in a proportion of these tumours which was intimately linked to better response to therapy and improved outcome. This molecular signature is combined loss of heterozygosity (LOH) of the short arm of chromosome 1 (1p) and the long arm of chromosome 19 (19q).

Identifying this marker of more favourable outcome, which in many respects may be a more powerful indicator of likely tumour behaviour than the standard morphological assessments which are described above, has transformed the approach to tumour diagnosis, with many centres now routinely assessing such gliomas for LOH 1p19q.

KEY TO FIGURES

P perivascular pseudorosette   **Ps** psammoma body   **T** tubule   **W** cellular whorl   **V** blood vessel

Fig. 23.13 **Ependymoma** (MP)

These tumours are derived from the ependymal cells which normally line the ventricular system. Histologically, the tumour cells are uniform and arranged around blood vessels, leaving a perivascular 'nuclear free zone' known as a ***pseudorosette* P**. In addition, areas of tumour form epithelial tubules **T** which recapitulate the structure of the central canal of the spinal cord.

Ependymomas are most commonly seen in the region of the fourth ventricle and are also the commonest intrinsic tumour of the spinal cord in childhood. Tumours range from low-grade lesions (WHO grade II) to high-grade, anaplastic ependymomas (WHO grade III). There is a propensity for tumour to spread via CSF pathways seeding the leptomeninges.

Fig. 23.14 **Meningioma** (MP)

Meningiomas are thought to arise from arachnoidal cells of the meninges and are common tumours in adults. The tumours are nearly always low grade and produce symptoms by slow compression of underlying brain or spinal cord. There are several histological patterns of meningioma, varying from epithelioid cell lesions to spindle-cell lesions.

This micrograph illustrates a meningioma composed of epithelioid cells arranged in whorls **W**.

At the centre of the whorls there may be areas of calcification termed ***psammoma bodies* Ps**.

In general, mitotic figures are not common in meningiomas. However, occasional meningiomas show increased mitotic activity and are then termed ***atypical meningiomas (WHO grade II)***. Such tumours are prone to local recurrence. Tumours with very high mitotic activity are rare and termed ***anaplastic meningiomas (WHO grade III)***.

Disorders of peripheral nerves

Diseases of the peripheral nerves (*peripheral neuropathies*) result in abnormal motor or sensory function in the territory of the affected nerve. There are two main patterns of disease. *Axonal neuropathies* are due to primary damage to axons, while *demyelinating neuropathies* are a result of primary damage to Schwann cells and the myelin sheaths they form.

Generalised peripheral neuropathies may be found in association with a variety of diseases, such as diabetes mellitus, lead poisoning, alcoholism, uraemia and some malignancies. Several specific peripheral neuropathy syndromes are associated with segmental loss of myelin. These include *post-infectious polyneuropathy (Guillain–Barré syndrome)* and a large group of *hereditary sensorimotor neuropathies*. Axonal degeneration underlies other causes of peripheral neuropathy, for example those due to toxins, trauma or ischaemia. As a world problem, an important cause of peripheral nerve disease is leprosy (see Fig. 4.9) in which nerve trunks are infiltrated by large numbers of macrophages filled with *Mycobacterium leprae,* with resulting loss of nerve fibres.

Tumours of peripheral nerve are common and are derived from Schwann cells (the cells forming peripheral myelin sheaths), fibroblasts and perineural cells. Examples are shown in Figures 23.15 and 23.16.

Fig. 23.15 Schwannoma (MP)

These tumours, derived from Schwann cells, typically arise in peripheral nerves and are usually solitary, rounded tumours found in relation to nerve trunks. They are benign and usually slow growing. Schwannomas arising from the eighth cranial nerve (occasionally referred to as *acoustic neuromas*) can be part of the syndrome of neurofibromatosis type 2 or may arise as solitary tumours.

There are two patterns of growth seen histologically. Compact or *Antoni A* **AA** areas are composed of spindle cells with pink cytoplasm forming characteristic palisades (*Verocay bodies* **Vb**), while degeneration in the tumour results in loosely arranged vacuolated tumour areas termed *Antoni B* **AB**.

Fig. 23.16 Neurofibroma (HP)

Neurofibromas are tumours of peripheral nerves consisting of a mixture of cell types including Schwann cells, fibroblasts and perineural cells. They may be solitary, but are frequently multiple, especially in the genetically determined disease *neurofibromatosis type 1* (NF1; von Recklinghausen's disease).

Histologically, the tumour is composed of loosely arranged spindle cells with varying amounts of intervening collagen. A frequent feature is accumulation of connective tissue mucopolysaccharides resulting in a gelatinous or myxoid tumour. In contrast to Schwannomas, neurofibromas expand the nerve trunks in a diffuse manner. Neurofibromas are benign tumours. However, malignant tumours arising from peripheral nerve or showing nerve sheath differentiation termed *malignant peripheral nerve sheath tumours (MPNST)* may be encountered, particularly in association with NF1.

KEY TO FIGURES
A atrophic fibres   **AA** Antoni A area   **AB** Antoni B area   **L** lymphoid infiltrate   **N** normal sized fibres
P phagocytosis   **Vb** Verocay body

Diseases of skeletal muscle present with weakness, wasting of muscle and/or pain, typically made worse by exercise. These symptoms and signs can be due to either primary disease of muscle (*myopathy*) or secondary to degeneration of or damage to the nerve supplying the muscle (*neurogenic*). For this reason, muscle diseases are commonly considered together with diseases of the nervous system. Histology often provides the only satisfactory method of distinguishing between myopathic and neurogenic muscle diseases (Fig. 23.17). Myopathies can be acquired (*inflammatory* or *toxic*) or genetically determined (*dystrophies*).

Inflammatory diseases of muscle are typified by muscle fibre inflammation and destruction. They may be subdivided according to whether the cause is unknown (*idiopathic*) or an infectious agent. A number of idiopathic inflammatory myopathies are recognised which are thought to be associated with immunologically associated muscle damage. The commonest amongst these are *dermatomyositis*, *inclusion body myositis* and *polymyositis* (Fig. 23.18).

The dystrophies are characterised by degeneration and regeneration of muscle fibres resulting in progressive muscle wasting and weakness. There are several syndromes differing in age and sex incidence, time of onset and clinical course. Many are due to mutations in genes coding for structural proteins in muscle, such as the dystrophin protein producing either *Duchenne* or *Becker muscular dystrophy* (Fig. 23.19).

Mutations in either mitochondrial DNA or the nuclear DNA encoding mitochondrial proteins, whether inherited or acquired, can result in a number of heterogeneous syndromes with particular predilection for the heart, central nervous system and skeletal muscle (*mitochondrial myopathy*; Fig. 23.20).

A number of systemic disease processes may also be associated with muscle weakness and wasting, such as Cushing's disease, thyrotoxicosis and carcinomatosis.

Fig. 23.17 **Neurogenic muscular atrophy** (HP)

Weakness and wasting of skeletal muscle may occur as a result of lower motor neuron damage rather than primary muscle disease. Histologically, neurogenic muscle atrophy affects groups of muscle fibres supplied by damaged motor neurons, in contrast to the haphazard pattern of atrophy seen in the muscular dystrophies.

In this micrograph, normal-sized fibres **N** contrast sharply with a large group of atrophic fibres **A** from a denervated motor unit. This is an example of *spinal muscular atrophy* in which there is loss of spinal anterior horn cells. Similar changes are seen in a variety of peripheral nerve diseases.

Fig. 23.18 **Polymyositis** (HP)

Patients with polymyositis present clinically with proximal muscle weakness and have an elevated serum creatine kinase level, reflecting ongoing muscle necrosis. As seen in this biopsy, the characteristic appearance is of necrosis of individual muscle fibres, a lymphoid infiltrate **L** and phagocytosis **P** of muscle fibre debris. The disease is believed to be autoimmune in origin and is usually treated by immunosuppression.

Dermatomyositis is another form of inflammatory myopathy with characteristic skin rashes and a strong association with systemic malignancy. The histology is similar to that of polymyositis, though with a preferential involvement of perifascicular fibres (*perifascicular atrophy*).

Inclusion body myositis most commonly presents in the elderly with a steroid resistant, asymmetrical, often distal muscle weakness. The distinguishing feature on microscopy is the presence of cytoplasmic vacuoles which may stain for Alzheimer-associated proteins (e.g. amyloid β).

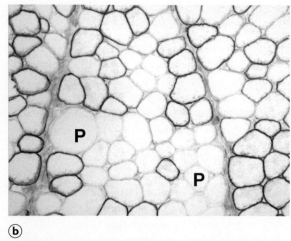

Fig. 23.19 Muscular dystrophy (a) HP **(b)** Immunocytochemistry for dystrophin protein (LP)

Dystrophin protein has a role in connecting the cytoskeleton of muscle to the extracellular matrix. Mutations in the dystrophin gene, located in the Xp21 region, are responsible for the two most common forms of muscular dystrophy, *Duchenne (DMD)* and *Becker (BMD) muscular dystrophies*.

Histologically, there is destruction of muscle fibres with replacement of muscle by fibrous tissue **F**. Residual fibres exhibit a markedly abnormal variation in fibre size, with atrophy of some fibres and hypertrophy of others.

As the disease progresses, the muscle becomes virtually replaced by fibrosis and, later, adipose tissue.

This gives rise to apparent swelling of the affected muscles and accounts for the *pseudohypertrophy* of calf muscles seen in DMD-affected children.

Immunocytochemistry can be used to reveal the pattern of staining with antibodies to dystrophin, which is normally ubiquitous on muscle fibres. As shown in micrograph (b), in this case there is abnormal patchy and pale staining of many fibres **P**.

DMD manifests in early childhood, has a relentless course and results in death in early adult life. In contrast, BMD symptoms develop at a later age and the disease has a less aggressive course.

Fig. 23.20 Mitochondrial myopathy (a) Gomori trichrome (HP) **(b)** Electron microscopy of mitochondrial inclusions

Mitochondrial myopathies may present in early adulthood with symptoms of muscle weakness, often involving proximal limb muscles and with prominent involvement of extraocular muscles. The muscle symptoms may form part of a complex of symptoms/signs including neurological symptoms and cardiomyopathy.

Morphologically, the most characteristic abnormality is aggregates of abnormal mitochondria, often in a subsarcolemmal location. These are best

appreciated using specialist muscle staining techniques. One such technique is illustrated in micrograph (a) where a section of skeletal muscle is stained with the Gomori trichrome stain. Here, abnormal accumulations of mitochondria appear as red-staining, subsarcolemmal deposits, with the affected fibres referred to as *ragged red fibres* **R**. Electron microscopy reveals mitochondria with abnormal crystalline inclusions often termed '*parking lot' inclusions* **PI**.

KEY TO FIGURES

F fibrous tissue   **P** patchy and pale fibres   **PI** 'parking lot' inclusions   **R** ragged red fibre

Fig. 23.21 Chapter review

PART 2

CHAPTER

23

Disorder	Main features	Figure
Vascular disorders		
Selective vulnerability	Neurons more vulnerable to hypoxic/ischaemic injury than glial cells. Shrunken, eosinohilic neurons in early stages, followed by phagocytosis of dead neurons and astrocytic proliferation	23.1
Infarction	Most a result of atheroma, thrombosis or embolism. Haemorrhagic or anaemic. Large infarcts heal with cavitation and gliosis	23.2
Haemorrhage	Primary intracerebral haemorrhage most often a complication of hypertension. Other causes – cerebral amyloid angiopathy, vascular malformations, aneurysms, tumours Other intracranial haemorrhages – extradural, subdural, subarachnoid	
Degenerative diseases		
Alzheimer's disease	Most common cause of dementia. Unknown aetiology. Typically in elderly. Amyloid plaques and neurofibrillary tangles on microscopy	23.3
Parkinson's disease	Idiopathic destruction of neurons in substantia nigra. Motor symptoms/signs. Inclusions (Lewy bodies) in surviving substantia nigra neurons	23.4
Dementia with Lewy bodies	Common cause of dementia. May be history of visual hallucinations, fluctuating cognition and parkinsonian symptoms. Inclusions in cortical and nigral neurons	23.5
Prion diseases	Transmissible via abnormal prion protein. Most common – sporadic Creutzfeldt–Jakob disease. Also iatrogenic, variant, familial. Neuronal loss, spongiform change and gliosis	23.6
Infections		
Bacterial meningitis	Acute, purulent exudates in meninges. Most common organisms – meningococcus, pneumococcus, *Haemophilis influenzae*	
Herpes simplex encephalitis	Most common acute necrotising encephalitis. Neuronal death, astrocyte proliferation, lymphocytes round blood vessels and necrosis	23.7
HIV encephalitis	Inflammation of white matter with clusters of mononuclear cells and occasional multinucleated cells	23.8
Demyelinating diseases		
Multiple sclerosis	Well-defined plaques of demyelination with relative preservation of neuronal elements and inflammatory cell response	23.9
Tumours of CNS		
Astrocytoma	Graded on histological features from grade I (lowest grade) to grade IV (highest grade, most aggressive; glioblastoma). Varied histological features	23.11
Oligodendroglioma	Typically sheets of cells with round nuclei and cleared cytoplasm, fine vessels and foci of calcification. Molecular diagnostics of value	23.12
Ependymoma	From ependymal cells lining ventricles. Perivascular pseudorosette arrangements of tumour cells and epithelial tubules	23.13
Meningioma	From arachnoidal cells of meninges. Cells arranged in whorls with some containing psammoma bodies	23.14
Peripheral nerves		
Leprosy	Nerve trunks infiltrated by macrophages filled with *Mycobacterium leprae*, with resulting loss of nerve fibres	4.9
Schwannoma	Derived from Schwann cells. Biphasic appearance with Antoni A (with occasional Verocay bodies) and Antoni B areas	23.15
Neurofibroma	May be solitary or multiple in association with NF1. Loosely arranged spindle cells with intervening connective tissue	23.16
Skeletal muscle		
Neurogenic atrophy	Result of damage to nerve innervating muscle. Clusters of atrophic fibres	23.17
Polymyositis	Inflammatory infiltrate with necrosis and phagocytosis of muscle fibres	23.18
Duchenne/Becker muscular dystrophy	Mutation of dystrophin gene on X chromosome. Muscle fibre destruction with replacement by fibrous tissue and wide variation in fibre size	23.19
Mitochondrial myopathy	Aggregates of abnormal mitochondria with trichrome stain (ragged red fibres) and mitochondrial inclusions in electron microscopy preparations	23.20

Appendix 1 – Notes on commonly used staining methods

■ **Haematoxylin and eosin (H&E)**
This is the most commonly used stain in histology and routine pathology. Haematoxylin is a dye which stains acidic structures a purplish-blue, and eosin a dye which stains basic structures pinkish-red. In the animal cell, most of the acidic structures reside in the nucleus due to nuclear DNA, whereas most of the cytoplasmic structures are basic. Thus nuclei stain purplish-blue and cytoplasm is pinkish-red, unless the cell contains abundant RNA, in which case there may be a purplish tint to the cytoplasmic staining (e.g., plasma cells – see Fig. 3.2).

The intensity of cell staining by H&E depends on many factors, including the particular formulation of the H&E stain (there are many recipes), but the thickness of the tissue section is most important: you will note that the staining intensity is greater when we have used thick sections for low-power pictures than when we have used very thin sections for very high-power pictures.

■ **PAS and DPAS (periodic acid–Schiff and diastase periodic acid–Schiff)**
The periodic acid–Schiff (PAS) reaction essentially demonstrates complex carbohydrates by staining them an attractive magenta colour. Not only does it stain pure complex carbohydrates such as glycogen, it also stains carbohydrates which are complexed with proteins and lipids. Many of these complexes are present in animal tissues as structural proteins, for example in basement membranes (see Fig. 15.9c), fungal cell walls (see Fig. 4.15), and mucins secreted by some epithelial cells. Staining due to glycogen can be eradicated by pre-treatment of the tissue section by the specific enzyme, diastase (amylase).

■ **Ziehl–Neelson and Wade–Fite stains**
These two stains are used to demonstrate bacteria belonging to the *Mycobacterium* group, which all possess a protective capsule containing lipids that affect the rate at which dyes move into and out of the bacterium during staining. Two dyes are used, basic fuchsin mixed with phenol, and methylene blue. The first dye (which is red) is forced into all the tissues in the section (including any *Mycobacteria*) by heating. The section is then exposed to acid and alcohol which wash the red dye out of everything except the *Mycobacteria*, which hold on to it because of the lipid capsule. All the other tissues are then free to take up the contrasting blue dye, but the *Mycobacteria* remain red against a blue background (see Fig. 4.10).

■ **Giemsa stain**
Although this stain is mainly used in a slightly modified form to stain red and white blood cells in blood and bone marrow smears, it can also be used to demonstrate some microorganisms.

■ **Gram stain**
This method is mainly used in smears of bacteria in diagnostic microbiology, but can also be used in histological sections to show whether any bacteria present are Gram-positive or Gram-negative (see Fig. 11.20b).

■ **Congo Red and Sirius Red**
These two dyes have a special affinity for proteins with a β-pleated sheet pattern, for example, amyloid. Amyloid stains red with both methods (see Fig. 5.3b), and shows an apple-green birefringence when examined by polarising microscopy.

■ **Van Gieson**
This is a method which uses two coloured solutions, picric acid (yellow) and acid fuchsin (red) as a mixture. The acid fuchsin stains collagen orangey-red, and all other tissues yellow (see Fig. 14.7c). Now rarely used on its own, it is more frequently combined with a stain for elastin (***elastic-van Gieson***). This method is particularly useful for the staining of arteries because it clearly distinguishes between the elastic lamina (black), the smooth muscle of the tunica media (yellow) and collagen (red) (see Fig. 11.15). It is also used to demonstrate the mixture of collagen and elastic fibres in the dermis of the skin.

■ **Perls' stain**
This old method is used to demonstrate the presence of ferric iron in tissues, usually at the site of old bleeding where the iron-containing pigment, haemosiderin (which is derived from local haemoglobin breakdown), accumulates. It is also used to demonstrate the excess

accumulation of iron in various tissues in the primary iron-storage disease, haemochromatosis (see Fig. 14.8).

▪ Goldner's trichrome

This method was developed for use in resin sections of undecalcified bone in the elucidation of metabolic bone disease such as osteomalacia and Paget's disease. It uses a combination of different dyes which distinguish between calcified bone (blue-green colour) and uncalcified osteoid (orange-red colour). Haematoxylin stains the nuclei of osteoblasts and osteoclasts, so that the level of cellular activity can also be assessed (see Fig. 22.2).

▪ Silver methods

Many histological staining methods use silver salts such as silver nitrate in solution to demonstrate a wide range of structures, including fungi and cells and fibres, particularly cells and fibres in the central nervous system. In general, these methods can be temperamental, and are becoming less popular. An example is shown in Fig. 4.16d.

▪ Loyez haematoxylin method

Haematoxylin is a very versatile dye, and in the past was used to demonstrate a wide range of specific structures. The Loyez method is an iron haematoxylin method which demonstrates myelin.

▪ Immunohistochemical and immunofluorescent methods

One of the great advances in histotechnology has been the development of these methods. The details are complicated, but basically a specific monoclonal antibody is raised against a specific chemical in the tissues. This is then applied to a tissue section and the antibody binds selectively to any of its specific antigen in the tissue. The site of this antibody binding is visualised using either a fluorescent or a coloured marker. Using techniques such as this, it is possible to localise substances such as insulin and other hormones, immunoglobulins, and a wide range of other substances within tissues (see Figs 13.13b, 15.7b and 16.6).

Appendix 2 – Glossary of pathological terms

Abscess – a localised collection of pus, formed from accumulation of dead and dying neutrophils and destruction of tissue

Acanthosis – an increase in the thickness of the stratum spinosum (prickle cell layer) of the epidermis

Acid- and alcohol-fast bacilli – pseudonym for *Mycobacteria*, derived from the fact that they retain staining with carbofuschin after treatment with acid and alcohol

Acidophilic – staining strongly pink with the acidic dye eosin (also known as *eosinophilic*)

AIDS – acquired immune deficiency syndrome, caused by infection with the Human immunodeficiency virus (HIV)

Amoeba – unicellular protozoan organism, important cause of diarrhoea worldwide

Amyloid – insoluble extracellular fibrillar protein, stains pink in routine H&E sections but best demonstrated using special stains, such as Congo red, or electron microscopy

Anaemia – deficiency of red blood cells in the blood stream

Aneurysm – abnormal dilatation of the wall of a blood vessel or the heart

Architecture – the organisation and arrangement of cells within a tissue

ARDS – adult respiratory distress syndrome, a severe form of lung disease with diffuse alveolar damage and formation of hyaline membranes in the alveoli

Asbestos – a mineral fibre used in industry and associated with development of lung fibrosis and malignant tumours, especially *mesothelioma*

Ascites – abnormal collection of fluid within the peritoneal cavity

Assman focus – focus of granulomatous inflammation in the apex of the lung, seen in secondary tuberculosis

Atypical mitosis – abnormal cell division usually seen in malignant tumours, described as 'tripolar' when the chromosomes appear to divide into three groups instead of the normal two

β-pleated sheet – unusual form of tertiary protein structure, typically seen in amyloid, making the protein insoluble and resistant to digestion by normal enzymes

Basophilic – staining strongly blue-purple with the basic dye haematoxylin (also known as *haematoxyphilic*)

Biphasic – with two different phases, sometimes used descriptively for tumours with two different growth patterns, e.g. mesothelioma, synovial sarcoma

Birefringence – the optical property of double refraction, splitting light into two perpendicular beams, useful in identifying crystals and other substances such as *amyloid*

Breslow depth – depth of invasion of malignant melanoma, measured in millimetres from the stratum granulosum to the deepest invading tumour cell, useful in assessing likely prognosis

Bronchiectasis – abnormal permanent dilatation of the bronchi due to chronic lung infection

Bulla – in skin, a large fluid-filled blister and in lung, a large cytically dilated airspace

Carcinoma – a malignant tumour of epithelial origin

Caseous necrosis – a form of tissue death, usually associated with tuberculosis, in which all cellular detail is lost, leaving soft, cheese-like material

Chancre – a painless ulcer which forms in the primary stage of syphilis infection

Chemokine – *cytokine* with chemotactic activity

Cirrhosis – end stage of many types of chronic liver disease, with regenerative nodules of hepatocytes and intervening bands of fibrous scar tissue

CISH – chromogen in situ hybridisation

Clark level – depth of invasion of malignant melanoma through the normal layers of the skin, from epidermis (level 1) through to subcutaneous fat (level 5)

Consolidation – solidification of tissue, usually used to describe lung when filled with exudate fluid in pneumonia

Councilman body – a small pink globule within the liver which is formed due to death of an individual hepatocyte, usually in acute viral hepatitis

Cribriform – sieve-like, often used to describe the architectural arrangement of cells in a tumour

Cryptogenic – term used to describe a disease of unknown origin (also called *idiopathic*)

Cytokine – small secreted molecules which control and modulate inflammation, the immune response and haematopoiesis

Cytology – the study of cells

Dermatitis – inflammation of the skin

Desmosome – a specialised form of intercellular junction, particularly numerous in stratified squamous epithelium and giving rise to the histological appearance of 'prickles' between the cells (also known as macula adherens)

Differentiation – the process by which a cell becomes more specialised, often used in tumour pathology to describe the extent to which a tumour resembles normal tissue

Dyskeratosis – abnormal maturation of squamous epithelial cells with premature formation of keratin

Dysplasia – abnormal cell maturation, commonly used to describe pre-cancerous changes seen in epithelium

Ectopic – in the wrong place

Effusion – a collection of fluid within a body cavity

Electrophoresis – a method of separating large molecules using electrical charge, commonly used to examine serum proteins

Emphysema – abnormal and permanent dilatation of airspaces within the lungs, resulting in progressive obstruction to airflow and impaired gas exchange

Empyema – a collection of *pus* in a body cavity, typically in the pleural cavity, but also used to describe pus within the gallbladder

Endarteritis obliterans – inflammatory process affecting blood vessels, with proliferation of the intima such that it blocks the lumen of the affected vessel

Eosinophilic – staining strongly with the pink dye eosin (also known as *acidophilic*)

Epidermotropism – migrating towards the epidermis, e.g. atypical lymphocytes in mycosis fungoides

Epithelioid – cells resembling epithelial cells that are not epithelial, i.e. round to ovoid cells with plenty of cytoplasm and round to ovoid nuclei, e.g. epithelioid smooth muscle cells in epithelioid leiomyoma

Epithelioid macrophages – activated macrophages with abundant pink cytoplasm, said to resemble epithelial cells and typically seen in *granulomas*

Erosion – loss of the superficial part of an epithelial or mucosal surface (see also *ulcer*)

Extramedullary haematopoiesis – formation of blood cells outwith the bone marrow, usually in the liver or spleen

Exudate – a protein-rich fluid which oozes out of damaged blood vessels, typically due to inflammation

Fascicle – a bundle, often used to describe the arrangement of smooth muscle cells in tumours

Fibrinoid – resembling fibrin, stains bright red with H&E

FISH – fluorescence in situ hybridisation

Fistula – an abnormal connection between two epithelial or endothelial surfaces

Grade – in tumour pathology, the extent to which the tumour resembles normal tissue (see also *differentiation*)

Granuloma – a collection of epithelioid macrophages and sometimes, but not always, multinucleate giant cells with or without necrosis

Haematemesis – vomiting of blood

Haematogenous – via the bloodstream

Haematopoiesis – formation of blood cells

H&E – haematoxylin and eosin, a standard histological staining method which stains cytoplasm pink and nuclei blue-purple in colour

Haematoxyphilic – staining intensely with the blue-purple stain haematoxylin (also known as *basophilic*)

Haemolytic anaemia – deficiency of red blood cells due to chronic red cell breakdown (lysis)

Haemoptysis – coughing up blood

Haemosiderin – a granular, brown substance containing iron, typically formed from breakdown of haemoglobin in the tissues

Hepatomegaly – enlargement of the liver

Histogenesis – differentiation of cells to form specialised tissues

HIV – Human immunodeficiency virus, the cause of AIDS

Hyaline – glassy and deep pink-staining

Hyperchromasia – dark staining, usually used to describe abnormal nuclei in tumours which contain excess nuclear DNA and so stain intensely with haematoxylin

Hyperplasia – adaptation with increase in the number of cells

Hypertrophy – adaptation with increase in the size of cells

Hyperuricaemia – increased blood level of uric acid, associated with development of gout

Idiopathic – term used to describe a disease of unknown origin (see also **cryptogenic**)

Immunohistochemistry – technique using specific antibodies to identify and stain tissue components (also known as immunocytochemistry and immunoperoxidase staining)

Induration – hardening of a tissue or organ, usually due to inflammation

Infarction – tissue death due to inadequate blood supply

Interface hepatitis – inflammation disrupting the *limiting plate* of hepatocytes around the edge of the portal area

Involucrum – in osteomyelitis, a covering of new bone around the dead bony *sequestrum*

Ischaemia – insufficient blood supply

Jaundice – yellow discoloration of the tissues due to accumulation of bilirubin

Koch's bacillus – old term for *Mycobacterium tuberculosis*

Koilocyte – an abnormal squamous cell due to infection by the Human papilloma virus (HPV), may be binucleate and typically with a clear halo around an irregular, raisin-like nucleus

Langhans' giant cells – multinucleate giant cells with the nuclei arranged in a horseshoe-like pattern, typically associated with tuberculosis but not *pathognomonic*

Leukaemia – malignant disease with excess numbers of circulating white blood cells

Lichenification – leathery thickening of the skin due to chronic scratching and rubbing

Limiting plate – the layer of hepatocytes around the edge of the portal tracts in the liver

Lymphadenopathy – enlargement of lymph nodes

Lymphoma – a malignant tumour of lymphoid tissue

MALT – mucosa-associated lymphoid tissue

Melaena – black, altered blood in the stool, usually due to bleeding from the upper gastrointestinal tract

Melanoma – a malignant tumour of melanocytes

Mesothelioma – a malignant tumour of mesothelial cells, usually affecting the pleura, strongly associated with previous *asbestos* exposure

Metaplasia – transformation of one type of differentiated tissue to another

Monoclonal – tumour or cellular proliferation derived from a single cell

Necrosis – death of cells in a living organism

NOS – not otherwise specified, a term usual to denote a tumour of the most usual or common type for that particular organ (also sometimes called NST – no special type), e.g. in the breast, the most common variant of malignant tumour is ductal carcinoma NOS, indicating that that it is not one of the rarer special types such as tubular carcinoma

Oedema – abnormal accumulation of fluid in the tissues

Oncocyte – epithelial cell packed with mitochondria, giving the cytoplasm a pink, granular appearance

Osteoid – uncalcified bone matrix produced by osteoblasts

Osteolytic – causing breakdown of bone, typically used to describe the effect of metastatic tumour in causing apparent 'holes' in the bone on X-ray

Osteosclerotic – causing excess deposition of bone, typically seen in cases of metastatic carcinoma from the prostate and showing areas of increased bone density on X-ray

Palisading – lining up, usually of cells or nuclei, giving the ordered appearance of a fence

Pannus – a membrane of fibrovascular granulation tissue seen in damaged joints, typically in rheumatoid arthritis

Papillary – forming finger-like projections, typically used to describe the arrangement of tumour cells in projections around fine vascular cores

Paraneoplastic syndrome – a non-metastatic systemic effect of tumour, usually due to production of hormones, antibodies or other factors by the tumour cells

Pathognomonic – a feature so characteristic of a particular disease that it is sufficient to make the diagnosis

Pleomorphism – variation in cell shape or nuclear shape, typically associated with malignant tumours

Pneumoconiosis – a chronic lung disease caused by dust inhalation

Pneumonia – inflammation of the lung parenchyma with *consolidation* due to inflammatory exudate within the air spaces (see also *pneumonitis*)

Pneumonitis – inflammation of the lung, usually used to refer to interstitial inflammation rather than inflammation within the air spaces (see *pneumonia*)

Pneumothorax – collection of air within the pleural cavity

Polyclonal – cellular proliferation derived from multiple different cells

Polyp – a growth which protrudes from an epithelial surface

Pott's disease – tuberculosis affecting the spine

Pseudoepitheliomatous hyperplasia – pattern of extreme epidermal hyperplasia which may mimic carcinoma

Purulent – containing pus

Pus – green material composed of dead and dying neutrophils

Pyogenic – pus forming

Sarcoma – a malignant tumour of mesenchymal origin

Sequestrum – a piece of dead bone, typically seen in osteomyelitis

Sinus – a blind-ended tract leading to a cavity (see also *fistula*)

Splendori–Hoeppli phenomenon – tissue reaction seen with certain infections, where organisms become encrusted with pink, proteinaceous material

Spongiosis – oedema of the epidermis, highlighting the spaces between keratinocytes with intervening 'prickles'

Stage – in tumour pathology, how far the disease has spread

Starling forces – osmotic and hydrostatic pressures which govern movement of fluid within the microcirculation

Steatosis – fatty change

Tingible body macrophage – a macrophage containing many fragments of apoptotic debris in its cytoplasm, typically seen in reactive germinal centres of lymph nodes or in other sites with high rates of cell turnover

Transudate – a fluid derived from plasma which has a low protein content

Ulcer – a full-thickness defect in an epithelial or mucosal surface (see also *erosion*)

Vertical transmission – transmission of an infectious disease from a mother to her newborn

Vesicle – a small fluid-filled blister in the skin

Viral inclusion bodies – large collections of virus particles within infected cells which can be seen using light microscopy

INDEX